Controlling Our Reproductive Destiny

New Liberal Arts Series

Light, Wind, and Structure: The Mystery of the Master Builders, by Robert Mark, 1990

The Age of Electronic Messages, by John G. Truxal, 1990

Medical Technology, Ethics, and Economics, by Joseph D. Bronzino, Vincent H. Smith, and Maurice L. Wade, 1990

Understanding Quantitative History, by Loren Haskins and Kirk Jeffrey, 1990

Personal Mathematics and Computing: Tools for the Liberal Arts, by Frank Wattenberg, 1990

Nuclear Choices: A Citizen's Guide to Nuclear Technology, by Richard Wolfson, 1991

Discovery, Innovation, and Risk: Case Studies in Science and Technology, by Newton Copp and Andrew Zanella, 1992

Controlling Our Reproductive Destiny: A Technological and Philosophical Perspective, by Lawrence J. Kaplan and Rosemarie Tong, 1994

This book is published as part of an Alfred P. Sloan Foundation program.

Lawrence J. Kaplan and Rosemarie Tong

Controlling Our Reproductive Destiny

A Technological and Philosophical Perspective

The MIT Press
Cambridge, Massachusetts
London, England

© 1994 Massachusetts Institute of Technology

Figures 1.1, 1.2, 3.1–3.15, 4.1, 4.4, 4.5, 5.1, 5.2, 6.1, 6.2, 7.1–7.4 © Robin Brickman

This book was set in Times Roman by Asco Trade Typesetting Ltd., Hong Kong and was printed and bound in the United States of America.

Library of Congress Cataloging-in-Publication Data

Kaplan, Lawrence J., 1943–
 Controlling our reproductive destiny : a technological and philosophical perspective / Lawrence J. Kaplan and Rosemarie Tong.
   p.   cm. — (New liberal arts series)
 Includes bibliographical references and index.
 ISBN 0-262-11176-4
 1. Human reproductive technology. 2. Human reproductive technology— Moral and ethical aspects. I. Tong, Rosemarie. II. Series.
 RG133.5.K37   1994
 176—dc20   92-38060
                                                                  CIP

To our parents
Betty Kaplan and to the memory of Hyman Kaplan
—L.J.K.

and

Joseph Behensky and to the memory of Lillian Ann Nedred
—R.T.

Without them we would not have been nor would we be who we are.

Contents

Series Foreword

The Alfred P. Sloan Foundation's New Liberal Arts (NLA) Program stems from the belief that a liberal education for our time should involve undergraduates in meaningful experiences with technology and with quantitative approaches to problem solving in a wide range of subjects and fields. Students should understand not only the fundamental concepts of technology and how structures and machines function, but also the scientific and cultural settings within which engineers work, and the impacts (positive and negative) of technology on individuals and society. They should be much more comfortable than they are with making calculations, reasoning with numbers and symbols, and applying mathematical and physical models. These methods of learning about nature are increasingly important in more and more fields. They also underlie the process by which engineers create the technologies that exercise such vast influence over our lives.

The program is closely associated with the names of Stephen White and James D. Koerner, both vice-presidents (retired) of the foundation. Mr. White wrote an internal memorandum in 1980 that led to the launching of the program two years later. In it he argued for quantitative reasoning and technology as "new" liberal arts, not as replacements for liberal arts as customarily defined, but as liberating modes of thought needed for an understanding of the technological world in which we now live. Mr. Koerner administered the program for the foundation, successfully leading it through its crucial first four years.

The foundation's grants to 36 undergraduate colleges and 12 universities supported a large number of seminars, workshops, and symposia on topics in technology and applied mathematics. Many new courses were developed and existing courses modified. Some minors or concentrations in technology studies were organized. A Resource Center for the NLA Program, organized at Stony Brook, published a monthly newsletter and a series of monographs, collected educational materials prepared at the colleges and universities taking part in the program, and continues to serve as a clearing house for information about the NLA program.

As the program progressed, faculty members who had developed successful new liberal arts courses began to prepare textbooks. Also, a number of the foundation's grants to universities supported writing projects of professors— often from engineering departments—who had taught well-attended courses in technology and applied mathematics designed for liberal arts undergraduates. It seemed appropriate not only to encourage the preparation of books for such courses, but also to find a way to publish and thereby make available to the widest possible audience the best products of these teaching experiences and writing projects. This is the background with which the foundation approached The MIT Press and the McGraw-Hill Publishing Company about jointly publishing a series of books on the new liberal arts. Their enthusiastic response led to the launching of the New Liberal Arts Series.

The publishers and the Alfred P. Sloan Foundation express their appreciation to the members of the Editorial Advisory Board for the New Liberal Arts Series: John G. Truxal, Professor Emeritus, Department of Technology and Society, State University of New York, Stony Brook, Chairman; Joseph Bordogna, Professor and Dean Emeritus, School of Engineering and Applied Science, University of Pennsylvania; Robert W. Mann, Whitaker Professor of Biomedical Engineering, Massachusetts Institute of Technology; Merritt Roe Smith, Professor of the History of Technology, Massachusetts Institute of Technology; J. Ronald Spencer, Associate Academic Dean and Lecturer in History, Trinity College; and Allen B. Tucker, Jr., Professor of Computer Science, Bowdoin College.

In developing this new publication program, The MIT Press was represented by Frank P. Satlow and the McGraw-Hill Publishing Company by Eric M. Munson. The first six books in the series were jointly published. Subsequent books have been solely published by The MIT Press, represented by Terry Ehling.

Samuel Goldberg
Alfred P. Sloan Foundation

Preface

This book is an outgrowth of a workshop in Bioengineering and Health Technology held at the Massachusetts Institute of Technology during the summer of 1984 and sponsored by the Alfred P. Sloan Foundation. The aim of the workshop's directors was to motivate liberal arts college professors to develop interdisciplinary courses that would use a variety of intellectual levels to focus on technological developments, particularly biomedical ones. We chose as our subject of concern the field of reproductive technology. Both of us were interested in the scientific, ethical, legal, and social implications of the reproduction-controlling (contraception, sterilization, and abortion) and reproduction-aiding (artificial insemination, in vitro fertilization) technologies, but each of us had very different perspectives on these matters. One of us was a biochemist, a man, and rather traditional with respect to marital and familial relationships. The other one of us was a philosopher, a woman, and a feminist in perspective. If anyone could construct a well-balanced course in reproductive technology, we believed that we could. As it turned out, our course captured the interest of many students at Williams College. It provided our humanities-oriented students with a background in science and technology, and our science-oriented students with an appreciation of the ethical, legal, and social consequences of scientific and technological developments. We enjoyed our collaborative teaching experience so much that we decided to write this text with the support of the Sloan Foundation.

We hope this book will prove useful to both humanists and scientists as they seek to keep the lines of communication between the worlds of "value" and "fact" open. Throughout this book, we aim to provide students with enough scientific background to fully understand the technologies we have selected for discussion. Science does not dwell in a theoretical realm separate from the practical realm in which technology supposedly abides. On the contrary, science and technology are symbiotic partners: knowing why something works is just as important as knowing how something works. Similarly, we consistently seek to provide students with enough legal cases, ethical principles, and social trends to analyze the risks and benefits, pros and cons, and "rights" and "wrongs" of the many reproductive technologies currently available and those which are sure to be developed in the future. Since we live in a pluralistic society, it is important for us to appreciate why some of us wholeheartedly approve of reproductive technologies, while others of us strongly disapprove of them. There may be ways for us to weave our reproductive destinies collaboratively despite our differing belief systems.

We thank all of the colleagues and reviewers who have aided in the production of this book. We also thank the students in our course who stimulated our thought and we particularly thank those individuals who assisted with the manuscript in different stages of development. In the early stages, Yoshika Fujita, Elyse Rosenblum, Nancy Gannon, Francine Davis, David Attisani, and Crescent Varonne made significant contributions. In the later stages, Erika Elvander, Kristin Garris, and Ruth Turner provided valuable assistance with various aspects of the manuscript. Throughout much of this project, Shirley Humphrey provided invaluable technical and editorial assistance, made insightful suggestions based on a number of critical readings of the entire manuscript, and prepared the index. Our thanks also to Robin Brickman, who creatively rendered the original artwork for the book. Finally, a special thank you to Katherine Arnoldi of MIT Press, who provided steady editorial guidance to bring this project to a successful completion.

1   Introduction

If we scan the newspapers, watch television, or listen to the radio, we are likely to read, view, or hear something daily about a reproduction-controlling technology (e.g., contraception, sterilization, or abortion) or a reproduction-aiding technology (e.g., artificial insemination or in vitro fertilization). In addition, we may know someone personally who uses contraception, has been sterilized, has had an abortion, is being treated for infertility with gamete intrafallopian transfer, in vitro fertilization, or artificial insemination, or is negotiating for the services of a contracted mother. Indeed, we ourselves may have already used one or more of these technologies.

The Procreative Options of the Fertile and Infertile

The ordinary result of sexual intercourse between fertile people used to be pregnancy. If fertile people wished to avoid pregnancy, then the only real choice they had was to refrain from sexual intercourse. Similarly, the almost inevitable result of infertility used to be childlessness. If infertile people wished to have children in their lives, their main options were adoption, foster parenthood, or being that special "aunt" or "uncle" in a child's life. Today sexually active fertile people do not necessarily have to have children, and infertile people do not necessarily have to remain genetically childless. Developments in reproductive technology have permitted an increasing number of people to control more successfully whether, when, and even how they are going to bear and beget children.

To be sure, not everyone is in a position to make such choices. Free and responsible choice requires *power* and *knowledge*. The empowered person is the person who is not repressed, oppressed, or suppressed by external constraints (e.g., chains, threats, taboos) or internal problems (e.g., depression, fatigue, anxiety). She or he is also a person with enough political power, economic advantages, and social stature to act on her or his decisions effectually. The knowledgeable person is the informed person, someone with enough knowledge to make responsible decisions about how to use or not use his or her procreative powers wisely. Because relatively few people are fully empowered and knowledgeable, reproductive choice is always a matter of degree. What also limits reproductive choice is the state of reproductive technology. After all, birth-control devices and sterilization techniques do fail sometimes, and fertility treatments are far from universally successful.

Not only are the reproduction-controlling and reproduction-aiding technologies limited; they have a paradoxical relationship. One half of our procreative story is about people who are fertile but who, for any number of reasons, cannot or should not have children. Infertile people who desire children are the other half of our procreative story, and they often are willing to endure many physical and psychological hardships and to spend much money to get pregnant. To appreciate fully these two procreative stories, we must understand many aspects of the basic science of reproduction, the details of the reproduction-controlling and reproduction-aiding technologies, and the social, political, legal, moral, ethical, and religious ramifications of these processes. We also must understand, however, that when we elect a specific option, such as hiring a surrogate mother, to improve our own situation, our actions have implications far beyond our lives and may have an impact on others for many generations.

We will discuss these complexities in detail in later chapters; for now, however, we will illustrate their many and profound ramifications with the single example of in vitro fertilization technology. Contrary to the situation just a few years ago when anyone of us had a mother and a father, it is now possible for a baby to have a genetic mother (who gave her eggs), a genetic father (who gave his sperm), a gestational mother (who provided her uterus), and a social mother and father (who raise the child). A recent case in which these factors were involved concerned a mother who was artificially inseminated with her daughter's husband's sperm so that her daughter and son-in-law could have a child genetically related to both of them. The woman was, therefore, both the child's mother and grandmother.

Historical Background of Reproduction

Currently, we regard our understanding of the process of reproduction as very advanced; we also regard our reproduction-aiding and reproduction-controlling technologies as highly sophisticated. With advancement and sophistication, however, come significant problems. Our modern technological developments frequently outstrip our ability to deal with them on a moral, legal, and political level. If we wish to close this potentially dangerous gap, it is helpful to see where we have been historically as well as to understand where we are. Hence, we will review some of the attitudes, beliefs, and scientific knowledge of past eras. Our aim is to learn both from our predecessors' valuable insights and their apparent mistakes.

In Neolithic times, human beings were ignorant of a man's role in procreation, making no connection between sexual intercourse and pregnancy. A woman's body seemed to ripen with children in the same way that a tree ripened with fruit. Over time, however, human beings came to understand the intimate connection between sexual intercourse and pregnancy. Men as well as women were recognized as having a procreative role, although no one was sure whether these roles were equal or unequal. At times, debates about whether men or women were the primary procreators led to heated arguments that now seem rather absurd. Nevertheless, by reviewing these past controversies, we can determine just how much science has improved our reproductive knowledge.

In ancient times, the Greek physician Hippocrates (460–540 B.C.) attempted to clarify the respective roles of the sperm and the egg in the procreative process. When he cut open a 24-hour-old chicken egg, he discovered a chick embryo in a recognizable shape. Startled by his discovery, Hippocrates proposed that the chicken egg contained a tiny, preformed chicken ready for development. While this seemed clear in the case of egg-laying chickens, the situation was not so obvious in the case of humans who did not seem to produce eggs. Impressed by their mentor's discovery, Hippocrates' students sought to apply it to human beings. Interestingly, however, they proposed not that the human *egg* but that the human *sperm* contains an outline for the parts of the body prior to birth.

The Greek philosopher Aristotle (384–322 B.C.) agreed with Hippocrates' students that the sperm is virtually all-important in human procreation. He described the process of reproduction as one in which the passive female principle waits to be molded by the active male principle. The male principle, he said, is active because it is potent. Originally derived from red blood, male semen has enough internal heat to transform itself from a diffuse red substance into a concentrated white substance. In contrast, female semen (which Aristotle identified with women's menstrual flow) remains always red because it is not hot enough to boil itself to the point of white perfection. Lacking heat, women also lack activity. In comparison to hot, active men, they are cold, passive creatures who contribute very little to the process of human reproduction.[1]

In the spirit of Aristotle, the physician Galen (129–circa 200 A.D.) claimed that the male seed is produced in the right testis (ovary) and then implanted in the right side of the uterus where it assumes active male characteristics. In contrast, the female seed is produced in the left testis (ovary) and then implanted in the left side of the uterus where it assumes passive female characteristics. Because Galen believed that the left side of the uterus was fed by impure, unheated blood, he concluded that women were deficient in heat. Since women are relatively cold, they cannot generate enough warmth to develop their bodily organs, including their sexual organs. As a result, cold-blooded women are able to produce only imperfect seed, which has less impact on reproduction than the perfect seed of warm-blooded men.[2]

Although arguments about the respective merits of the female and male reproductive cells continued into modern times, by then scientists were using empirical data rather than speculation to support their theoretical claims. After many painstaking observations, the English physician William Harvey (1578–1657 A.D.) announced that "all animals reproduce by eggs!"[3] Harvey rejected earlier proposals that the "male semen becomes part of the fetal body and even that it finds access to the uterus."[4] He considered the egg far more important than the sperm in the production of new animal organisms, regarding the sperm as a catalyst that simply

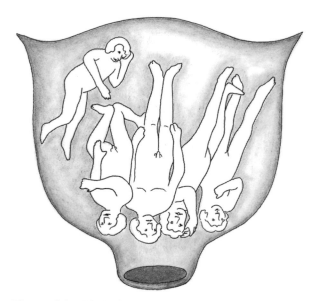

Figure 1.1 Birth figures representing the fetus preparing to emerge from the uterus as envisioned in the medieval age. (Redrawn from B. Rowland, trans., *Medieval Woman's Guide to Health* Kent, OH: Kent State University Press, 1981)

triggers the egg to begin development. Working with a primitive microscope and a lively imagination, the Italian anatomist Marcello Malpighi (1628–1694 A.D.) later claimed that Harvey was correct to emphasize the role of the egg in animal procreation. The animal egg, said Malpighi, contains a minuscule form of the adult animal waiting to be triggered into production, as depicted in figure 1.1.[5]

A swing back in the direction of emphasizing the role of the sperm in animal procreation took place when the Dutch histologist Anton van Leeuwenhoek (1632–1723 A.D.) used his microscope to study semen samples. To his amazement, he discovered a great quantity of living "spermatic animalcules" in the semen.[6] Subsequent analysis led the embryologist Hartsoeker to insist that tiny preformed beings, or homunculi, could be seen if a spermatozoon were viewed without its covering, as illustrated in figure 1.2.[7] This was a complete turn around from the proposals that the egg contained the preformed being. Now the egg was seen as little more than the nourishment for the male seed.

The egg-sperm debate did not end with these discoveries. The controversy raged on. Those that advocated the theory that the egg was the crucial element in procreation and those that supported the homunculus, or little-man-in-the-sperm, theory each proposed more and more imaginative explanations to support their claims. Given the spirited manner in which these claims and counterclaims were made, it is easy to forget that the sperm was not discovered until 1677 by van Leeuwenhoek and that the mammalian egg was not properly identified until 1827 by Karl Ernst von Baer.

Unfortunately, the egg-sperm controversy, fueled more by ignorance than by knowledge, has continued until the present time. Its flames have been fanned by folklore and fable, mystery and superstition. As we do not wish to add to this nonsense, we intend to discuss the respective roles of the egg and the sperm in more dispassionate terms. There is no need to valorize either the egg's or the sperm's reproductive role because, as things stand (though this could change), both are necessary for procreation and neither alone is sufficient. The process of reproduction is complicated enough without permitting cultural lenses to distort biological facts.

Sex Preselection Then and Now

As is well known, the sex of a child is determined by the nature of the sperm cell that fertilizes the egg. If the sperm is a male type, it has the Y chromosome and, if it is a female type, it has the X chromosome. For

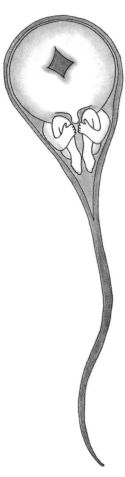

Figure 1.2 The homunculus, or "tiny man" in the human sperm as pictured by the early microscopists.

centuries, many have tried to select preferentially one type of sperm over the other to ensure the birth of a child of a particular sex. Aristotle proposed a method that involved making love in the north wind for a male child and in the south wind for a female child. Hippocrates suggested tying a string around the right testicle to stimulate the production of the "male sperm" and tying the left one to stimulate the "female sperm." Alchemists in medieval times offered this bizarre proposal: Drink the blood of a lion and then have intercourse under a full moon to ensure a male child. In Scandinavian countries, the sex of the child was believed to depend on which side of the bed a man hung his pants before engaging in intercourse. Although these theories and myths have largely been dismissed with the controversies about the superiority of one seed over the other, the desire of many prospective parents to influence the reproductive process in order to produce a child of a specific sex remains fairly constant.

Over the past three decades, many scientists have tried to apply new information about the reproductive process to develop sex preselection techniques that work. In the 1960s, Dr. Landrum Shettles claimed that a child's sex could be influenced by the timing of sexual intercourse and the acidity or alkalinity of the female reproductive tract. He proposed that sperm carrying X chromosomes (for a female) would have an advantage in the acidic environment that exists just prior to ovulation and that sperm carrying Y chromosomes (for a male) would have an advantage in the alkaline environment that exists at the time of ovulation. He also proposed to increase the chances by having the woman douche with vinegar if a female child was wanted and with baking soda if a male was wanted. Shettles's views have not been substantiated and this method is not recommended by doctors, although the method is still practiced by hopeful couples. In fact, a few years ago, ProCare Industries Ltd. marketed a home test kit called *GenderChoice*, based on this method. The kit contained literature describing the role of acidity and alkalinity in sex preselection and the need for timing intercourse with ovulation; it also included a thermometer to determine the basal body temperature and paper tissues for mucus samples.

One of the most recent proposals for sex preselection takes advantage of the assumption that sperm carrying the Y chromosome move faster than sperm carrying the X chromosome. To increase the chances of a male child, semen is collected and placed in a test tube on the top of a dense solution of the protein albumin. The more vigorous Y-chromosome carrying sperm swim through the dense solution toward the bottom of the tube, where they are collected. After washing and concentrating the Y-chromosome carrying sperm, a woman can be artificially inseminated with them.

Other methods of separating the Y-carrying sperm from the X-carrying sperm have as their the goal increasing the chances of engendering a girl. One method for obtaining sperm carrying the X chromosome involves a filtration system on the separation material called *Sephadex*; during filtration, the heavier X-chromosome carrying sperm reach the bottom of the system first. Sex preselection is a very active area of reproductive research, and undoubtedly many more developments are just around the corner.

Reproductive Health and Reproductive Choices

Though we are about to discuss advances made in the reproduction-aiding and reproduction-controlling technologies, we must remember that technology is not a substitute for the kind of appropriate reproductive practices that help ensure good reproductive health. It is unwise to rely on reproductive technology to correct problems that could be avoided with reasonable care and safe sexual practices. Our future reproductive health depends on our current reproductive behavior.

In this book, we try to provide in-depth coverage of the scientific, ethical, political, and legal issues that surround the technologies of reproduction. We cannot, however, be completely comprehensive in a work of this length. Nor can we be completely up-to-date. The ethics, politics, and law of reproduction are changing as rapidly as the science and technology of reproduction. New moral insights, political interpretations, and legal rulings about reproduction appear daily. What is considered morally good, politically correct, and legally advisable at the time a couple chooses to use a reproductive technology may be just the opposite by the time the woman delivers a baby.

Although we realize that many of our readers will be interested in how they themselves can use one or more of the currently available reproductive technologies, this book is not intended to be a "how-to" manual for either the reproduction-controlling or the reproduction-aiding methods. Many fine manuals that deal in some detail with contraception, abortion, and sterilization, as well as hormone treatment, in vitro fertilization, and embryo transfer are available.[9] Since new developments are being announced almost weekly, those interested in using such modalities should consult widely with medically trained personnel so their decisions are based on the latest information. This week's scientific miracle may prove to be next week's health disaster.

2 An Ethical and Legal Framework: Toward an Evaluation of the Reproduction-Controlling and Reproduction-Aiding Technologies

In the introduction, we mentioned the paradoxical relationship between fertile people who may use a reproduction-controlling technology to avoid having children and infertile people who may use even a physically taxing and stress-inducing reproduction-aiding technology because they want children very much. Fertile people choose not to procreate for diverse and complex reasons: Some are too unhealthy; others are too immature; still others are too poor. Then there are those people who are healthy, mature, and financially secure, but who simply do not want to parent children. Their work is all-consuming, or their intergenerational skills are limited, or their life-style is too free-form. Finally, there are those people who are ideologically opposed to childbearing. They are concerned about overpopulation, or they are worried about bringing a child into a self-destructive world.

Significantly, the healthier and the wealthier of these fertile people will also tend to have the most reproductive options. Just because society recognizes a woman's right to have an abortion, for example, does not mean that it feels obligated to fund one for her. Recently, *Time* magazine published an article on abortion's "hardest cases." Among these cases was that of a seventh-grader named Pamela (a pseudonym) who was raped by her stepfather. When her mother discovered what had happened, she took Pamela to a Planned Parenthood clinic to arrange for an abortion. Told that Medicaid would not pay the $400 cost of an abortion, Pamela's mother, who works two jobs but clears less than $600 a month, exclaimed that she simply did not have $400. Planned Parenthood officials subsequently softened and agreed to perform the abortion for $100 because it seemed too cruel to force a 12-year-old girl to carry her stepfather's child to term.[1] Under similar circumstances, a rich preadolescent would have fared much better. Her mother would have been able to pay $400 or even more to secure the services of a private physician for her.

Equally complex is the procreative situation of many infertile people. A variety of critics wonder whether infertile couples who want children act wisely when they assume all of the hardships and expenditures that accompany the use of some of the reproduction-aiding technologies. Pro-choice feminists worry that infertility is a problem largely because society continually signals to women that unless they have children, their lives will prove to be ultimately meaningless. Pro-life conservatives also believe that infertility is a problem, but they think there is a simple solution for it. They suggest that fertile girls and women should simply carry their *unwanted* fetuses to term so that infertile couples can adopt them. But to ask a girl such as Pamela to carry her pregnancy to term so an infertile couple can adopt her child is to ask her to bear an extraordinarily heavy psychological as well as physical burden. Similarly, to ask an infertile couple to forego the possibility of begetting a child genetically related to them in favor of adopting Pamela's infant is to ask them to make a personal sacrifice that relatively few fertile couples would choose to make. Clearly, it is unrealistic to believe that either Pamela or the infertile couple who are pressured to adopt her infant would be well-served by this accommodation.

It is also unrealistic to believe that fertile and infertile people can avoid entirely the kinds of misunderstandings that will inevitably arise between them: (1) How can you have an abortion? I'd do anything to get pregnant! (2) How can you justify spending thousands of dollars trying to get pregnant when there are babies just waiting to be adopted? Sure, they may not look at all like you, but they still deserve to be loved. (3) In this country if you're rich, your money can buy you procreative freedom; but if you're poor, procreative freedom is not an option. If you're fertile, you'll probably wind up with more kids than you can handle; and if you're infertile, you can forget about having kids—rich people are not going to pay the bills for poor people to get pregnant.

To prevent this kind of stone casting and name calling, we first need to understand what motivates it. Misunderstandings usually arise because people are different. Some people are rich; others are poor. Some belong to the so-called majority; others are members of an ethnic or racial minority group. Some are men; others are women. Everywhere issues of class, ethnicity, race, and gender intersect, helping to explain why some people are adamantly opposed to various reproductive technologies, whereas others wholeheartedly endorse them.

People's different social backgrounds do not explain entirely their positions on contraception, sterilization, abortion, in vitro fertilization, and artificial insemination, however. Their diverging ethical viewpoints also shape their attitudes toward these technologies. In the West, ethics is dominated by three major traditions: a virtue-oriented tradition, a social-utility tradition, and an individual rights-oriented tradition.

The Virtue-Oriented Tradition

Perhaps the most well known of all *virtue-oriented ethicists* is the ancient Greek philosopher Aristotle (384–322 B.C.). According to Aristotle, we all desire personal happiness (*eudaimonia*), or "a state of well-being, thriving, or flourishing";[2] and we become happy persons by exercising our distinctively human capacities of thought and action. A happy person, says Aristotle, is a reflective person—that is, a person who is able to establish an order of priority among his or her personal, professional, and political activities.

What enables the happy person to act rationally, notes Aristotle, is the virtue of practical wisdom—that is, the ability to strike consistently a rational midpoint between emotional excesses or defects. Without practical wisdom, we act rashly or timidly instead of courageously, or ostentatiously or niggardly instead of generously, or arrogantly or obsequiously instead of with proper self-respect.

Unfortunately, it is one thing for us to recognize our need for practical wisdom and quite another for us to cultivate this virtue. In fact, Aristotle repeatedly cautions that acting in a practically wise manner is no easy achievement:

It is the expert, not just anybody, who finds the center of the circle. In the same way, having a fit of temper is easy for anyone; so is giving money and spending it. But this is not so when it comes to questions of "for whom?" "how much?" "when?" "why?" and "how?" This is why goodness is rare, and is praiseworthy and fine.[3]

Given that goodness is so hard to achieve, critics understandably object that an ethics of virtue is an impractical guide for action in a society that is both heterogeneous and individualistic. People have different values, and they often insist on marching to the beat of their separate moral drummers. They increasingly reject practical wisdom—the ability to determine what is worth wanting—in favor of mere cleverness—the ability to get what one wants simply *because one wants it*. For example, an individual may not care whether it is good, in general, for infertile couples to pay fertile women for their gestational services. Instead she or he may judge the so-called rightness or wrongness of this practice (called *contracted* or *surrogate motherhood*) solely in terms of how much the infertile couple want a child genetically related to them. For this reason alone, say the critics, we cannot afford to guide our actions by subjective ideals; we must instead guide them by objective rules. Unless everyone's rights, general responsibilities, and specific duties are precisely delineated, too much will be left to individual judgment.

But is it really the case that ideals should play no role in our moral lives? *Virtue-oriented ethicists* respond that no matter how heterogeneous a society is, it should have room for ideals as well as rules. The moral life is more than a matter of following rules. Indeed, if all we ever do is what we are told to do, we will forever remain moral infants—safe, secure, and smug in our obedience to moral laws but with small souls capable of no great thoughts or actions. In contrast, if we require ourselves to live up to some self-imposed ideals, we will be able to become the moral equivalents of giant redwoods as opposed to tiny bonsai trees. Thus, virtue-oriented ethicists urge a woman contemplating abortion to consider the fabric of her entire moral existence, with particular attention to the texture of her relationships. Will her decision to abort enable her and those to whom she is related to flourish as human beings? Will it enhance or detract from her image of herself as a basically good person? Although rules may help this woman decide rightly, virtue-oriented ethicists ask her to consult her deepest ideals as she struggles to be as good as she can be under an extraordinarily difficult set of circumstances.

The Social-Utility Tradition

In contrast to virtue-oriented ethicists, who focus on the moral requirements for individual character, *social-utility ethicists* focus on the moral requirements for group happiness. They argue that what makes an act right is that it maximizes aggregate utility, or the overall happiness of the group that is affected by the consequences of a particular action. A person who wants to do the right thing should consider which one of a set of possible actions is likely to produce the most good for the most people and then perform that action. For example, if a person is trying to decide whether to use contraceptives, she or he should estimate how much good is likely to be produced by using contraceptives as compared to how much good is likely to be produced by not using them. If this person happens to be a sexually active teenage girl, she will probably produce more overall good by using contraceptives than by not using them. One of the distinguishing features of utilitarian thought, then, is the fact that whether or not the sexually active teenage girl wants to use contraceptives, she is morally required to use them if she will thereby serve the group's good. *Group* happiness, not personal happiness, is the ultimate goal of utilitarian action.

Another distinguishing feature of utilitarian thought is its apparent willingness to sacrifice an individual's rights in order to serve the group's well-being. For example, if the only way to eliminate a deleterious gene from the gene pool is for the state to sterilize involuntarily all carriers of it, then utilitarians will endorse this course of action as a regrettable, but nonetheless necessary, violation of some individuals' procreative rights.

The Rights-Oriented Tradition

To be sure, *rights-oriented ethicists* concede that since no right is absolute, there may be some circumstances that warrant, for example, the state's interference with an individual's procreative liberty. However, they insist that such circumstances are very rare and that it is misguided, in any event, to base the rightness of an action solely on the good consequences it produces for the aggregate. What makes an action right, they insist, is not its consequences but the reasons for which it is done. An act is right if its doer (1) believes that not only he or she but everyone would be permitted to do it under the same circumstances; (2) gives equal respect and consideration to the interests (desires, needs, wants) of everyone who will be affected by it; and (3) does it not because other people told him or her to do it or because he or she feels like doing it but because it is the right thing for anyone to do under the same set of circumstances.[4] For example, it is right for one woman to have an abortion only if (1) all women may have an abortion under the same circumstances; (2) the mother's, the father's, the fetus's (assuming it is a person, or at least a potential person), and all other affected persons' interests have been equally and respectfully considered; and (3) the woman decides to have the abortion because she *herself* is convinced that any rational person may, or even must, have an abortion under the same circumstances.

Moral Diversity

The fact that ethicists disagree among themselves about what makes an action right and what makes a person good can be disconcerting. How can we hope to formulate laws about abortion, to regulate the dissemination of contraceptives conscientiously, and to set high standards for in vitro fertilization clinics and sperm banks, for example, if morality is relative, subjective, and even arbitrary? Certainly, all of us have heard someone, perhaps ourselves, make a comment to the following effect: I listen to expert X's view and it seems to make sense. But then I listen to expert Y's view and expert Z's view, and they make sense too. I may as well do whatever I please!

Philosopher Alasdair MacIntyre sympathizes with this particular reaction to moral diversity. He claims that, as it now stands, for example, human reason cannot choose rationally between the three major moral arguments presented by abortion's opponents and proponents:

1. Everybody has certain rights over his or her own person, including his or her own body. It follows from the nature of these rights that at the stage when the embryo is essentially part of the mother's body, the mother has a right to make her own uncoerced decision on whether she will have an abortion or not. Therefore abortion is morally permissible and ought to be allowed by law.

2. I cannot will that my mother should have had an abortion when she was pregnant with me, except perhaps if it had been certain that the embryo was dead or gravely damaged. But if I cannot will this in my case, how can I consistently deny to others the right to life that I claim for myself? I would break the so-called Golden Rule unless I denied that a mother has in general a right to an abortion. I am not of course thereby committed to the view that abortion ought to be legally prohibited.

3. Murder is wrong. Murder is the taking of innocent life. An embryo is an identifiable individual, differing from a newborn infant only in being at an earlier stage on the long road to adult capacities and, if any life is innocent, that of an embryo is. If infanticide is murder, as it is, abortion is murder. So abortion is not only morally wrong but ought to be legally prohibited.[5]

For at least three reasons, says MacIntyre, each of these competing arguments makes considerable sense to us. First, each argument is based on a set of premises which, though fundamentally different from those in the other arguments, are equally compelling to a rational person. We cannot deny the force of an argument based on rights, nor one based on the principle of universalizability, nor one based on the value of human life, since all of these values are of vital importance to us. It is impossible for us to choose between such conceptually incommensurable values.

Second, each argument is made as impersonally as possible. We strive to be objective when we are debating the morality of abortion, for example. We try to screen out considerations that are related to our gender, race, ethnicity, religion, and social class. Yet no matter how much we struggle to be neutral, we fear that there may be no way to avoid the blinding lights of our own subjectivities. The more we realize how difficult it is to transcend our unique particularities, the more we begin to fear with MacIntyre that ultimately ethical arguments may be nothing but "a class of antagonistic wills, each will determined by some set of arbitrary choices of its own."[6]

Third, each argument has a distinctive, historical origin. MacIntyre notes that "a concept of rights which has Lockean antecedents is matched against a view of universalizability which is recognizable Kantian and an appeal to the moral law which is Thomist."[7] MacIntyre stresses the history behind ethics because he believes that human beings create the ethical systems that bind them. Moral principles and concerns do not descend on human beings from on high; rather human beings pull them out of the historical ground that roots them in a particular spatiotemporal nexus.

MacIntyre's third point is particularly important. Living in a pluralistic community, we realize that our conceptions of the good are multiple, and so we design our social and political institutions to enable us to reach as much consensus as possible about the things that matter the most to us. We agree that we should follow certain procedural rules when we are asked a difficult question such as, "Should the state be permitted to sterilize women who give birth to cocaine-addicted babies?"

First, we try to get straight on the facts: Is it possible for a cocaine-addicted woman to overcome her addiction? How long-lasting and serious are the consequences of coming into the world addicted to cocaine? Second, we appeal to the values that are embedded in the three major ethical systems that have shaped the Western moral point of view. We ask ourselves whether a woman's right to procreate is so fundamental that it cannot be abrogated under any circumstances or whether it is a right that not only may be but must be abrogated when her baby's well-being is affected deleteriously. Moreover, we seek to ask these questions in a respectful manner that aims to avoid the excess of arrogance as well as the defect of obsequiousness. Just because *I* believe something is right does not make it right. However, it does not make it wrong either. Any bona fide moral point of view is worthy of everyone's respect and consideration, but if we want to achieve the kind of consensus that permits people to live together in relative harmony, we need to regard our particular moral points of view as ones that are subject to revision by others as well as by ourselves.

Of course, consensus is not always possible, but there is no way of knowing for certain, before actual dialogue commences, whether our moral differences are going to be irreconcilable in any particular instance. It is this fact, that we cannot know in advance whether our attempts at consensus are destined for success or failure, that motivates us to communicate with one another. During the process of sharing information and revealing ourselves, we may change our minds and even shift our points of view. Such changes and shifts are not harmful compromises or spineless accommodations on our part. Rather, they are a sign that we are actively engaged in the process of constructing a set of common moral values. We make our moral values in dialogue with other human beings rather than discovering them ready-made.

Legal Principles

Unfortunately, moral dialogue is not easy. It can be disturbing, exhausting, rambling, and contentious, as well as exciting, creative, productive, and satisfying. Perhaps this is why so many people prefer the impersonality of the law to direct, eyeball-to-eyeball moral discussion. Admittedly, turning to the law can be good insofar as it permits people to articulate certain principles with which almost everyone can agree. But it can also be bad when people fail to realize that the law is not a seamless web. Within it are contained many of the contradictions, confusions, inconsistencies, and incoherences, and much of the incompleteness that plague morality.

Although much of our reproductive policy is based on the almost universally accepted harm principle (a person's liberty may be restricted only to prevent physical or psychological injury to other specific individuals), some of it is based on other, more controversial principles. Among these principles, says philosopher Joel Feinberg, are those of (1) legal paternalism (a person's liberty may be restricted to protect himself or herself from self-inflicted harm or even to confer a benefit on him or her); (2) legal moralism (a person's liberty may be restricted to protect other specific individuals, or society as a whole, from immoral behavior, where the word *immoral* means neither "harmful" nor "offensive" but something like "against the rule of a higher authority" (God) or "against a social taboo"); and (3) the offense principle (a person's liberty may be restricted to prevent offense to other specific individuals, where *offense* is interpreted as behavior that causes feelings of shame, outrage, or disgust in those against whom it is directed).[8]

The harm principle is most forcefully stated in John Stuart Mill's *On Liberty*. According to Mill, if a human being is a competent adult, then "the sole end for which mankind [is] warranted, individually or collectively, in interfering with the liberty of action of any of their number is self-protection."[9] In other words, unless a competent adult threatens to harm either an individual or society in general, that person is permitted, for example, to use whatever reproduction-controlling or reproduction-aiding techniques she or he wants.

Whatever its virtues, the harm principle is nonetheless plagued with problems of definition. Harm is, after all, a concept that expands and contracts with frustrating ease. On the one hand, if we define *harm* narrowly as physical abuse and assault only, then whole categories of psychological damage will not count as harm. On the other hand, if we define *harm* broadly so as to include every imaginable psychological distress, then the person who would do no harm had best move to a deserted island for fear of traumatizing, disquieting, or unsettling another human being. To be sure, the correct definition of *harm* lies between these extremes but, even if we identify this midpoint today, it is likely to change tomorrow as we recognize new human rights and interests.

Whereas the harm principle aims to prevent harm to others, the principle of legal paternalism aims to prevent harm to self. The argument in favor of restricting a person's liberty—and we are speaking of adults here —often begins with an analogy to the parent-child relationship. Just as children sometimes make the wrong decisions about their own best interests and must be ruled by their parents, so too do adults sometimes need to be ruled by their guardian, the state. This analogy is most plausible when an adult is unable to act voluntarily because she or he is ignorant of crucial information or is blocked by some form of internal or external coercion. It is least plausible when an adult knows what he or she is doing and is under no coercive force to do it. Whereas most adults want to be saved from making mistakes they regard as foolish or forced —that is, mistakes made in ignorance or under duress—they do not also want to be stopped from making the kind of "mistakes" that reflect their own idiosyncratic priorities.

When it comes to state interference with competent adults' decisions to act in what is perceived as less than their own best interests, cases can be made both against and for such interference. Antipaternalists argue, for example, that if a competent woman wants to smoke in the privacy of her own home, or if a competent man wants to drink in the privacy of his own home, then the state has no right to interfere. Although smoking and drinking present health hazards to each of these individuals respectively, antipaternalists insist that it is not the state's prerogative to force people to be as healthy as possible. If a person values short-term creature comforts more than long-term health benefits, it is that person's prerogative to add some health risks to his or her life. After all, of what significance is free expression if the only things that a person can express freely are those that have the state's seal of approval?

But even if most persons believe that the decision to harm themselves is their own to make, paternalists point out that, under certain circumstances, almost everyone is willing to limit his or her right to self-determination. Competent adults may decide at time t to precommit themselves to a future course of action at time $t + 1$ that will prevent them from indulging in self-harm then.[10] Among the reasons competent adults may give for limiting their own liberty are the following. First, a person may know that she or he cannot trust herself or himself at time $t + 1$ to do what it is she or he agreed to do at time t. For example, so that he will take his much-needed but hated medicine at time $t + 1$, Joe gives Jane his bottle of pills at time t, instructing her not to go out with him unless he takes one of them. Second, a person may find it advantageous that others know that she or he has precommitted herself or himself to a certain course of action. Returning to our example, if Jane knows Joe does not want to change his mind at time $t + 1$, the actual time for him to take his medicine, about a decision he made at time t to take it, Jane will not have to feel in anyway apologetic when she refuses to go out with Joe until he first takes his medicine.

As desirable as it may be to protect one's self from one's own future irrationalities, it may be even more desirable to protect one's self from the future irrationalities of the groups to which one belongs. In *Managing the Commons*, Garrett Hardin describes a classic case of group irrationality.[11] A town has one common sheep pasture that is rapidly becoming overcrowded. Reasoning that "just one more sheep won't hurt," each citizen irresponsibly continues to add sheep to the pasture until no more grass is left for any of the sheep to eat, with the obvious disastrous consequence. Had the citizens been bound by an agreement made at time t setting an upper limit on the number of sheep allowed in the pasture at any future time including time $t + 1$, then they would not have been able to keep on adding sheep to the pasture. In other words, such an agreement would have enabled the citizens to act in their *real* best interest at time $t + 1$, that of preserving a common sheep pasture, when tempted to act in their *perceived* best interest, that of adding more sheep to the common pasture.

Restriction-of-liberty cases have been made not only for and against people who harm either others or themselves but also against those who act immorally, where the term *immoral* is not the equivalent of the term *illegal*. A particular action may be considered immoral without being illegal. For example, lying to friends may be morally wrong, but no legislature is likely to enact laws against it. Conversely, some illegal actions may be morally acceptable; for example, refusing to serve in an unjust war is not immoral and yet it is illegal. Nevertheless, despite the difference between law and morality, these two realms of behavior control do intersect. Indeed, if we examine typical laws against homosexual relations, prostitution, gambling, drugs, drinking, euthanasia, suicide, and obscenity, we will find that they are often based on beliefs about God's commandments, nature's laws, or society's traditions. Currently, because an increasing number of people no longer view God, nature, or society as binding authorities, there is a growing conviction that the law, especially the criminal law, should not forbid an activity simply because it is immoral.

One of the clearest statements of the view that the criminal law's true function is to prevent harmful and not simply immoral conduct was that of the Wolfenden Committee. In the 1950s, this committee was established in England to review laws concerning homosexuality and prostitution. The committee decided that a firm line should be drawn between the public and private realms—that is, between the area in which our actions affect the community as a whole and the realm in which our actions affect only, or primarily, ourselves. Whereas the criminal law has roles to play in the public realm—preserving "public order and decency," protecting "the citizen from what is offensive or injurious," and providing "sufficient safeguards against exploitation or corruption of others, particularly those who are specially vulnerable because they are young, weak in body or mind or inexperienced"[12]—it has no role to play in the private realm. What consenting adults do to each other in the privacy of their own homes is their own business.

If applied to matters other than the ones it scrutinized, the findings of the Wolfenden Committee suggest, for example, that so long as a reproductive decision between a man and a woman remains within the private realm, it is not the law's concern. However, if such a reproductive decision enters into the public realm—for example, by affecting a third party in a harmful way—then the law has a right, and perhaps an obligation, to restrict the freedom of the involved individuals. For example, whether a couple decides to have 2 or 20 children is ordinarily its own business, but if a community is suffering from so much overpopulation that its very survival is at stake, then the state may be not only permitted but also required to regulate the number of children people have.

However, not everyone agrees with the Wolfenden Committee's conclusion that morality should not be legislated. Lord Patrick Devlin has argued that the law may be used to preserve morality just as it may be used to safeguard anything essential to the existence of society. Devlin argues that conformity to moral prescriptions (in his view, Judeo-Christian moral prescriptions) is just as necessary for social stability as is obedience to legal codes. Without common morality as well as common legality, the fabric of society will weaken and fray.[13]

Although Devlin's opponents concede that the continuance of a society is a good thing, they caution that there are exceptions to this rule. Philosopher H. L. A. Hart observes that not all societies are worth continuing:

We might wish to argue that whether or not a society is justified in taking steps to preserve itself must depend both on what sort of society it is and what the steps to be taken are. If a society were mainly devoted to the cruel persecution of a racial or religious minority, or if the steps to be taken included hideous tortures, it is arguable that what Lord Devlin terms the "disintegration" of such a society would be morally better than its continued existence, and steps ought not to be taken to preserve it.[14]

Moreover, even if the continuance of a certain society is desirable, it is not any *specific* morality that is required for its continuation but only *some* morality. Thus, in a period of rapidly changing moral opinions, a society may have several factions representing new, ascendant moralities as well as several factions representing the old, descendant morality. Far from being a problem, this kind of moral evolution is a necessary feature of any progressing or changing society. Devlin's argument is, according to his critics, extremely conservative in that he would have us maintain the current morality, no matter what that might be, in order to preserve our society's stability, even if that very "stability" is suffocating and stultifying us.

As debatable as it is to restrict immoral behavior simply because it is immoral, it is even more debatable to restrict so-called offensive behavior. The offense principle is similar to the harm principle in that it protects others from the consequences of a prohibited action, and it is similar to legal moralism in that the prohibited action is often said to violate God's, nature's, or society's norms. However, we can readily distinguish the offense principle from these other principles. For example, in Kurt Vonnegut's short story, *Welcome to the Monkey House*, people react to public eating in much the same way that we currently react to public defecating. Although no one in the Monkey House is actually harmed by watching someone else eat and no one considers eating in public immoral, there are, nonetheless, laws against public eating because everyone is seriously offended by what they regard as disgusting, animalistic behavior.[15]

In our own society, the offense principle has most often been directed against pornography—that is, sexually explicit representations. According to philosopher Joel Feinberg, it has been urged that the state has a right to restrict offensive material if it is universally offensive (likely to cause almost anyone, irrespective of his or her gender, race, ethnicity, or religion to feel shame, embarrassment, or disgust) and if it is virtually unavoidable (so pervasive that a person would have to be both blind and deaf not to notice it).[16] But even if the state has a right to restrict universally offensive and virtually unavoidable sexually explicit representations, opponents of the offense principle point out that very rarely is anything universally offensive and virtually unavoidable. With respect to the claim that pornography is universally offensive, critics note that whereas most people are disgusted by *thanatica* (sexually explicit representations that show people engaged in the destruction of the human body), few people are disgusted by *erotica* (sexually explicit representations that show people engaged in a celebration of the human body). Likewise, with respect to the claim that pornography is virtually unavoidable, critics point out that there are many ways to keep pornography confined to the private realm in this era of home videos and that no society that calls itself free may have as one of its legitimate aims "unithink." The fact that what we think influences what we say and do does not give the state a warrant to control our thoughts so that we will all say and do approximately the same thing.

Given these latter two considerations, it is unlikely that the offense principle will be used on its own to justify restrictions on the development or use of reproductive technology. Although many people used to find offensive the ideas of sex without procreation and procreation without sex, their number is decreasing. Yesterday's unaccepted behavior can become today's accepted behavior. For example, when the protagonist in Marge Piercy's feminist science fiction novel, *Woman on the Edge of Time*,[17] is shown a baby-brooder in which seven human embryos are suspended upside down, each in a sac of its own inside a larger fluid receptacle, her stomach slowly turns upside down as well. Before long, her tour guides realize that their visitor from another time and place is sickened by a sight they now find beautiful but that they too used to find ugly. When something offends us, we must ask ourselves both *why* it offends us and whether it *should* offend us. To fail to ask these questions is to give reason no role to play in the life of our emotions.

Conclusion

Nonetheless, even if we all agreed that only the harm principle should shape our reproductive policies, we would still have some hard work ahead of us. The fact that a court rules that a law is (un)constitutional or a legislative body votes unanimously for a bill does not mean that the law or bill is right, and any retreat from the willingness to do our own moral thinking is particularly irresponsible when it comes to technological developments that control or assist a process as important as human reproduction.

Frequently, we express the concern that technology advances faster than ethics. We worry that our reproductive technologies are developing without humane guidance and that we are going to use them whether or not we comprehend their moral implications. Yet our reproductive technologies have the capacity not only to create new moral challenges and problems but also to resolve some old moral challenges and problems. For example, if researchers develop the artificial placenta, they will solve the abortion dilemma in one major respect: Fetal extraction will no longer have to result in fetal extinction. Of course, were the artificial placenta developed, both sides of the abortion debate would need to ask themselves some previously unasked questions. For example, when a pregnant woman chooses abortion, is it only fetal extraction or also fetal extinction that is her goal? Similarly, when a person claims that she or he wants to save "babies" from being aborted, is she or he ready to commit billions of dollars to the maintenance of fetuses in artificial placentas so that every one of them can come to term? What if this particular expenditure caused health care to consume not simply 12 percent of the gross national product, as it does now, but 24 or even 36 percent of it? These are hard questions because no one wants to think that human love is limited or that human life is anything less than the ultimate value and yet, unless we ask ourselves the hard questions, we are acting in a largely irresponsible manner.

The cumulative knowledge of scientists, technologists, ethicists, lawyers, and concerned citizens certainly benefits us, but it also burdens us. The more we know about reproduction-controlling and reproduction-aiding technologies, the more responsible we become to make them serve such fundamental human values as freedom, happiness, and justice. These technologies can liberate people to make decisions about whether to become parents; they can bring happiness to the aggregate, depending on how wisely they are used; and they can bring justice to individuals, depending on how widely they are distributed. On the other hand, these technologies can enslave people, make them very unhappy, and violate their rights. The initial choice belongs to each of us, the ultimate consequences to all of us.

3 The Human Reproductive System

In chapter 2, we discussed some ethical systems, legal principles, and social perspectives in order to appreciate the ways in which reproduction-controlling (contraception, sterilization, and abortion) and reproduction-aiding technologies (artificial insemination, in vitro fertilization, and embryo transfer) affect our world for better or for worse. In this chapter, we discuss the human reproductive system to comprehend how these technologies work in and through our bodies. As we see it, it is equally as important to understand how we reproduce as it is to understand why or whether we should reproduce. To be informed about reproductive technologies is to know as much about them as possible, from the perspective of the natural scientist as well as from those of the social scientist and the humanist.

General Principles of Sexual Reproduction

During sexual reproduction, specialized reproductive cells called *gametes* combine to form a zygote destined to develop into a new individual. The characteristics of these two gametes, the ovum and the sperm, enable them to execute the functions that are unique to them as well as those that they share in common. In many ways, the reproductive work that the sperm and the ovum do together represents a highly successful division of labor.

Sexual reproduction begins when the primordial gametes migrate to the developing zygote's gonads (ovaries in women, testes in men). There the production of the mature gametes, the egg and the sperm, begins. In tracing the development of the egg (oogenesis) and sperm (spermatogenesis), we will notice that they develop in distinctive ways that permit them to communicate the correct amount of genetic information to the zygote.[1] When somatic (or body) cells divide, each new cell must have all the genetic information of the parent cell, information that is transmitted through the process of mitosis (see the appendix). But when gametes, or germ cells, divide, each new cell must have only half the information of the parent cell, information that is transmitted through meiosis (see the appendix). In humans, the diploid (or parent) cells contain 46 chromosomes composed of 23 homologous pairs of chromosomes, one individual of each pair coming from the mother and the other from the father. In contrast, the haploid cells contain 23 chromosomes (that is, 23 *individual* chromosomes, not 23 *pairs* of homologous chromosomes), obtained neither exclusively from the mother nor exclusively from the father.[2] Rather, due to so-called genetic shuffling, these 23 individual chromosomes are selected in random fashion partly from the maternal diploid cell and partly from the paternal diploid cell.[3] Since new combinations of genes are constantly being created first through meiosis and then through the fusion of the egg cell and sperm cell,[4] human individuality is not at risk. No one of us will look entirely like his or her mother or father.

Thus far we have been discussing human sexual reproduction in general terms, focusing neither on the sperm nor on the eggs. If we are to appreciate the complexity of this process, however, it is necessary to understand fully the nature and production of the sperm and the egg separately. For each of these two gametes, we will first describe the cell, then discuss the mechanism and hormonal control of its production, and finally describe the reproductive tracts (the male tract and the female tract) through which the gametes are transported and in which both the gametes and the developing offspring are housed and nourished.

Male Reproductive System

Description of the Sperm Cell

Interestingly, in direct contrast to the egg, which is one of the largest cells in our bodies, the sperm is the smallest. A human sperm, which looks and acts like a tadpole, is only 0.06 mm long. The sperm has two functions: to deliver its set of genes to the egg and to stimulate the egg to begin development. The sperm, shown in figure 3.1 consists of a head, a midpiece, and a tail section, each with a specialized function.

The head of the sperm, which contains the nucleus with its haploid chromosome, is capped by a small compartment called the *acrosomal vesicle* that contains hydrolytic enzymes. When the egg and the sperm come together, these enzymes are released. By digesting the outer coat of

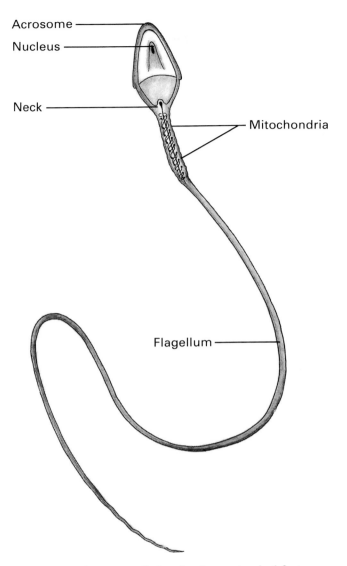

Acrosome

Nucleus

Neck

Mitochondria

Flagellum

Figure 3.1 A sperm cell showing its anatomical features.

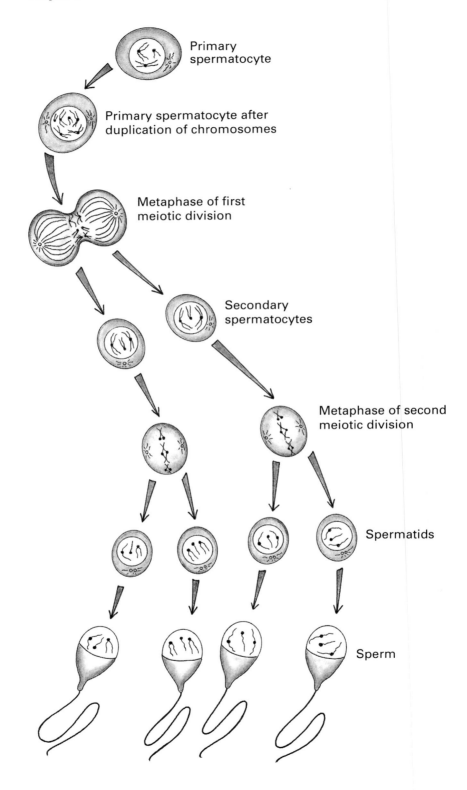

Primary spermatocyte

Primary spermatocyte after duplication of chromosomes

Metaphase of first meiotic division

Secondary spermatocytes

Metaphase of second meiotic division

Spermatids

Sperm

the egg, the enzymes enable the sperm to penetrate to the egg's plasma membrane.

A sperm cell is very compact and ideally shaped to deliver the paternal chromosomes to the egg. The midpiece contains a large number of mitochondria (organelles that provide energy to the cell), and the long flagellum (a motile tail) wags vigorously to propel the sperm toward the egg.

Evidence increasingly indicates that the egg releases chemicals that direct the sperm to swim up the female genital tract toward it. This journey is a difficult one because the female glands release fluids that tend to push down on the sperm even as it swims upstream. Influenced by temperature and acidity, so-called male-producing sperm and female-producing sperm apparently swim at different rates of speed in the female genital tract, a fact that partially explains why a higher percentage of boy babies are conceived at certain times of a woman's menstrual cycle and girl babies at others.

Development of the Sperm

After their initial development in the embryonic gonads, the immature male germ cells, or spermatogonia, are mostly dormant in the testes until the onset of puberty. At this time, the production of the sperm, or spermatogenesis, takes place when the spermatogonia begin to mature.[5] The spermatogonia, located in numerous tiny tubules contained in the testes, undergo a period of proliferation by mitosis, and then some of the spermatogonia differentiate into the primary spermatocytes. Each diploid primary spermatocyte produces two daughter cells, the secondary spermatocytes. In turn, each of the two secondary spermatocytes produces two haploid spermatids. A lengthy period of maturation then takes place during which the spermatids are transformed from spherical cells into the characteristic streamlined shape of the sperm cells. The overall process is shown in figure 3.2.

Two special features that characterize human spermatogenesis are the distribution of the chromosomes and the incomplete division of the cytoplasm. In spermatogenesis, however, the daughter cells are not all identi-

Figure 3.2   The cellular stages in the production of mature sperm cells. The primary spermatocyte has a diploid chromosome number and each chromosome is double-stranded. After the second meiotic division, the spermatids are haploid with single-stranded chromosomes. Further development (see figure 3.3) leads to a mature sperm cell.

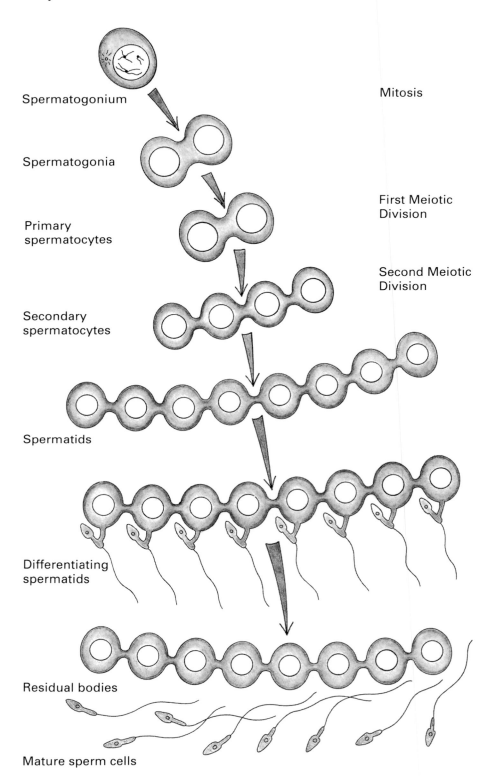

Spermatogonium

Mitosis

Spermatogonia

First Meiotic Division

Primary spermatocytes

Second Meiotic Division

Secondary spermatocytes

Spermatids

Differentiating spermatids

Residual bodies

Mature sperm cells

cal in chromosomal makeup. One important difference in the chromosomal makeup of the resulting cells involves the distribution of the "sex chromosome." Of the 46 chromosomes (23 matching or homologous pairs) in each human cell, one pair, the sex chromosomes, is specially involved in sex determination. Since there are two types of sex chromosomes, they are not always a homologous pair. One is a medium-sized chromosome called the *X chromosome*; the other is a smaller chromosome called the *Y chromosome*. Normally, a female possesses two X chromosomes and a male possesses one X and one Y chromosome. The other 22 chromosome pairs are similar in both sexes. Since pairs of homologous chromosomes are separated during meiosis, of the four spermatids produced during spermatogenesis, two contain the haploid X chromosome and two contain the haploid Y chromosome.[6]

Another characteristic of spermatogenesis is that the cytoplasm of the developing germ cells does not separate completely to produce individual cells during the stages of mitosis and meiosis. Due to this incomplete separation, the daughter cells are connected by cytoplasmic bridges that remain until the final stage of sperm differentiation (figure 3.3). During this procedure, a great deal of the mass of the cell is discarded and only a small amount of cytoplasm is incorporated into the functional sperm cell, with the chromosome tightly packed inside. It is not until the sperm cells are separated from the residual bodies that they become mature sperm, obtaining the streamlined shape needed to move in the female reproductive tract.

Hormonal Control of Sperm Production

To regulate the amount of sperm present at any time, the rate at which spermatogenesis occurs must be carefully controlled. Obviously this depends on a number of factors, including the sexual activity of the male. Spermatogenesis is hormonally regulated to ensure a well-controlled sperm production. The hormonal mechanisms that regulate sperm production are based on the principle of negative feedback. In a negative feedback system, an increase in an element's output causes its production to decrease. One of the best ways to understand a negative feedback

Figure 3.3 The maturation of sperm cells showing how the progeny of a single spermatogonium remain connected via the cytoplasmic bridges through the primary and secondary spermatocyte stages and through the spermatid stage until the mature sperm cells separate from the residual bodies, which contain the majority of the cytoplasm.

mechanism is to consider the operation of a thermostat that has been set to maintain room temperature at a certain degree. When the room cools below the set point, the thermostat causes the furnace to turn on and to produce heat, and when the room warms above the set point, the thermostat causes the furnace to shut off and to cease heat production. The various hormones involved in both the male and female reproductive systems function very much like the negative feedback mechanism of a furnace. The more we understand how these hormones ordinarily regulate reproduction, the more we will understand the workings of methods of birth control that interrupt these normal hormonal processes.

Testosterone usually is thought of as the male hormone, but it alone does not regulate the production of sperm. Two other hormones, produced by the pituitary gland located at the base of the brain, are necessary for sperm production and maturation. These hormones, called *gonadotropins* because of their effect on the gonads, are follicle-stimulating hormone (FSH) and luteinizing hormone (LH). These hormones initially were identified in the female, and their names reflect their effect in the female reproductive system. Later they were found to play comparable roles in the male, but the original names have largely been retained (although LH is sometimes called interstitial cell–stimulating hormone [ISCH] in men).

The blood carries these two gonadotropins from their site of synthesis in the pituitary to their site of action in the testes. In the testes, FSH and, to a lesser extent, testosterone are both needed to stimulate sperm production in the large number of seminiferous tubules present, as shown in figure 3.4. LH is also required for sperm production insofar as it stimulates the secretion of testosterone from the surrounding cells and plays a role in the maturation of the sperm. Finally, gonadotropin-releasing hormone (GnRH), which is produced by the hypothalamus (a gland located at the base of the brain and attached to the pituitary gland by means of a stalk), is required for sperm production because it regulates the production of both FSH and LH (see figures 3.5 and 3.6).[7]

With this in mind, we can compare the regulation of the hormones testosterone, FSH, LH, and GnRH with the negative feedback mechanism described earlier. When the concentration of testosterone in the blood becomes elevated, it not only inhibits the release of LH from the pituitary gland; it also inhibits the release of GnRH from the hypothalamus. In the absence of GnRH, no LH or FSH is released; and in the absence of these hormones, no more testosterone is released. Consequently, sperm production is decreased. In sum, when too much testosterone is produced, its further production is inhibited until its level in the blood drops. No sooner does the concentration of testosterone in the blood begin to drop, how-

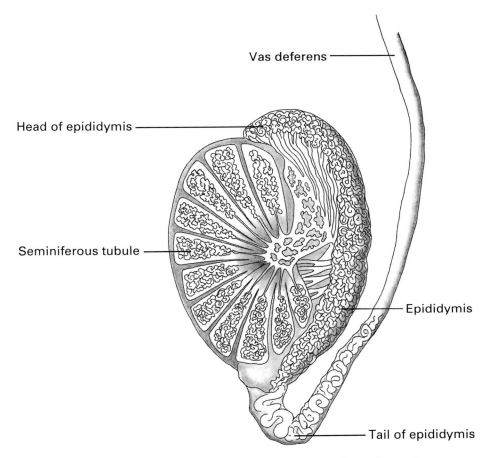

Vas deferens

Head of epididymis

Seminiferous tubule

Epididymis

Tail of epididymis

Figure 3.4 A cross-section of a human testis, showing the regions where sperm production and maturation take place.

ever, then its inhibiting effect on GnRH is lost. As GnRH levels rise, LH is again secreted which, in turn, stimulates the production of more testosterone, leading to the production of more sperm.[8]

In addition to GnRH, a substance called *inhibin* regulates FSH. Inhibin is released from the testes and, as its concentration increases, it inhibits both the secretion of FSH from the pituitary gland and the production of GnRH in the hypothalamus. Just as LH is not secreted until the level of testosterone drops, so too FSH is not secreted until the level of inhibin drops due to a decreased sperm production. In both cases, increased levels of secretion of LH and FSH result in the increased production of sperm.

Clearly, the production of sperm is no chance matter; it depends on a delicate interplay of hormones whose overproduction or underproduction can effectively inhibit a man's capacity to reproduce. In addition to the

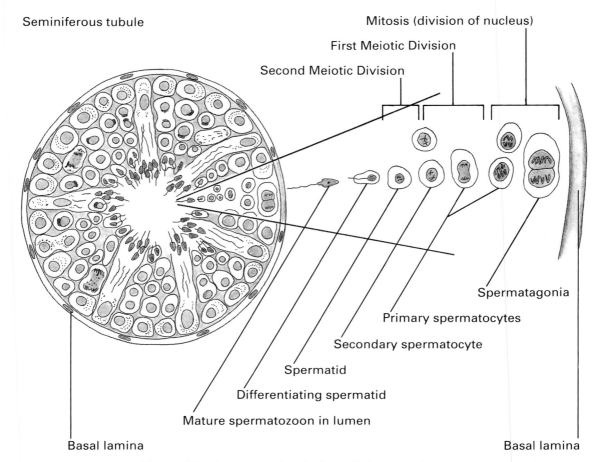

Seminiferous tubule

Mitosis (division of nucleus)

First Meiotic Division

Second Meiotic Division

Spermatagonia

Primary spermatocytes

Secondary spermatocyte

Spermatid

Differentiating spermatid

Mature spermatozoon in lumen

Basal lamina

Basal lamina

Figure 3.5 A cross-sectional view of the seminiferous tubules in the human testis, showing the location of the stages of sperm maturation.

hormonal regulation of sperm, many other factors may significantly influence spermatogenesis. For example, because the hypothalamus, the gland that produces GnRH, seems to be controlled directly by the brain, some scientists speculate that stress and the psychological factors related to it can negatively affect sperm production.

The Sperm Tract and the Production of Semen

From its site of production in the testes, the sperm must travel through the sperm tract to reach the outside of the body. As it does so, the various components that make up the seminal fluid are added to the sperm. The sperm tract, illustrated in figure 3.7, consists of a number of ducts including the epididymis, the vas deferens, the ejaculatory duct, and the

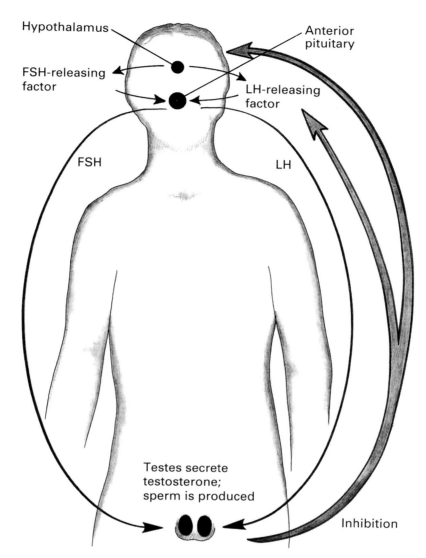

Figure 3.6 Hormonal control of spermatogenesis showing, the interaction among the hypothalamus, the anterior pituitary, and the testis. FSH, follicle-stimulating hormone; LH, luteinizing hormone.

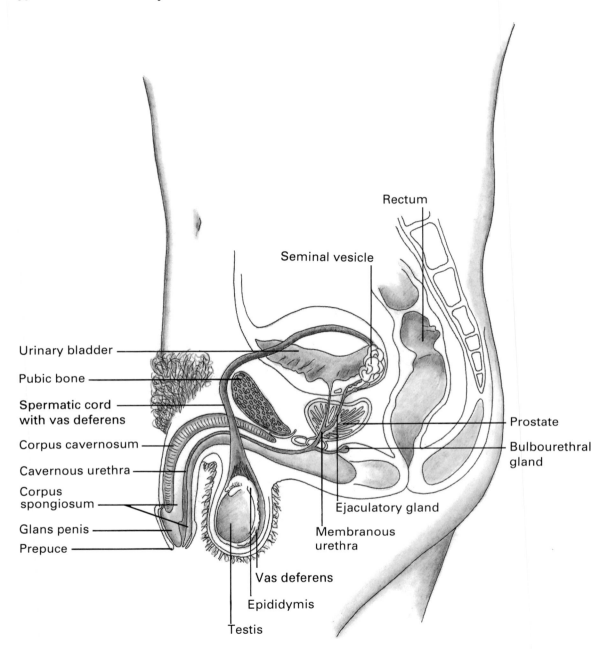

Figure 3.7 The male reproductive system, showing the relative location of the testis and the other glands that secrete fluids to make up the semen.

urethra. In addition, a number of glands that secrete various fluids join the sperm tract through a series of small ducts.

After being produced in the seminiferous tubules, the sperm are stored in the epididymis, which is a highly coiled, interconnected network of seminiferous tubules lying in the upper part of the testes. As the sperm mature in the epididymis, they become capable of movement as the neck of each sperm becomes flexible.

The vas deferens carries the sperm from the epididymis to the ejaculatory duct. At this point, the ducts of the seminal vesicles join the sperm tract and provide a viscous, alkaline secretion containing fructose and prostaglandins. The fructose, a sugar, is a source of energy for the sperm; the prostaglandins stimulate uterine contractions and help the sperm move to the female's fallopian tubes where fertilization takes place. The prostate gland surrounds the ejaculatory duct at the place where it becomes the urethra. It secretes a milky fluid that aids in sperm motility. The fluid contains, among other things, a large concentration of bicarbonate ions that gives the semen its alkaline pH. The alkaline nature of the seminal vesicle fluid and the prostate gland fluid reduces the acidity present in the urinary system, which is joined to the sperm tract at the urethra. This is particularly important since sperm motility is adversely affected by an acidic environment. Finally, the bulbourethral glands (Cowper's glands) secrete a mucuslike substance that provides lubrication for the urethra.

The secretions just described are called *seminal fluid*, and the combination of sperm and seminal fluid is called *semen*. Since there frequently is confusion as to the distinction between sperm and semen, it is worthwhile to point out that while sperm are under the careful hormonal control previously described, the seminal fluid is produced by the body as needed and is not affected by hormonal levels. Also important is the fact that the semen contains an antibiotic substance called *seminalplasmin*. Were it not for seminalplasmin, seminal bacteria would almost always infect women's vaginas, making sexual intercourse a routine health hazard.

Female Reproductive System

Description of the Egg Cell

From one perspective, the egg is a highly specialized cell with a single function—namely, the generation of a new individual. From another perspective, the egg is developmentally the least restricted cell in an animal

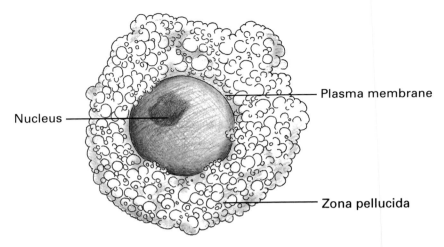

Nucleus — Plasma membrane — Zona pellucida

Figure 3.8   An egg cell, showing the anatomical features.

because, if fertilized, it can give rise to every cell type in the organism. Although it is barely visible with the naked eye, the egg is very large when compared to a typical body (somatic) cell. For example, a human egg is approximately 0.13 mm in diameter, a size 10 times the diameter and 1000 times the volume of most other human body cells. The egg is large so that it can adequately nourish the embryo until a connection is made between it and the mother.

In addition to its size, there are a number of structural features specific to the egg cell (figure 3.8). Whereas most cells have an external surface called the *plasma membrane*, the egg has a special structure called the *outer egg coat* or *zona pellucida*. Consisting of a jellylike extracellular matrix composed mostly of glycoprotein molecules, the outer egg coat protects the egg from mechanical damage. It is also the site of specific receptors that enable same-species sperm (and *only* same-species sperm) to recognize the egg and, in the presence of certain conditions, to interact with it.

When such interaction does occur—that is, when a sperm cell actually does penetrate an egg cell—cortical granules, a set of specialized secretory vesicles located in the outer area of the egg's cytoplasm, release their contents and, in so doing, immediately alter the egg's outer coat so that no other sperm will be able to fuse with the egg.[9]

Development of the Egg

The development of mature egg cells is called *oogenesis*.[10] There are several important differences between egg production and sperm production. The initial stage of oogenesis occurs when the primordial germ cells

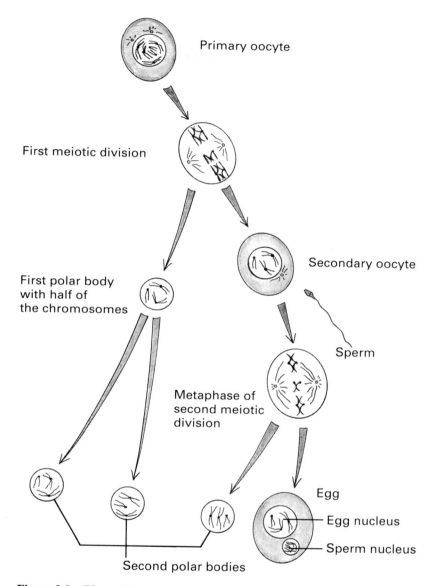

Primary oocyte

First meiotic division

First polar body with half of the chromosomes

Secondary oocyte

Sperm

Metaphase of second meiotic division

Egg

Egg nucleus

Sperm nucleus

Second polar bodies

Figure 3.9 The cellular stages in the production of mature egg cells. The primary oocyte has a diploid chromosome number and each chromosome is double-stranded. After the second meiotic division, which does not occur until after the sperm enters the egg, the oocytes are haploid with single-stranded chromosomes. Notice the loss of relatively little cytoplasm in the polar bodies.

migrate to the zygote's developing ovaries and differentiate into oogonia (figure 3.9). At approximately 5 gestational months, when the production of new oogonia stops never to resume again, the embryo has nearly 6 to 7 million oogonia. By the time the girl is ready to be born, these oogonia, now called *primary oocytes*, will have started the process of meiosis (see the appendix), which will be completed for individual oocytes between puberty and menopause.

After the girl reaches puberty, the remaining steps of the first stage of meiosis take place for individual oocytes just before each ovulation. At this time, the cytoplasm of the primary oocyte divides asymmetrically into a larger cell called the *secondary oocyte*, which contains essential genetic information, and a smaller cell called the *first polar body*, which eventually degenerates. When the follicle on the surface of the ovary ruptures during ovulation, the secondary oocyte together with the polar body and some follicle cells are released.[11]

Only if the secondary oocyte is fertilized by a sperm does it undergo the second meiotic stage. When this happens, the cytoplasm of the secondary oocyte again divides asymmetrically to produce a large mature egg and a small polar body. The mature egg now contains a haploid number of single chromosomes and, because of the two asymmetrical cytoplasmic divisions, a large amount of cytoplasm. Instead of the four haploid cells produced during spermatogenesis, only *one* functional mature egg is produced from each primary oocyte in order to provide the developing embryo with food and energy until its mother is able to do so.

Oogenesis is an enormously wasteful system.[12] During the first months of human embryonic development, approximately 1700 primordial germ cells migrate to the developing ovaries. After several months of mitotic division, these oogonia number approximately 7 million. Of these oogonia, however, only 400,000 or so will develop into primary oocytes. During the 40 years or so of a woman's reproductive life, relatively few of these primary oocytes will mature into secondary oocytes. Indeed, only 400 to 500 secondary oocytes are ultimately released from the ovaries at a rate of approximately 1 per month.

Production of Eggs

The eggs, which develop in the ovaries, pass through the fallopian tubes to the uterus (figure 3.10). The actual path of the egg will depend on whether it is fertilized. Because of the cyclical nature of the maturation and release of the eggs and because of the different conditions that prevail on fertilization, the female reproductive system is more complicated and

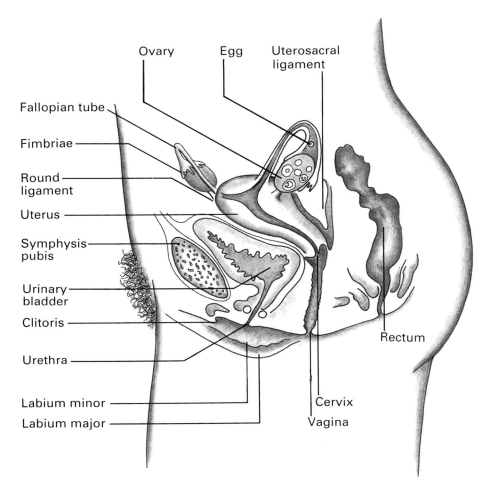

Ovary Egg Uterosacral ligament

Fallopian tube

Fimbriae

Round ligament

Uterus

Symphysis pubis

Urinary bladder

Clitoris

Urethra

Labium minor

Labium major

Rectum

Cervix

Vagina

Figure 3.10 The female reproductive system, showing the relative location and orientation of the ovaries, the fallopian tubes, and the uterus.

under more hormonal control than the male system. The ovaries have two purposes: releasing eggs on a regular monthly cycle and producing female sex hormones.[13] Contained in the cortex of the ovaries are hundreds of thousands of ovarian follicles in different stages of development. Each follicle consists of one primary oocyte surrounded by layers of follicular cells. As illustrated in figure 3.11, only one of these follicles per month ordinarily reaches maturity, ruptures, and releases an egg into a funnel-shaped structure called the *infundibulum* that covers each of the fallopian tubes (oviduct). Initially, cilia (see the appendix) and muscular contractions sweep the egg down the fallopian tubes, but their sweeping motion soon slows down. Owing to this slowdown, it takes the egg several days to reach the uterus, the pear-shaped organ located at the end of the

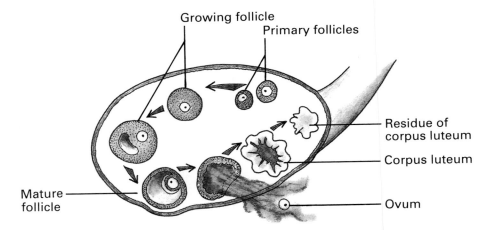

Figure 3.11 Cross-sectional view of the ovary, showing the maturation of the follicles.

fallopian tubes. Because the egg is capable of being fertilized for only 10 to 15 hours after ovulation, fertilization must take place in the fallopian tube, if it is to occur at all.

Under hormonal regulation, the lining of the uterus (endometrium) is prepared monthly for the possible implantation of a fertilized egg. If implantation does not take place, the endometrium is sloughed off (menstruation) and the monthly cycle is repeated. If implantation does take place with a resulting pregnancy, the uterus houses, nourishes, and protects the developing embryo and fetus.[14]

Hormonal Regulation

Because hormones regulate two coordinated cyclical systems in woman—the ovarian cycle and the uterine cycle—hormonal regulation is more complicated than in man (figure 3.12). As we shall see, success or failure of several reproduction-aiding technologies for women depends on the careful regulation of the hypothalamic hormone GnRH, the pituitary hormone FSH, and the ovarian hormones estrogen and progesterone.

Ovarian Cycle

Follicular Phase

When the hypothalamus gland secretes GnRH, the pituitary gland responds by secreting FSH and LH. FSH stimulates the primary oocyte to increase in size and surrounding follicle cells to increase in number

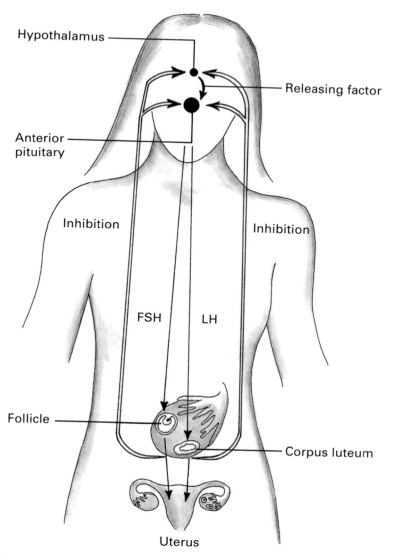

Figure 3.12 Hormonal control of oogenesis, showing the interaction among the hypothalamus, the anterior pituitary, and the ovary. The releasing factor from the hypothalmus stimulates the production of follicle-stimulating hormone (FSH) and luteinizing hormone (LH) which, in turn, stimulate follicle and egg production in the ovary. LH also stimulates estrogen production, which not only stimulates follicle and egg development but inhibits the production of releasing factor and LH and FSH.

as they mature. As a result of both FSH stimulation and the presence of LH, these other follicle cells begin to produce and secrete estrogen. Consequently, the primary oocyte matures into the secondary oocyte, proceeding through the rest of the phases of the first meiotic stage. After approximately 14 days, FSH secretion decreases and estrogen reaches maximal levels. At this point, for reasons unknown, there is a rapid rise in the LH level as the secondary oocyte follicle approaches full size. Having reached full size, the follicle bursts and the egg is released into the fallopian tubes.[15]

Luteal Phase

After the follicle ruptures, estrogen levels decrease slightly. The ruptured follicle then undergoes a transformation into a new cellular structure called the *corpus luteum* (literally, "yellow body") that produces high levels of progesterone and estrogen in the woman's body. The increased levels of progesterone and estrogen act as a negative feedback mechanism to inhibit the production of LH and FSH, thereby preventing the maturation of another primary oocyte and follicle as long as the corpus luteum remains functional—usually between 10 and 14 days if fertilization does not take place. As the corpus luteum degenerates, estrogen and progesterone levels drop, causing FSH and LH levels to rise. The increased FSH and LH levels then promote the initiation of a new follicular phase.

Uterine Cycle

Proliferation Phase

During the hormonal cycle (figure 3.13), the uterus undergoes several profound changes. For example, at the beginning of the follicular phase of the ovarian cycle, the lining of the uterus (the endometrium) is in a state of disintegration from the previous cycle. As estrogen starts to stimulate the endometrium during the follicular phase and until ovulation, however, it will regenerate, growing thick and glandular and becoming conducive to implantation.

Secretory Phase

After ovulation and the formation of the corpus luteum, the secreted progesterone and estrogen act on the uterine wall to induce further glandular development and to sensitize the uterus for contact with the early

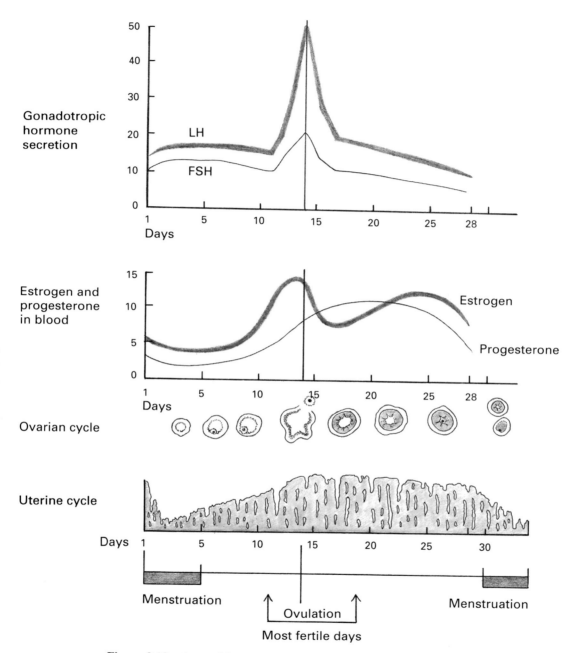

Figure 3.13 A graphic representation of the correlation of the hormonal stages and the physical events that take place in the menstrual cycle.

embryo or blastocyst. A great deal of glycogen is secreted into the tissue as a source of energy, the number of blood vessels increases, and various enzymes accumulate. All these factors help to create an ideal uterine environment for the implantation of a fertilized egg. This secretory phase of the uterine cycle corresponds with the luteal phase of the ovarian cycle. A summary of these interdependent cycles is presented in table 3.1.

If fertilization and implantation do not take place, the corpus luteum degenerates. As the levels of progesterone and estrogen drop, the process of menstruation begins with the gradual disintegration of the endometrium. Many tiny blood vessels are ruptured, and the blood passes to the outside of the woman's body through the vagina.

Table 3.1 Summary of the hormonal, ovarian, and uterine changes that take place during the menstrual cycle

Days:	1 2 3 4 5 6	7 8 9 10 11 12	13 14 15 16	17 18 19 20 21 22 23 24	25 26 27 28
Ovarian phase:	Follicular		Ovulation	Luteal	
Uterine phase:	Menstrual	Proliferation		Secretory	

Hormonal changes

Follicle-stimulating hormone	Increasing	High, then declining	Low	Low	Increasing
Luteinizing hormone	Low	Low, then large increase	High	Decreasing	Decreasing
Estrogen	Low	Increasing	High	Decline, then increase to high	Decreasing
Progesterone	None	Very little	Very low	Increasing to high	Decreasing
Ovarian changes	New follicle begins to develop Old corpus luteum degenerating	Growth and maturation of follicle Meiosis occurring in primary oocyte	Follicle ruptures and egg is released into oviduct	Corpus luteum formed and secreting actively	Corpus luteum begins to degenerate
Uterine changes	Degeneration and sloughing of thickened and glandular endometrium	Development of new endometrial layer	Continued	Active secretion by glandular endometrium; high vascularization	Endometrium begins to degenerate

From J. J. Nagle, Heredity and Human Affairs, 3rd edition (St. Louis: Mosby, 1984) 130.

If fertilization does take place and a blastocyst (a ball of 60 to 100 cells) reaches the uterus, the outer cells of the blastocyst secrete the hormone human chorionic gonadotropin (HCG). This hormone has the same effect as LH and acts to maintain the corpus luteum which, in turn, continues to secrete progesterone. Under the influence of the elevated levels of progesterone, no other follicles begin the maturation process. In addition, the uterus is maintained in a thickened, glandular state, and menstruation does not occur. The secretion of high levels of HCG continues through the twelfth week of pregnancy and then declines. At this time, the placenta begins to produce enough progesterone to sustain the pregnancy.[16]

Some Comparisons and Contrasts

Clearly, the processes of spermatogenesis and oogenesis are similar to each other, but they do differ from each other in several important ways. First, from the time of puberty, primary spermatocytes are constantly entering the meiotic cycle and undergoing differentiation to become mature sperm, whereas the primary oocytes enter this phase on a cyclical (monthly) schedule. Second, whereas four mature gametes are produced for each of the primary spermatocytes that begins meiosis, only one mature gamete is produced from each of the primary oocytes. Third, it takes much longer for eggs to mature than for sperm to mature.

Because we have already explained the first and second differences, we need to focus here only on the third one. The overall time period for the production of mature sperm is approximately 64 days. It takes nearly 16 days for the spermatogonia to mature into primary spermatocytes. An additional 32 days is required for meiosis to occur, during which time the primary spermatocytes first become secondary spermatocytes and then spermatids. Finally, it takes 16 more days for the spermatids to develop into fully mature sperm. At any given time, a large number of cells are going through all the stages of spermatogenesis. This ensures that sperm are constantly being produced in large quantities. Indeed, spermatogenesis is an enormously wasteful process. Although the male produces millions of sperm, only one is needed to fertilize the egg.

By the time the female fetus is 6 months old, the oogonia in her embryonic ovaries will have differentiated into primary oocytes. They will remain suspended in this early stage of meiosis until the girl reaches puberty. The mature woman will never have any more primary oocytes than she had as a 6-month-old fetus. With the onset of puberty, one primary oocyte becomes a secondary oocyte approximately every 28 days. When a woman ovulates, she is ovulating not a mature egg but a secondary oocyte. In fact, unless that secondary oocyte is fertilized by a sperm, it will not develop into a mature egg. However, if it is fertilized, it will mature in less than 1 day, completing its development before the fusion of its nucleus with that of the sperm. Whereas it takes 64 days for the sperm to mature completely, it takes anywhere from 12 to 50 years for the egg to mature completely, with each egg actually being older than the woman producing it—if we count her age from the time of birth.

Fertilization

All the hormonal mechanisms, physiological processes, and anatomical structures described thus far are designed to accomplish one thing: the production of mature gametes under conditions such that they may come together to produce a new individual and perpetuate the species. The result of the production of the egg, with its intricate hormonal regulation, however, is not only its formation within the ovary but also its release into the female reproductive tract. In contrast, the hormonal control and physiological production of the sperm leave it in the testes and do not provide a mechanism for its introduction into the male reproductive tract. Through sexual intercourse, the sperm is released from the testes into the male reproductive tract and then is introduced into the female reproductive tract where it may interact with the egg.

If the interaction between the gametes is successful and results in the fusion of the egg and sperm in a process called *fertilization*, the sexual reproductive process is completed and the development of a new individual begins.[17] Specifically, on fertilization the egg is activated to begin its developmental process and, through the fusion of the nuclei of the two gametes, the new genetic makeup of the individual is established. If fertilization does not take place, the sperm and egg die within hours of their release into the human reproductive system.

Fertilization can be viewed as consisting of four steps. First, the sperm must specifically recognize the egg so that it does not fuse with other cells present in the female reproductive tract. It is also important that the fusion be species-specific so that fertilization of an egg by the sperm of another species will not take place.[18] Second, a carefully controlled regulation of the entry of only one sperm cell is necessary so that the genetic material of only one paternal cell is present. Third, the sperm must trigger the dormant metabolic and developmental processes of the egg. Finally, the nucleus of the sperm must fuse with the nucleus of the egg so that the full complement of chromosomes is present in the new individual.[19]

Both the egg and the sperm have specific mechanisms to ensure that the appropriate interactions take place for proper fertilization.[20] The egg is surrounded by the zona pellucida through which only sperm of the same species can pass.[21] In addition, mammalian sperm are unable to fertilize an egg until they undergo a process called *capacitation*. Capacitation, involving the removal of the sperm from the seminal fluid, is induced in vivo by the secretions in the female genital tract. Capacitated sperm are able to bind specifically to the zona pellucida.[22] On binding, the sperm undergo an acrosomal reaction that alters the plasma membrane in their tips and releases the contents of the acrosomal vesicle.[23] The contents contain digestive enzymes that enable the sperm to dissolve a hole in the layers surrounding the plasma membrane of the egg (figure 3.14). Once the sperm is in contact with the plasma membrane of the egg, the plasma membranes of the two cells fuse into a single continuous layer that becomes progressively larger until the sperm is entirely incorporated into the egg.[24]

Immediately following the fusion of the plasma membrane of the sperm with the plasma membrane of the egg, a series of events takes place to block the entrance of another sperm cell.[25] Although many sperm may bind to the egg through interaction with the numerous receptors, if more than one sperm fuses with the egg (polyspermy), too much DNA will be present and a nondiploid cell will result, with the consequence that development stops and the fertilized egg degenerates. The events that block polyspermy consist of changes in the plasma membrane of the egg and release of the contents of the cortical granules.[26] The cortical reaction alters the glycoprotein in the zona pellucida so that it can no longer bind sperm or activate them to undergo the acrosomal reaction.[27]

The next step in the fertilization process is activation of the egg to begin metabolism and development. Before fertilization, the egg is metabolically quiescent. It does not synthesize DNA, although it synthesizes RNA and protein at very low rates. There is only minor transport of substances into and out of the cell. On fertilization, the metabolic activity of the egg increases and DNA synthesis begins. The actual mechanism of activation is unknown, but it seems clear that the sperm serves only as a trigger of a system present in the egg. In fact, the sperm itself is not required for activation, which can be achieved by a variety of nonspecific chemical or physical treatments. Of course, if activation occurs in the absence of sperm, the resulting embryo contains only half the proper number of chromosomes and usually does not survive. Many studies indicate that an increase in the cytosolic Ca^{2+} concentration initiates the development of the egg.[28] There also is a rise in the intracellular pH and

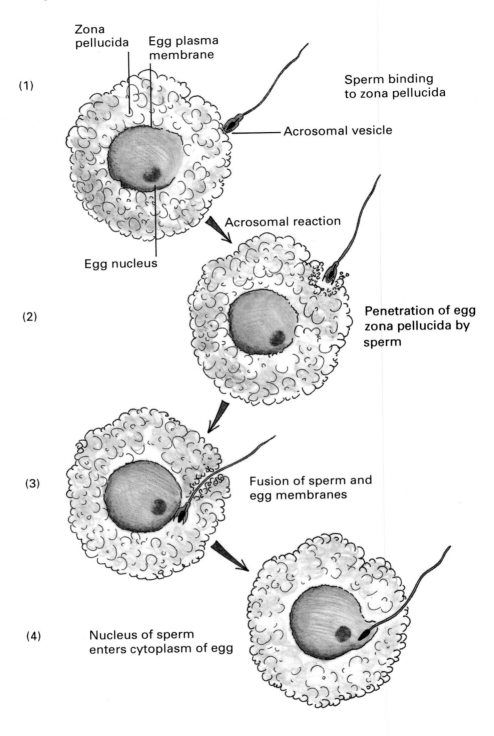

(1) Zona pellucida

Egg plasma membrane

Sperm binding to zona pellucida

Acrosomal vesicle

Egg nucleus

Acrosomal reaction

(2) Penetration of egg zona pellucida by sperm

(3) Fusion of sperm and egg membranes

(4) Nucleus of sperm enters cytoplasm of egg

an influx of Na^+, which are associated with an increase in protein and RNA synthesis and eventually lead to DNA synthesis, resulting in DNA replication.[29]

The final step of fertilization involves the fusion of the nuclei (at this stage called *pronuclei*) of the sperm and egg. Once the sperm enters the egg, its nucleus rotates 180 degrees and migrates toward the nucleus of the egg. Approximately 30 minutes after the plasma membranes of the two cells fuse, the paternal and maternal nuclei fuse to recreate the diploid nucleus.

Embryonic Development

As mentioned earlier, during the final stages of fertilization, the egg's 23 chromosomes combine with the sperm's 23 chromosomes to reconstitute the 46 chromosomes of the diploid cell. The fertilized ovum, or zygote, undergoes several mitotic divisions known as *cleavage*. As the zygote travels down the oviduct, it divides many times, producing a solid ball of cells called a *morula*. It takes approximately 3 days for the morula to travel to the uterus. The morula continues to develop as it floats in the fluid of the uterus for several days. In the uterine cavity, the morula undergoes a cellular rearrangement to form a hollow ball called the *blastocyst*.[30] By the end of the first week, the 60- to 100-cell blastocyst (figure 3.15) consists of an outer layer of cells called the *trophoblast* that eventually will produce the embryonic membranes, an inner cell mass that is destined to form the embryo, and a cavity called the *blastocele*. Further differentiation takes place until, toward the end of the second week of development, the outer cell layer makes contact with the uterus and the blastocyst enzymatically digests its way into the endometrium where it is totally encapsulated.[31] This process is called *implantation* and is the point at which pregnancy begins.[32]

After implantation occurs, a series of events takes place to ensure that the embryo has sufficient contact with the mother to provide a supply of nutrients (including oxygen) and disposal of its metabolic waste (including

Figure 3.14 The penetration of the sperm into an egg is shown starting with (1) the binding of the sperm to the zona pellucida and the dissolution of the acrosomal membrane to release the acrosomal enzymes and continuing with (2) the enzymatic digestion of the zona pellucida and penetration of the sperm through the zona pellucida and (3) binding of the sperm to the egg through the fusion of their membranes; (4) finally, the nucleus of the sperm enters the egg.

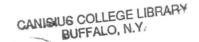

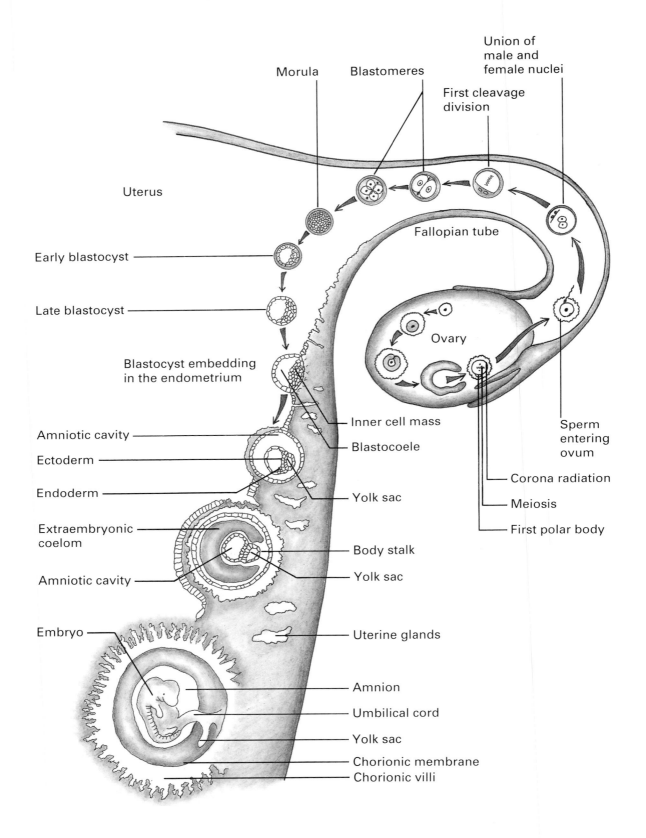

Morula

Blastomeres

Union of male and female nuclei

First cleavage division

Uterus

Fallopian tube

Early blastocyst

Late blastocyst

Ovary

Blastocyst embedding in the endometrium

Inner cell mass

Blastocoele

Amniotic cavity

Ectoderm

Endoderm

Yolk sac

Sperm entering ovum

Corona radiation

Meiosis

First polar body

Extraembryonic coelom

Amniotic cavity

Body stalk

Yolk sac

Embryo

Uterine glands

Amnion

Umbilical cord

Yolk sac

Chorionic membrane

Chorionic villi

Figure 3.15 The events leading up to the implantation of an embryo into the wall of the uterus. (1) The egg is released from the follicle on the ovary and (2) is swept into the fallopian tube. (3) The first stage of meiosis releases a polar body. (4) Sperm penetrates the egg and triggers the second stage of meiosis with release of another polar body. (5) The nuclei of the sperm and the egg fuse. (6) The first cell division takes place. (7) The embryo continues to divide and (8) further division leads to the morula. (9) An early blastocyst is formed and (10) approximately 4 days after fertilization, a late blastocyst is formed. (11) About 7 days after fertilization, the blastocyst begins to implant into the wall of the uterus. (12) The wall of the uterus begins to engulf the blastocyst and (13) the blastocyst differentiates into specialized areas. (14) The placenta begins to form from the wall of the uterus and the outer part of the embryo. (15) Once implantation is complete, the amnionic sac, the chorionic membrane, and the chorionic villi, which allow for the exchange of nutrients between the embryo and the mother, develop.

carbon dioxide). As the trophoblast grows, branches, and extends into the tissue of the uterus, embryonic blood vessels develop, and the vascularized, membranous structure is known as the *chorion*. The chorionic membrane contains a number of fingerlike projections, called *chorionic villi*, which project into the uterine wall and provide a firm attachment for the embryo. This intimate and extensive region of attachment between the chorion and the uterus, called the *placenta*, serves as the embryo's nutritive, respiratory, and excretory organ. A second membrane called the *amnion* forms between the developing embryo and the chorion. The amnion is filled with the amniotic fluid in which the embryo floats and provides a protective environment for the embryo and, later, for the fetus. The extensive mass of tissue and blood vessels that develop at the placenta are connected to the embryo by the umbilical cord. With all of the tissue that develops to provide for the maintenance of the embryo, there is no actual blood flow and no nerve connection between the mother and the embryo.

4 Contraception

For some couples, pregnancy and reproduction are largely a matter of chance. Others avoid having children or regulate the times when they do have children by using one or more contraceptive methods. Generally speaking, *contraception* is any intentional action aimed at artificially preventing the fertilization or implantation of the human egg.[1] It is increasingly difficult to distinguish contraception from two other reproduction-controlling technologies, sterilization and abortion. What, after all, is the difference between a reversible sterilization and a long-lasting contraceptive such as Depo-Provera, which works for 3 months?[2] And what, if anything, is the difference between a very early abortion and the use of a drug such as RU 486? One of the drug's developers, French physician Dr. Etienne-Emile Baulieu, refers to RU 486 as a "contragestive." Just as a contraceptive acts against conception, a contragestive acts against gestation.[3] Nevertheless, given the present state of technological development, contraception is still a *less* permanent means of birth control than is sterilization and a *more* preventive (as opposed to remedial) means of birth control than is abortion.

Although birth-control methods have been available for centuries, effective ones have been available for only approximately 50 years. A good way to classify modern contraceptive techniques is according to their differing modes of actions. No catalogue of contraceptives is complete, then, unless it includes methods that (1) stop intercourse before the man ejaculates, avoiding transmission of the sperm into the vagina (coitus interruptus); (2) adjust the time of intercourse to correspond with the woman's least fertile periods (rhythm); (3) interfere with the union of the sperm and the egg by some physical or chemical barrier (condom and diaphragm); (4) prevent implantation of the fertilized egg (intrauterine device [IUD]); and (5) interfere with production of the sperm and the egg (birth-control pill and gossypol). Some of these methods are illustrated in figure 4.1.

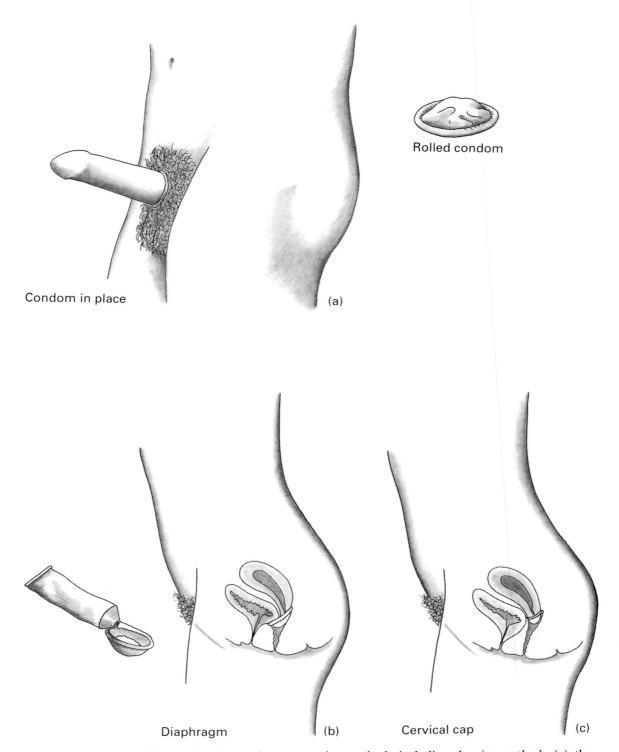

Rolled condom

Condom in place

(a)

Diaphragm

(b)

Cervical cap

(c)

Figure 4.1 Assorted contraceptive methods including: barrier methods (a) the condom, (b) the diaphragm, (c) the cervical cap, (d) the contraceptive sponge; spermicides (e) female condom, (f) foams and jellies; and (g) the intrauterine device.

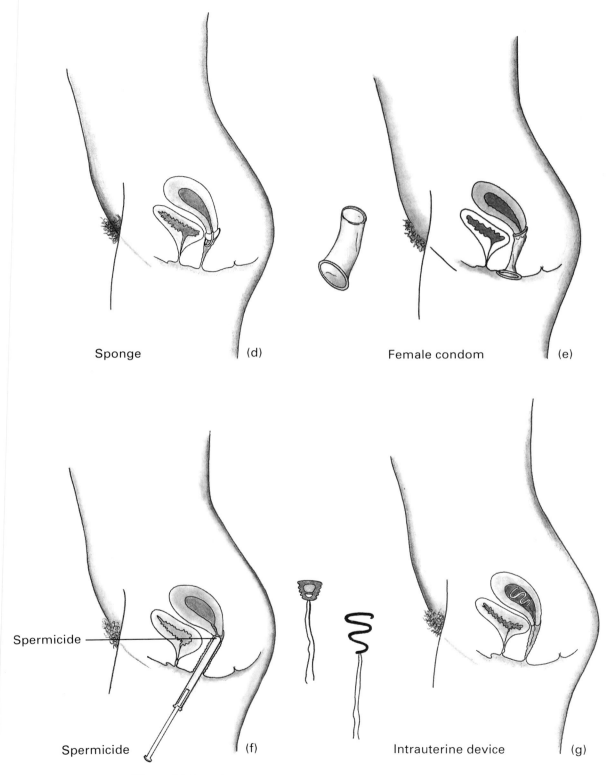

Sponge (d)

Female condom (e)

Spermicide

Spermicide (f)

Intrauterine device (g)

Figure 4.1 (cont.)

Contraceptive Methods

Coitus Interruptus

Perhaps the oldest recorded method of birth control is coitus interruptus, the withdrawal of the penis from the vagina just before the ejaculation of the sperm. Because some semen usually leaks from the penis before ejaculation, and because many men find it difficult to withdraw at the appropriate moment during sexual intercourse, coitus interruptus results in approximately 18 pregnancies per 100 women per year.[4] Nevertheless, coitus interruptus is used extensively worldwide with some notable exceptions, including the United States where only approximately 2 percent of couples trust so-called withdrawal methods.[5]

The Rhythm Method

The rhythm method is a mode of contraception based on a couple's awareness of the fact that fertilization can take place only within approximately 15 hours of ovulation. If a couple becomes attuned to the rhythm of the woman's month-long reproductive cycle, the couple can abstain from sexual intercourse during the woman's fertile days. The advantage of this mode of contraception is that it enables the couple to learn a great deal about how the female body works. But this knowledge is not easily obtained. A woman must be systematic enough to observe and record data about her reproductive cycle. Moreover, a couple must be disciplined enough to act consistently on this information. Indeed, several studies have found that accidental pregnancies among rhythm method–using couples are usually the result of failed abstinence and not of some inability to master one of the three methods devised for determining fertility: the calendar method, the basal body temperature method, and the mucus pattern method.

The Calendar Method

A woman who uses the calendar method keeps track of her fertility cycle for at least 8 months. She charts the beginning and ending of each menstrual cycle and the occurrence of each ovulation (usually on the fourteenth day of the cycle). By subtracting 18 days from the total length of her shortest menstrual cycle, the woman can estimate the beginning of her fertile period and, by subtracting 11 days from the total length of her longest menstrual cycle, she can estimate the end of her fertile period. As soon as the woman knows she is entering her fertile period, she and her partner should abstain from sexual intercourse until it is safe for them to resume sexual relations.

Basal Body Temperature Method

A woman who uses the basal body temperature (BBT) method takes her temperature every morning for 3 to 4 months. She does this in order to pinpoint the days on which her temperature drops slightly and then increases. The BBT of most women drops slightly before ovulation and increases by $0.4°F$ to $0.8°F$ between 1 to 3 days after ovulation. Since the days between ovulation and the temperature rise are a woman's most fertile days, she and her partner should avoid sexual intercourse during that time.

Mucus Method

A woman who uses the mucus method examines her cervical mucus throughout her menstrual cycle and records changes in it. Before and after ovulation, cervical mucus is viscous and yellow. Because of a drop in saline content and a rise in estrogen during ovulation, however, the cervical mucus becomes thinner, clearer, and more elastic with a consistency similar to that of an egg white. By charting the changes in her cervical mucus over several months, the woman will be able to estimate her time of ovulation. She and her partner should avoid sexual intercourse during and around this unsafe period.

Even when a couple practices one or more of these fertility-awareness methods conscientiously, the rhythm method remains relatively unreliable since the precise time of ovulation is often very difficult to pinpoint. A couple may think that they have entered the safe, postovulatory period when they have not; and even if the partners have correctly identified the time of ovulation and avoid sexual intercourse during it, a woman may still become pregnant if one of her eggs joins with a sperm that has survived in her reproductive tract from a prior act of sexual intercourse.[6] A failure rate of approximately 20 percent confirms just how difficult it is not only to predict ovulation accurately but also to control human sexual desire.

Physical Obstruction of the Union of Sperm and Egg

More reliable than coitus interruptus and the rhythm method are contraceptive methods such as the condom, the diaphragm, the cervical cap, and the sponge, which provide physical or chemical barriers to prevent the sperm from reaching the egg. In general, these methods work well with virtually no dangerous side effects, but they are not very convenient.

The Condom

The most popular barrier method is the condom, which is a thin sheath placed over the erect penis before intercourse. Commentators tell two stories about the introduction of this contraceptive device to the modern world. According to the first story, Dr. Condom, physician to Charles II of England (1660–1685), developed the contraceptive for his royal patient. While the condom allegedly solved the king's problem of fathering too many illegitimate children and won knighthood for Dr. Condom, the eminent doctor is probably more of a mythological character than a historical figure.[7] According to the second story, thin sheaths were used centuries ago to prevent the spread of sexually transmitted disease (STD) —hence the term *prophylactic* ("protecting against disease"). Until the introduction of the oral contraceptive, at which time their use declined, condoms were the most widely used contraceptive device. Recently, latex condoms have gained new popularity because they provide protection against STDs including the acquired immunodeficiency syndrome (AIDS).

Originally made of linen or animal intestines, the condom today is a thin rubber sheath that one partner (either, the man or the woman) places over the male's erect penis before engaging in intercourse (figure 4.1a). The closed end of the condom is either plain or tipped with a nipple to contain the ejaculated sperm so that it does not enter the female reproductive tract. "Rubbers," as condoms are commonly called, are simple, inexpensive, and available without a prescription or visit to the doctor's office. They are also approximately 86 percent effective in preventing pregnancy. Most failures occur owing to tears in the rubber or accidental slippage during intercourse. Some men and women claim that condom use reduces sensation and therefore overall sexual pleasure but, with the advent of natural-skin, textured, or lubricated condoms, this problem has been alleviated. Unfortunately, natural-skin condoms allow passage of viruses and therefore do not provide protection from STDs. The latex condom's ability to prevent transmission of the AIDS virus and other

STDs, especially when it is used in conjunction with a spermicide, makes it a wise contraceptive choice for people with multiple sexual partners.

The Diaphragm

The diaphragm is a physical barrier that prevents entry of sperm into the uterus after being released into the vagina. Fitted to the contours of a particular woman's body by a physician, the diaphragm is a dome-shaped rubber cup with a flexible rim, as shown in figure 4.1b. Up to 6 hours before intercourse, the woman folds and inserts the diaphragm into her vagina at the cervix. There the diaphragm unfolds, its springy rim holding the cup tightly against the walls of the vagina to block the opening to the uterus. No less than 6 to 8 hours after intercourse, the woman removes the diaphragm from her body and washes it for use during subsequent acts of sexual intercourse.[8]

In addition to a slightly heightened risk of urinary tract and bladder infections,[9] the only other notable risk of diaphragm use is a very low incidence of toxic shock syndrome (10 cases per 100,000 women). Given that the diaphragm is a relatively safe contraceptive, it is surprising that only 1 percent of women use it.[10] Women's perception that the diaphragm is not as effective as the contraceptive pill or the IUD may account for its relative unpopularity. But the fact remains that a properly fitted diaphragm is up to 94 percent effective when the woman uses it consistently and inserts it correctly.[11] In contrast, when her diaphragm is improperly fitted or when she uses it incorrectly or inconsistently, a woman's risk of pregnancy increases to approximately 17 percent per year.[12] There is some reason to believe that young, sexually active women are not particularly good candidates for diaphragm use because the failure rate for women younger than 25 years who have sexual intercourse four or more times weekly approaches 20 to 25 percent.[13]

The Cervical Cap

Although the cervical cap has existed for centuries, the U.S. Food and Drug Administration (FDA) only recently approved it as a legitimate reproduction-controlling device.[14] Like the diaphragm, the cervical cap (shown in figure 4.1c) is made to fit tightly over the cervix, thereby preventing the entry of sperm into the uterus. The effectiveness of the cervical cap, when used in combination with a spermicide, is very similar to that of the diaphragm but, when it is used inconsistently or incorrectly, it approaches a failure rate of 8 to 27 percent, with young, sexually active women experiencing the most problems.[15]

The main advantages of the cervical cap are that it is small ($1\frac{1}{2}$ inches in diameter) and can be worn for twice as long as the diaphragm (48 hours compared to 24). Unfortunately, the cervical cap is more difficult to insert than the diaphragm, it dislodges more readily, and some women report abnormal Papanicolaou's (Pap) tests when they begin to use the cervical cap. Because an abnormal Pap test could signal an infection or even the beginning of cervical cancer, the FDA recommends that women have a Pap test after using the cervical cap for 3 months and that they immediately stop using the cap in the event of abnormal Pap test results.[16]

The Contraceptive Sponge

Yet another physical barrier contraceptive is the polyurethane sponge, approved for general use by the FDA in 1983. Outfitted with a small loop for easy removal, the sponge (shown in figure 4.1d) contains a spermicide that is released slowly at the cervix. After the woman inserts the sponge into her vagina against her cervix, it blocks, absorbs, and kills sperm for approximately 24 hours. Sponges are 91 to 94 percent effective if used in strict accordance with instructions, but only 72 to 82 percent effective if used inconsistently or incorrectly.[17] The sponge has several advantages compared to other barrier methods: It does not require fitting, it comes already permeated with spermicide, and it lasts 24 hours no matter how many times sexual intercourse takes place. Its major disadvantage is that it can be used once only.

The Female Condom

Another physical-barrier contraceptive has recently been approved by the FDA. While the female condom has many of the general features of the male condom, it is worn internally by the woman and completely covers the inside of the vagina (see figure 4.3e). A flexible ring on each end of the condom holds it in place. One ring is worn internally, like a diaphragm, and fits over the cervix while the other ring is outside. Since the 7 inch long sheath is made from polyurethane, it is not as effective against viruses as the male latex condom. The female condom has a projected failure rate of 5 percent (compared to 2 percent for the male condom), but that increases to 21 percent due to inconsistent use.

Chemical Barriers

In addition to physical barrier methods, chemical prevention is also available. Jellies, foams, creams, aerosols, and suppositories that are inserted into the vagina before intercourse act chemically to prevent the meeting of the sperm and egg by immobilizing or even killing the sperm. When a couple uses one of these chemical barriers (as shown in figure 4.1f) in conjunction with a condom or diaphragm, the device's contraceptive effectiveness is increased to approximately 97 percent.[18] The greatest advantages of these chemical contraceptives are their safety and availability over the drugstore counter. Their messiness is probably their greatest disadvantage. Another disadvantage is that after their application, a couple must wait 10 to 15 minutes before beginning intercourse.

In many modern products, the active spermicidal ingredient is nonoxynol-9. As a surfactant (surface-active agent), it directly attacks the lipid-containing layer of the sperm's cell membrane. By preventing the metabolism of fructose, which is necessary for the activity and survival of the sperm, nonoxynol-9 either immobilizes or kills the sperm.[19] Spermicides also advantageously reduce the incidence of infection by coating the walls of the vagina and preventing the entrance of infectious agents. Therefore, couples who use condoms or vaginal barrier methods (diaphragms, caps, and sponges) in conjunction with a spermicide are using the only contraceptives available that both prevent unwanted pregnancies and guard against infectious STDs.[20]

Shortcomings of Barrier Methods

Despite their basic simplicity and relatively high success rates, however, all these barrier methods suffer from the same major defect. They require the couple to plan ahead or to interrupt sexual intercourse at times when rational thought may not be as strong as the desire for sexual gratification and when the necessary contraceptive products may not be immediately available. These methods fail fairly frequently not because their design is fundamentally flawed but because couples fail to employ them when they should.

Prevention of Implantation of the Fertilized Egg

The intrauterine device is even more effective than the barrier methods. So ancient is the IUD that nearly 2000 years ago Hippocrates detailed its use.[21] For centuries, Arabian and Turkish camel drivers placed objects such as small pebbles in the uteruses of their camels to prevent pregnancies during long desert caravan trips. Among the main twentieth-century developers of the IUD was a Berlin physician, Dr. Graefenberg. His 1928 intrauterine ring of silkworm gut, which was held in shape by a silver- and copper-alloyed wire, has been improved over the years. Nevertheless, it bears a striking resemblance to the stainless-steel ring currently worn by approximately 40 to 45 million Chinese women.[22]

Although there is still considerable debate about just how the IUD works, the growing consensus is that it works as a type of irritant. As a foreign body in the uterus, it causes an inflammatory response that either destroys the blastocyst and sperm or prevents blastocyst implantation. IUDs come in a variety of sizes, shapes, and materials (figure 4.1g), but apparently the most effective IUDs are large and progestin-releasing or copper-laden.[23] The progestin-releasing IUDs (e.g., Progestasert-T) cause the cervix to produce a sticky, thick mucus that blocks the sperm from entering the uterus. The copper-laden IUDs (e.g., ParaGard Copper T), which release small amounts of copper into the uterus, act as infertility agents by affecting intrauterine enzymes and increasing inflammatory reaction.

With a use-effectiveness rate of 93 to 97 percent (most failures are due to undetected IUD dislodgment), the IUD is a fairly reliable reproduction-controlling device.[24] Another feature that counts in the IUD's favor is its convenience. After a physician inserts an IUD into a woman's uterus, it will protect her reasonably well from unwanted pregnancies for anywhere from 1 to 6 years. There is no evidence that IUDs cause uterine cancer and, in fact, regular IUD checkup examinations may help detect and treat cancer at an early stage. In general, IUDs seem to work better and stay in place with fewer side effects in women who have previously given birth. Women and their sexual partners are able to engage in sexual intercourse spontaneously and romantically; they do not have to take time out from their intimate exchanges to put on a condom, insert a diaphragm, cap, or sponge, or apply a cream, jelly, or foam.

Unfortunately, IUDs have negative as well as positive features. Among their inconvenient and sometimes painful side effects are (1) spotting, bleeding, hemorrhaging, and anemia; (2) cramping; (3) undetected expulsions; (4) lost strings (most IUDs come with a string so the woman can check for expulsion of the IUD); and (5) painful insertion and difficult removal. In addition to these negative side effects, the IUD is associated with several less frequent but even more serious risks: (1) uterine or cervical perforation, (2) uterine embedding, (3) pelvic inflammatory disease (PID), and (4) pregnancy. Because both perforation of the uterus and PID may lead to hospitalization, infertility, or death, physicians usually treat these conditions aggressively in addition to switching their patients immediately to other forms of contraception.

More dangerous still is pregnancy. As most reproductive researchers see it, even if a pregnant IUD user wishes to continue her pregnancy, a physician should remove the IUD for at least three reasons. First, if the IUD is left in place, there is a 50 percent chance of a spontaneous abortion, whereas the chance of spontaneous abortion if the IUD is removed is only 25 percent. Second, up to 95 percent of IUD users who abort show signs of infection. Third, if the IUD is left in place, the woman runs a 50 times greater risk of dying from septic abortion.[25] To be sure, some women deliver their IUDs together with their healthy babies; but the fetus and the IUD do not typically make for congenial "wombmates" and are best separated as soon as possible.

Despite reports of infection, hemorrhaging, and spontaneous abortions, many women in the United States used to believe that the IUD's risks did not outweigh its benefits of relative effectiveness and certain convenience. Then a heated controversy broke out with respect to one type of IUD, the Dalkon Shield. This devise was shaped like a crab, with little spines and a multifilament tail-string to minimize the possibility of expulsion and to maximize the opportunity for monitoring its position in the uterus. Unfortunately, the Dalkon Shield's crablike qualities also made it difficult and painful to insert, wear, and remove; and its filamentous string also made it easy for infectious bacteria to pass into the uterus. Indeed, studies showed that Dalkon Shield users were five times more likely to suffer from PID than women who wore other IUDs available on the market;[26] moreover, many of these studies also showed that Dalkon Shield users were at a much higher risk for septic abortions than were women wearing other kinds of IUDs. Over the years, twenty-one deaths, hundreds of cases of septic abortion, and thousands of cases of PID, many of them resulting in infertility, were reported to the FDA by Dalkon Shield victims or their survivors. Eventually, these women or their families filed a class-action suit against the A. H. Robins Company, manufacturers of the Dalkon Shield, alleging that the company continued marketing the device even after it was aware of its dangers. After paying $378.3 million in 9230 lawsuits, A. H. Robins filed for bankruptcy in 1985; nevertheless, the company survived dissolution and is currently fiscally sound.[27]

Apparently, the Dalkon Shield controversy was enough to deter many women from using IUDs. Currently, only 5 percent of U.S. women use IUDs,[28] despite the fact that studies indicate other types of IUDs—Lippes Loops, Saf-T-Coils, the Copper-7 200, and especially the Progestasert-T[29]

—do not present the same degree of health hazards as did the Dalkon Shield. Medicated Cu-T380A (ParaGard Copper T) is the newest IUD to be approved by the FDA. It is safer than previous models since its T shape conforms to the shape of the uterus. It also can be retained for at least 4 years, and perhaps even 6, because it contains more copper than previous models.

Although many kinds of IUDs are available worldwide, and although a number of IUDs bear the FDA's stamp of approval, U.S. manufacturers have withdrawn all IUDs except the Progestasert-T and Medicated Cu-T380A (ParaGard) from the market. Since manufacturers are not always able or even willing to risk the financial costs associated with being sued for the manufacture, distribution, and sale of faulty contraceptives, women who favor the IUD must use whatever a cautious market is willing to offer them.

Contraceptive Methods that Avoid or Suppress Ovulation

Made available to U.S. women in 1960, oral contraceptives rapidly became the most widely used method of contraception in the United States. The primary reasons for their popularity were their convenience and their effectiveness (97–99 percent). From 1965 until 1976, between one-fourth and one-third of the married women in the United States who were using contraceptives used oral ones. Since then, oral contraceptives have become less popular owing to a series of articles linking their use to an increased risk of heart attack, stroke, high blood pressure, and certain forms of cancer. Consequently, only approximately 13.8 million U.S. women currently use oral contraceptives,[30] even though today these agents are much safer than their predecessors.

The Structure and Action of the Steroid Hormones

To understand the action of oral contraceptives and their various side effects, we must first understand the chemistry of steroids and one of their particular subgroups, the steroid sex hormones. The steroids are members of the class of biochemical compounds called *lipids* (see the appendix for an introduction to this class of compounds). Steroids can exist in the free state or bond to other compounds such as fatty acids or carbohydrates. They are found in relatively large quantities in the nerve tissues, in cell membranes, in the reproductive organs and tissues, in the bile, and in the blood. Perhaps the best-known steroid is cholesterol, first discovered in gallstones. Because it is best known as the chemical that contributes to heart disease, cholesterol's role as a starting point in the synthesis of the steroid sex hormones is frequently overlooked.

The structural framework shared by all steroids is the *steroid nucleus*. As illustrated in figure A.6, it consists of four rings of carbon fused together in such a way as to make a very rigid, largely planar structure. For purposes of identification, the rings are lettered *A*, *B*, *C*, and *D*, and the position of each carbon is numbered as shown. This makes it easy to locate the various functional groups that are attached to the steroid nucleus. The basic biochemical activity of a steroid depends on where and how such groups are attached.

In figure A.6, which shows the structure of cholesterol, the basic steroid nucleus has been modified in three ways:

1. There is a hydroxyl (−OH) group at position 3 of the A ring.

2. There is a double bond between the carbon atoms at positions 5 and 6 of the B ring.

3. There is a long carbon chain (eight carbons long) attached to position 17 of the D ring.

From this relatively simple structure, the body can synthesize a wide variety of compounds. For example, the bile acids are synthesized from cholesterol in the liver, and cortisone is synthesized from cholesterol in the adrenal glands (located on top of the kidney).

The three major steroid sex hormones are progesterone, testosterone, and estradiol (see figure A.6). Figure 4.2 shows the relative positions of these hormones as intermediates in the series of metabolic reactions beginning with cholesterol. They are related to each other by both their structure and their metabolism.

Progesterone

Progesterone is a steroid that is synthesized in the corpus luteum, an endocrine tissue formed in the ovaries (recall the discussion of the female reproductive system). Progesterone is often called the *pregnancy hormone* because it helps promote the development of the uterine wall into which the fertilized egg implants. If pregnancy occurs, it acts as a built-in birth-control agent by preventing further ovulation. For this reason, compounds related to progesterone are the main components of oral contraceptives.

Testosterone

The major end product of the metabolism of cholesterol in the testes is testosterone. Testosterone and related androgens are responsible for the characteristics associated with masculinity such as muscle strength, a deep

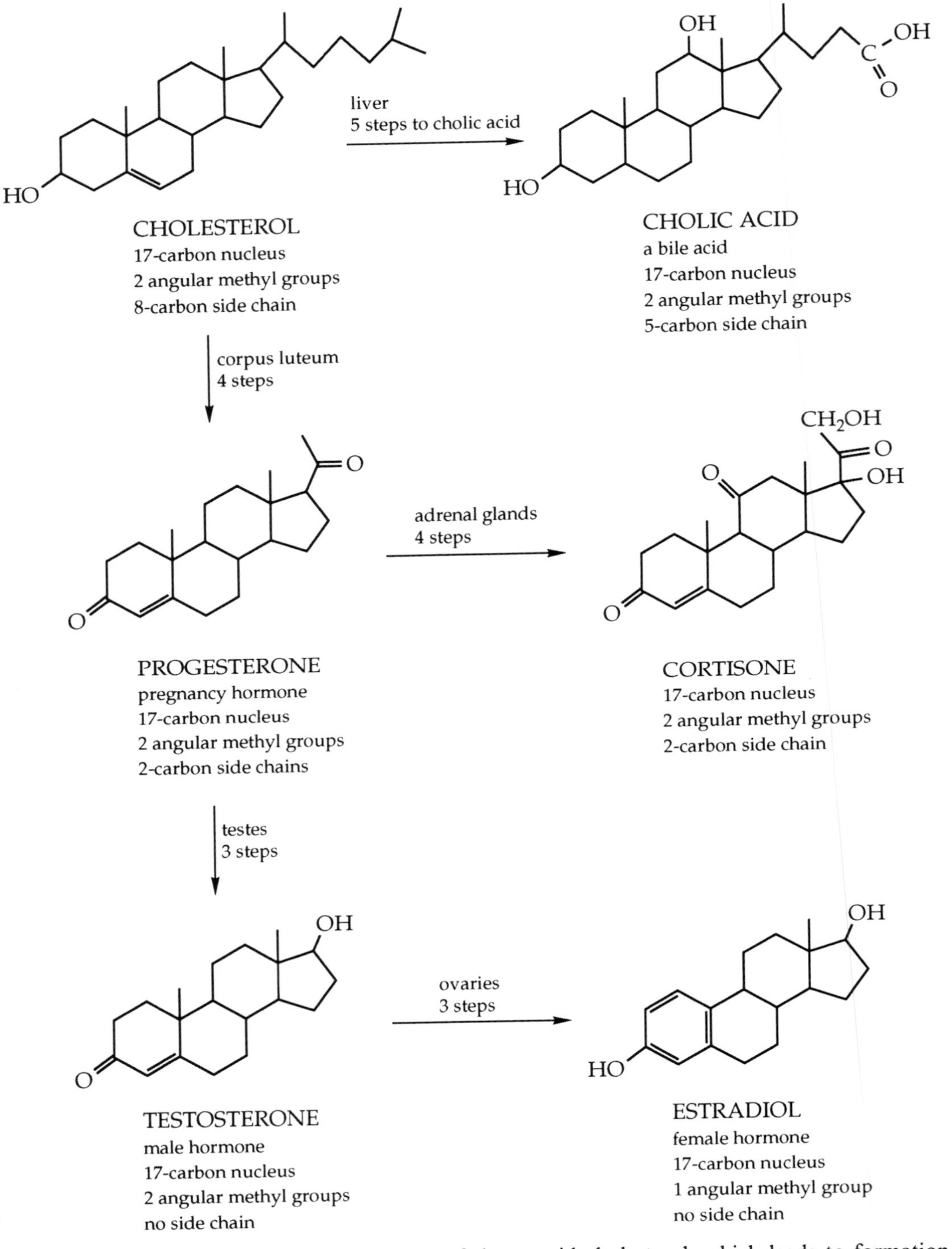

liver
5 steps to cholic acid

CHOLESTEROL
17-carbon nucleus
2 angular methyl groups
8-carbon side chain

CHOLIC ACID
a bile acid
17-carbon nucleus
2 angular methyl groups
5-carbon side chain

corpus luteum
4 steps

adrenal glands
4 steps

PROGESTERONE
pregnancy hormone
17-carbon nucleus
2 angular methyl groups
2-carbon side chains

CORTISONE
17-carbon nucleus
2 angular methyl groups
2-carbon side chain

testes
3 steps

ovaries
3 steps

TESTOSTERONE
male hormone
17-carbon nucleus
2 angular methyl groups
no side chain

ESTRADIOL
female hormone
17-carbon nucleus
1 angular methyl group
no side chain

Figure 4.2 The metabolism of the steroid cholesterol, which leads to formation of the sex hormones, progesterone, estradiol, and testosterone. In the corpus luteum, cholesterol is transformed into progesterone; in the testes, it is converted into testosterone but one of the intermediates is progesterone; and in the ovaries, cholesterol is converted into estradiol after being transformed into the intermediates progesterone and testosterone.

voice, and facial hair. Testosterone plays a vital role in the formation of sperm.

Estradiol

Estradiol is one of a class of female steroid hormones called *estrogens*. These hormones stimulate the growth of female tissue such as the breast and, in conjunction with progesterone, the lining of the uterus (the endometrium). The estrogens are synthesized from cholesterol in the ovaries. However, since cholesterol is first metabolized into progesterone and then testosterone before it is metabolized into estradiol in the ovaries, a woman who suffers a malfunction in this particular pathway may experience a buildup of male hormones and subsequent masculinization.

Birth-Control Pills

Oral contraceptives contain a number of synthetic steroids that were developed beginning in the early 1950s. Those synthetic steroids that are based on the structure of the progesterone molecule and that have the same hormonal properties are called *progestins*. The term *estrogen* applies to both the natural and synthetic forms of the estrogen molecule. Although the basic steroid structures are the same, the active ingredients of a variety of oral contraceptives are determined by the presence of different groups at position 3 in the estrogens and position 20 in the progestins.

For many years, scientists recognized the ability of these compounds to interrupt the menstrual cycle, but not until scientists developed a way to administer progestin and estrogen orally to women without having these compounds break down in their livers did these hormones become widely used. Scientists were able to block the initial metabolic step that occurs when the $-OH$ group at position C-17 is converted to the $=O$ group with the ethinyl group $-C\equiv C-H$ at position 17. The presence of this ethinyl group in oral contraceptives protects their effectiveness when taken orally. Figure 4.3 shows the structures of the most commonly used birth-control steroids, and figure 4.4 illustrates the differing modes of action of three categories of oral contraceptives known as (1) the combination birth-control pill, (2) the sequential birth-control pill, and (3) the minipill.

The combination birth-control pill

Developed in the late 1950s, each tablet of the combination pill contains a constant amount of estrogen and progestin. Although there is no single best way to take the combination pill, a standard way is for a woman to start her packet of pills on day 5 of her menstrual cycle, to take them faithfully for 21 days, and then to wait until day 5 of her next menstrual

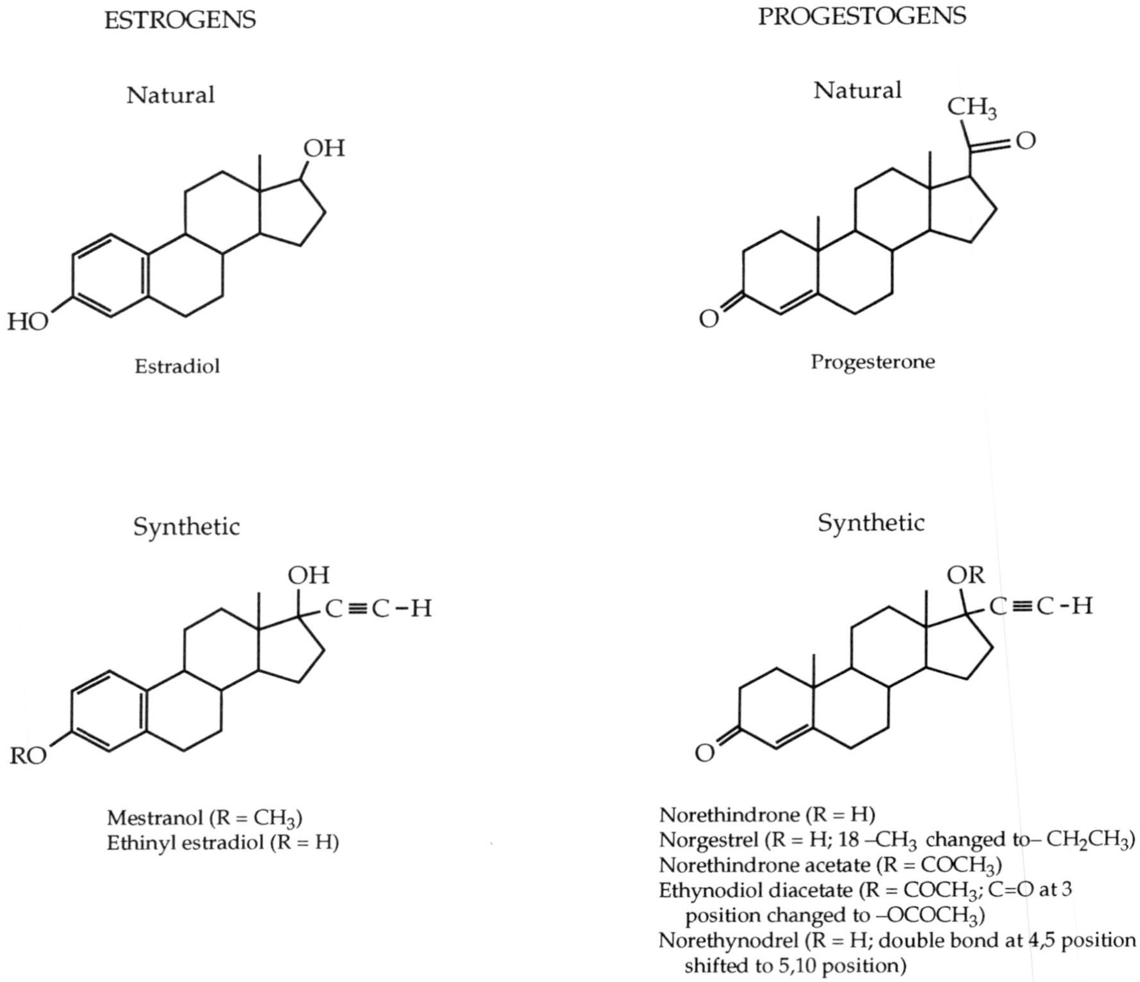

ESTROGENS

Natural

Estradiol

Synthetic

Mestranol (R = CH_3)
Ethinyl estradiol (R = H)

PROGESTOGENS

Natural

Progesterone

Synthetic

Norethindrone (R = H)
Norgestrel (R = H; 18 –CH_3 changed to– CH_2CH_3)
Norethindrone acetate (R = $COCH_3$)
Ethynodiol diacetate (R = $COCH_3$; C=O at 3
   position changed to –$OCOCH_3$)
Norethynodrel (R = H; double bond at 4,5 position
   shifted to 5,10 position)

Figure 4.3   The chemical structures of the natural female sex hormones and some of the common synthetic steroid hormones used in birth control pills

cycle before she starts her second packet of pills. Some combination pill packets contain 28 pills, some of which are placebos. The advantage of this system is that it is easier to remember to take a pill every day than to remember to take one intermittently.

With estrogen and progestin administered in this manner, menstruation continues even though ovulation stops. In other words, the uterine cycle, during which the endometrium is first built up and then broken down, is virtually unaffected by the combination pill, whereas the ovarian cycle is dramatically affected by it. The constant high level of estrogen and progestin in the blood stream inhibits the release of follicle-stimulating hormone (FSH) and luteinizing hormone (LH), respectively, thereby sup-

Combination pills   Sequential pills   Minipill

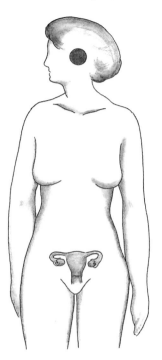 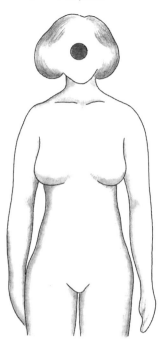 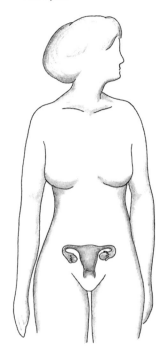

Areas affected:
pituitary and hypothalamus
are inhibited; ovulation is
prevented; cervical mucus
forms a barrier to sperm

Areas affected:
pituitary and hypothalamus
are inhibited; ovulation
is prevented

Areas affected:
ovulation is normal, but the
cervical mucus forms a
barrier to sperm

Figure 4.4 A simplified representation of the modes of action of the oral contraceptives: (a) with the conventional pill, ovulation is prevented by inhibiting the pituitary/hypothalmus, and the cervical mucus forms a barrier to the sperm; (b) the sequential pill prevents ovulation by inhibiting the pituitary/hypothalmus; (c) in many women the minipill allows normal ovulation but promotes the formation of cervical mucus to form a barrier to the sperm.

pressing ovulation. In addition, progestin increases the amount and thickness of the cervical mucus, thereby inhibiting the transmission of sperm from the vagina to the uterus. Thus, the overall effect of the combination pill is that "the sperm are unable to reach an ovum, and there is none there anyway."[31]

Significantly, the concentration levels of the two hormones in the combination pill have been reduced considerably since it was first introduced. Originally, the average pill contained 10 mg of progestin and 2 mg of estrogen. Today the average pill contains only a fraction of these amounts —1 mg of progestin and 0.05 mg of estrogen.

The sequential birth-control pill

Owing to the undesirable side effects associated with the original overly potent combination pill, reproductive researchers developed a sequential birth-control pill in 1965. With the sequential pill, the woman begins taking estrogen-only pills on the fifth day of her menstrual cycle and continues to do so for 16 days. She then takes a combination estrogen-progestin pill for an additional 5 days. Like the combination pill, the sequential pill disrupts the ovarian but not the uterine cycle. However, with the sequential pill, the high estrogen level is responsible for the inhibition of both FSH and LH. The sequential pill also has the same effect on the lining of the uterus, which builds up and is then sloughed during menstruation. The major difference between the sequential and combination pills is the effect each has on the cervical mucus. Since there is no progestin in the early part of the sequential pill cycle, the fluid in the cervix remains clear and thin so that the sperm can penetrate and reach the uterus. Thus, the overall effect of the sequential pill is that "the sperm are now able to reach an ovum, but none is there."[32]

The minipill

In a further attempt to minimize the harmful side effects of the combination pill, reproductive researchers concluded that estrogen, not progestin, was the primary problem. They then developed a progestin-only oral contraceptive, the so-called minipill, which produces fewer side effects.

Women who take the minipill ingest it every day of the year without the 5-day break during menstruation. Most notable about the minipill is that it usually does not disrupt the ovarian cycle, though it sometimes disrupts the uterine cycle.[33] Since there is no estrogen in the minipill, FSH and LH are usually not inhibited and ovulation frequently occurs normally. However, the constant, although low, dose of progestin in the minipill causes the cervix continually to produce sticky, thick mucus that blocks the sperm from reaching the egg. Thus, in many women, the overall effect of the minipill is that "the sperm are unable to reach an ovum that is available for fertilization."[34]

In addition to the minipill, the contraceptives Norplant and Depo-Provera contain only a progestin. The exact mechanism of action of these contraceptives is dependent upon the chemical nature of the synthetic progestin and its dose. As a general rule, a steady level of estrogen is extremely effective in suppressing ovulation, and while a steady level of progestin also may block ovulation it is considerably less effective.

Biphasic and triphasic pills

Additional attempts to simulate women's physiology have resulted in the production of the biphasic (two-phase) and triphasic (three-phase) birth-control pill. While there are variations in dose and timing with the various brands, the daily hormone dosage is altered within a single cycle with these pills. The triphasic pills now in use have three different progestin doses for different parts of the cycle and some also have different estrogen doses. The main advantage of triphasic pills is that they have a lower amount of progestin in a cycle than the combination birth-control pill.

Norplant

Contraceptive implants containing the progestin levonorgestrel in either Silastic capsules or covered rods have been developed for the long-term administration of this birth-control steroid, which functions by inhibiting ovulation. Subdermal implants provide a continuous and stable release of the drug and avoid the periods of elevated dose that occur with intermittent administration such as with the pill or the injection. The capsules are made by filling Silastic tubing with steroid crystals and then sealing the ends of the tube. The covered rods contain steroid crystals homogeneously dispersed in a polymer and covered with a thin Silastic membrane.[35]

These implants are marketed in products that take one of two forms. Norplant-1 consists of six capsules, each 3.4 cm in length containing a total of 220 mg of levonorgestrel. Norplant-2 consists of two covered rods, each 4.4 cm long and containing a total of 140 mg of levonorgestrel. With Norplant, the plasma levels of levonorgestrel remain at approximately 0.28 ng/mL during the first 5 years of use.[36]

Norplant is not meant to be self-administered. A physician implants the six rubbery matchstick-size rods just beneath the skin of a woman's upper arm (figure 4.5). There they continually release the small amounts of progestin into the blood stream.

Perhaps the greatest advantage of Norplant is that its failure rate in preventing pregnancy is only 0.2 percent. Norplant use also permits sexual spontaneity and the return of fertility by the next menstrual cycle after removal. Most of its disadvantages are similar to those of some oral contraceptives: menstrual irregularities, weight gain, mood changes, and headaches. However, Norplant has the added disadvantage that it must be *surgically* inserted and removed by a physician. A woman cannot remove it at will from her body without harming herself. Nevertheless, some women in the Third World, who live far away from their physicians, have attempted self-surgery, with the expected deleterious consequences.[37]

Used in some 15 countries worldwide, Norplant was recently approved for use in the United States based on an application made to the FDA in August 1988. The approval has sparked controversy, however. Although

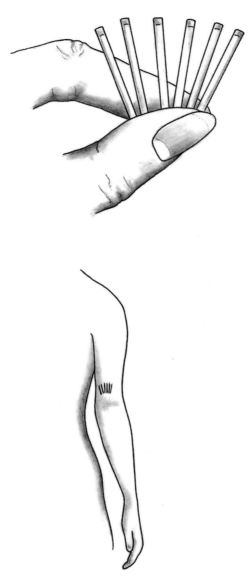

Figure 4.5 Norplant. The six small capsules and their location in the upper arm after implantation.

many women immediately contacted their gynecologists to determine whether they were good candidates for Norplant, some medical ethicists worried that Norplant could become an involuntary form of birth control —one that, for example, a judge might impose on a drug-addicted woman as a condition of her release from prison.

The morning-after pill

As long as our contraceptive technology is imperfect and human behavior is imperfect, there will be a need for postcoital contraception. Researchers have shown that pills containing 0.5 mg of *dl*-norgestrel and 0.05 mg of ethinyl estradiol (marketed in the United States as Ovral) work well in preventing pregnancy subsequent to unprotected midcycle intercourse. When used as morning-after pills, two Ovral tablets are taken within 72 hours (preferably within 12–24 hours) of coitus, and two more tablets are taken 12 hours later. Most women begin bleeding within 21 days following this regimen. The overall effect of the Ovral postcoital regimen appears to be related to luteal phase dysfunction, out-of-phase endometrial development, and disordered tubal transport of the fertilized ovum.[38] Ovral is 99 percent effective and has few side effects, the most common being nausea. Although the FDA has not approved Ovral (or other postcoital contraceptive methods) as a morning-after pill, many physicians have used it to treat women who have engaged in unprotected midcycle intercourse.

Side Effects

Because steroids are so potent and have so many functions within the body, it is not surprising that an artificial surplus of them causes some side effects. The risks associated with oral contraceptives vary in seriousness and include weight gain, hypertension, depression, an increased risk of blood clots, psychological disturbances, gallbladder disease, benign liver tumors, and urinary tract infections. Because estrogen is the cause of most of these problems, the dosage of this steroid has been significantly decreased in today's pill. In addition, the sequential pill is no longer marketed, not only because the first 16 pills in the sequence contain only estrogen as the active ingredient but also because it lacks overall effectiveness. The minipill is marketed, but physicians prescribe it for only 5 to 10 percent of women who use oral contraceptives as its effectiveness is reduced if it is taken even a few hours late 1 day; it causes more irregular bleeding than the combined pill; and it increases the risk of ectopic pregnancy and of benign ovarian cysts.[39]

For young, healthy, nonsmoking women, the pill is relatively safe. Women who are older than 35 years, smoke, or have a history of high blood cholesterol or triglycerides, high blood pressure, or diabetes, however, are at some risk for blood clotting, strokes, and heart attacks. From time to time, concerns have been raised about the carcinogenic effects of the pill, but a 10-year World Health Organization review published in December 1990 showed no link between oral contraceptives and breast, cervical, or liver cancer.[40]

Significantly some benefits as well as risks have been linked to the pill. The combination pill and minipill apparently offer women some protection from both ovarian and endometrial cancer. They may also protect women from PID although not from STDs.[41]

Each woman must consider her individual situation. She must weigh the health risks of using certain contraceptives against the consequences of engaging in unprotected sexual intercourse. Although contraceptives

Table 4.1 Putting risks into perspective: A comparison of the risks associated with using various birth-control methods, abortion, and non-reproductive activities

Risk	Chance of Death in Year per 100,000 Women (U.S.)
Having sexual intercourse (pelvic inflammatory disease)	2
No fertility control method (birth-related)	10
Oral contraceptive—nonsmoker	1.6
Oral contraceptive—smoker	6.3
Using intrauterine device	1
Using barrier method (birth-related)	1–2
Sterilization by tubal ligation	1.5
Sterilization by hysterectomy	62.5
Nonlegal abortion	33
Legal abortion	
Before 9 weeks	0.2
Between 9 and 12 weeks	1.5
Between 13 and 16	4
After 16 weeks	11.5
Smoking	500
Automobile driving	17
Using tampons	0.3

Data adapted from *The Physicians Desk Reference*, 45th edition (Medical Economics, New Jersey, 1991) 1600; and R. A. Hatcher, F. Stewart, J. Trussell, D. Kowal, F. Guest, G. K. Stewart, and W. Gates, *Contraceptive Technology 1990–1992*, 15th edition, (Irvington, New York: 1990) 146.

pose certain levels of risks to women, table 4.1 suggests that these are statistically less significant than several other risks that many people voluntarily accept.

New Contraceptives

No contraceptive is 100 percent effective, 100 percent safe, entirely convenient, and aesthetically pleasing. The rhythm method and coitus interruptus depend on the willpower of a couple either to abstain from or to interrupt sexual intercourse at certain times; the condom, diaphragm, cervical cap, and sponge depend on the ability of a couple not to get "swept away" in a moment of passion and disregard the protection kept handy; and the negative side effects of IUDs and oral contraceptives range from the irritating to the harmful. Given this state of affairs, many reproductive researchers are working to develop contraceptives that are even more effective, simple, and safe.

Depo-Provera

Among the newest of these contraceptives is the controversial Depo-Provera, an injectable contraceptive constituted of a synthetic progesterone called depot medroxyprogesterone acetate.[42] It works by mechanisms similar to the other progestin-only contraceptives. Because Depo-Provera contains no estrogen, a woman does not have to worry about cardiovascular risks; and because a single 150 mg injection lasts at least 3 months, she does not have to worry about forgetting to take it. The drug is injected into the arm or buttock and has been shown to be 99 percent effective in preventing pregnancy. It has been used since 1960 in many countries but was only approved for use in the United States as a prescription drug in October 1992 and became available in January 1993.

Despite the apparent advantages of Depo-Provera, the FDA did not approve its use earlier as a contraceptive in the United States for a number of reasons. First, Depo-Provera's biggest bonus—its long-lasting effect—also may be one of its most significant drawbacks. The drug's effectiveness involves the suppression of ovulation by affecting the hypothalamus, a suppression that may last from 6 months to 1 year after a woman has stopped receiving injections. A related problem is the risk to the fetus if a woman somehow does get pregnant while taking Depo-Provera. Because there is no way to withdraw the injection's 3-month effects, the fetus will be exposed for up to 3 months to progestins that may harm it.[43] Second, some reproductive researchers have shown that

Depo-Provera has its share of negative side effects, including irregular or prolonged menstruation, headaches, severe weight gain, acne, hair loss, and nausea.[44] Third, other reproductive researchers have established that large doses of Depo-Provera cause breast cancer in beagles and cancer of the endometrium in rhesus monkeys. Although there were no reports of these cancers in human Depo-Provera users in 90 countries worldwide, the FDA decided to adopt a cautious approach and kept Depo-Provera off the U.S. market[45] until recently.

The FDA approval came as a result of recent studies with humans which indicated that there appeared to be no increased risk of breast cancer in women. The cancer risk study show a slight increase in the risk of breast cancer for women younger than 35, but no increased risk of cervical, ovarian, or endometrial cancer for these younger women.[46]

Another, less popular injectable contraceptive contains norethisterone in a 200 mg dose given every 60 days.[47]

RU 486

In the autumn of 1988, RU 486 (mifepristone) became available to women in France as an abortifacient (refer to chapter 6 for a further discussion). As an antiprogesterone, RU 486 resembles progesterone and binds tightly to progesterone receptors in cells, with an affinity three times that of progesterone. Instead of evoking the hormone's usual effect of maintaining pregnancy, however, this progesterone antagonist blocks it.[48] The steroid nucleus enables RU 486 to bind to progesterone receptor sites, and the presence of a group at position 11 imparts the antagonistic action (figure 4.6). Unlike many hormones that act at the cell membrane, the synthetic steroid RU 486 enters the cell and binds to receptors in the nucleus where it acts as a blocking mechanism, perhaps as shown in figure 4.6.

In France, where RU 486 is approved for use, it is administered in conjunction with prostaglandins. Forty-eight hours after taking the RU 486 tablets, the woman receives a small dose of prostaglandin. Uterine contractions begin that expel an embryo within 24 hours. The 80 percent success rate of RU 486 administered alone is increased to 96 percent when administered in conjunction with a prostaglandin.

RU 486 is carefully regulated by French law and administered only under the supervision of a physician following a four-step process.

1. The woman goes to an authorized clinic for a pregnancy test and counseling, after which she must wait 1 week before having an abortion.

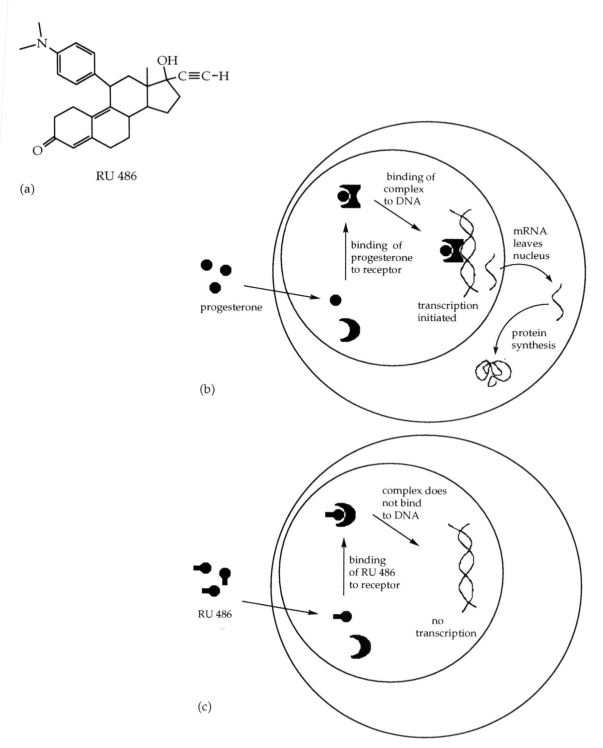

(a) RU 486

(b) binding of complex to DNA · binding of progesterone to receptor · progesterone · transcription initiated · mRNA leaves nucleus · protein synthesis

(c) complex does not bind to DNA · binding of RU 486 to receptor · RU 486 · no transcription

Figure 4.6 (a) The chemical structure of RU 486; (b) a schematic representation of the action of progesterone; and (c) the inhibition of the action of progesterone by RU 486.

2. She returns to the clinic and swallows three pills. (A single dose of 600 mg produces the best results.)[49]

3. Two days later the woman must have a dose of prostaglandin to induce contractions. In the method commonly used, the woman goes back to the clinic for an injection of prostaglandin. She waits approximately 4 hours after the injection for the embryo to be expelled. During this time she is monitored for hemorrhaging, which occurs in 4 to 5 percent of the women who use RU 486. If the embryo is not expelled in what the clinic considers a reasonable length of time, the woman is sent home to wait for the expulsion there. Approximately 47 percent of the women who are given RU 486 by injection, however, do abort before they leave the clinic, the rest doing so shortly after returning home. In a new variation on this method, the prostaglandin is administered orally[50] using a commercial product called Cytotec. This enables the woman to abort by swallowing a combination of pills (the RU 486 and the prostaglandin). It also increased the percentage of women who abort within 4 hours to 61 percent.

4. To ensure the abortion is complete, 1 week later the woman returns to the clinic for a final checkup. The 4 percent who have failed to abort are advised to have a surgical abortion.[51]

The law in France limits the use of RU 486 to the first 7 weeks of pregnancy. Many women prefer RU 486 to other forms of abortion because it is less invasive as well as more private, safer, and cheaper than surgical abortion. Already RU 486 has shown promise as a contraceptive that prevents ovulation, as a treatment for endometriosis that suppresses hormone production, as a breast cancer treatment that removes the progesterone stimulus, and as a labor enhancer that helps to soften and dilate the cervix.

New Contraceptive Methods for Women

To give women more control over the contraceptives in their bodies, reproductive researchers are working on a few new methods, including a progesterone-laced vaginal ring, a steroid-filled bracelet, a "pregnancy vaccine," and a birth-control battery. A woman would insert the ring into her vagina in a fashion similar to the diaphragm. There it would release a small, steady amount of progestin, sometimes in combination with estrogen, inhibiting ovulation and thickening the cervical mucus. Without diminishing the overall contraceptive effect of the ring, a woman could remove it to permit the easy flow of blood during menstruation or to permit the easy penetration of the penis during intercourse.

The bracelet is designed to fit snugly around the woman's upper arm, where the progestin would be absorbed into her skin slowly but constantly until she decided to remove it to become pregnant.[52]

Another method under development is a pregnancy vaccine that could come in a variety of forms. Currently, reproductive researchers are working on a vaccine containing antibodies specific for the hormone human chorionic gonadotropin (HCG), which is present only in pregnant women. By secreting HCG into the uterus, the newly implanted embryo stimulates other hormones that maintain it during the early stages of pregnancy. Although the HCG molecule is very similar to the LH molecule, it is differentiated by the beta-subunit of HCG. Researchers have developed a vaccine containing antibodies to this subunit that effectively makes a woman immune to pregnancy. The body rejects the ingredient essential for maintaining the corpus luteum without affecting the LH hormone involved in the menstrual cycle. Unfortunately, researchers are not certain how to reverse this process of immunization (one vaccination would last indefinitely), although several possibilities are being tested.[53]

Another contraceptive method being developed involves the effects of electricity on fertility. A miniature battery would be inserted into the cervix where it would give off a constant, very low stream of electricity capable of immobilizing sperm on their way to the uterus. Reproductive researchers claim that the battery appears to avoid the harmful side effects associated with the IUD.[54]

Developing Contraceptive Methods for Men

Since female birth control is so problematic, reproductive researchers have begun to turn their attention to male birth control. To be effective, a male contraceptive must do one of three things: stop the production of sperm, hinder the maturation of the sperm, or stop the transmission of sperm. To date, researchers have found ways to do each of these tasks, but in an imperfect manner.[55]

Stopping sperm production

Although antimetabolic agents and estrogen both serve very effectively to stop the production of sperm, antimetabolic agents are toxic and estrogen tends to cause a loss in libido, breast enlargement, and thromboembolic disease. Researchers are trying to temper estrogen with testosterone to neutralize estrogen's demasculinizing effects, but their efforts have not yet been successful. Researchers have had more success with progestin: When coupled with androgens, progestin avoids most of the demasculinizing effects associated with estrogen. Unfortunately, progestin is not as effective in blocking sperm production as are antimetabolic agents and estrogen.[56]

Gonadotropin-releasing hormone (GnRH) analogues are compounds modeled after the structure of the GnRH hormone, which plays a critical role in the reproductive cycles of both men and women. Researchers have discovered that, when taken either nasally or by injection, GnRH analogues are capable of halting the function of the entire male reproductive system, including sperm development.[57] Unfortunately, GnRH analogues also kill the male sex drive completely. Once again, researchers hope to neutralize this negative effect by combining GnRH analogues with testosterone, and some success has been achieved.[58]

Hindering sperm maturation

Researchers have discovered that gossypol, GnRH analogues, cyproterone acetate, and "belly jelly" impair sperm maturation and, therefore, egg fertilization. The Chinese have been using gossypol, a yellowish, phenolic compound derived from cottonseed oil, as a male contraceptive for some time. This drug blocks the action of the lactate dehydrogenase X enzyme, found only in sperm or testicular cells. By blocking this enzyme, gossypol hinders sperm maturation and mobility. However, the drug, which is 99.89 percent effective and very inexpensive to make, has several disadvantages. It causes potassium deficiencies, hair discoloration, and listlessness, and it seems to be particularly problematic for men with subclinical varicose veins in the testicles.[59] It may also cause impotence and, in some instances, permanent infertility.[60]

Researchers also believe that cyproterone acetate may impair the sperm so that they cannot penetrate the cervical mucus. Until researchers complete their tests on this drug, however, they cannot be confident about its full effects.[61]

Finally, researchers have developed a product called *belly jelly* that effectively inhibits sperm production. Belly jelly is a salve that is rubbed on the abdomen or the chest of the man immediately before intercourse. The combination of testosterone and estradiol in the cream is able to stop fertility without depleting the male libido. The trouble with belly jelly is that it can cause increased male characteristics in the female partner of the user: It often causes hair to sprout on the inner thighs or the upper lip of women who come in contact with it and, although a solution to this problem is being sought, belly jelly is not currently marketable.[62]

Stopping sperm transport

To stop the transport of sperm, researchers are working on methods of altering the vasectomy procedure to consist of a completely reversible vas occlusion. The traditional vasectomy operation involves cutting and tying off each end of the vas deferens so that the sperm can no longer pass through. Although the operation can be reversed in some cases, reversal certainly is not guaranteed. To achieve the reversible vas occlusion, instead of actually cutting the vas deferens, a surgeon would block it with a plug or a clip, which later could be removed to restore normal sperm transport.[63]

The Ethics of Contraception

Although contraception is currently standard practice nearly worldwide, discussion of its morality continues to elicit disagreement. Some religious thinkers regard contraception as a violation of the reproductive system; others accept it as a God-given means to regulate better our life here on Earth. A similar range of opinion is manifested in the legal realm. Some foreign legislative bodies base their contraceptive policies on national population statistics, requiring contraception if the population is too high and forbidding it if it is too low, or simply permitting it if the nation is at no serious risk. Although U.S. legislative bodies have not sought to impose an outright ban on contraceptives, in recent years they have sought to regulate contraceptive use among certain segments of the population (e.g., adolescents). They have also occasionally sought to require their use among certain segments of the population (e.g., cocaine-addicted women of childbearing age). Finally, social questions about contraceptive policy continue to be raised by liberals committed to personal freedom, by conservatives wedded to family traditions, and by feminists focused on women's reproductive rights.

Contraception and the Natural Law

Most ethicists either permit or require the voluntary use of contraceptives. However, ethicists who work within the natural-law tradition, which is associated primarily with the Roman Catholic Church, are opposed to the voluntary use of contraceptives even within marriage. Philosopher Michael Bayles summarizes the natural-law argument against contraception as follows:

1. Good ought to be pursued and evil avoided.

2. Good ends are those toward which people are naturally inclined.

3. People are naturally inclined to sexual intercourse.

4. A natural purpose of sexual intercourse is reproduction.

5. Therefore, reproduction ought to be pursued in sexual acts.

6. To act intentionally against the good of reproduction is evil and ought to be avoided.[64]

Although each one of this argument's premises is debatable (e.g., is an end rendered good simply because people are naturally inclined toward it?), premises 5 and 6 are particularly controversial.

For several centuries, natural-law theorists debated whether procreation is *the* purpose or simply *a* purpose of sexual intercourse. Initially, the consensus stressed the procreative function of human sexuality. In fact, the thirteenth-century theologian St. Bonaventure argued that marital relations were good only "if motivated solely by the desire to have children."[65] But because many married couples confessed that they usually focused on pleasure rather than procreation during sexual intercourse, theologians found it increasingly difficult to defend the view that sex is for procreation only.

Currently, most natural-law theorists maintain that marriage has two aims: (1) a conceptual aim, directed toward the conception of children, and (2) a relational aim, directed toward bringing husbands and wives together in a network of pleasure and love.[66] They insist, however, that the conceptual aim of marriage is primary, whereas the relational aim is secondary. Each and every act of sexual intercourse must, in principle, remain open to the transmission of life. Thus, most natural-law theorists forbid all forms of birth control that deliberately frustrate conception, permitting only those forms of birth control that work with, rather than against, the natural reproductive cycle. Among these approved natural methods is rhythm, intentionally abstaining from sex during the periods when pregnancy might result.

Not everyone within the natural-law tradition finds that the distinction between so-called unnatural and natural methods of birth control makes a moral difference, however. Roman Catholic commentator Michael Novak writes:

I do not understand why it is "unnatural" to block the spatial flow of sperm so that it does not fertilize the ovum—to block it by diaphragm, or condom, say (however disagreeable such devices are)—and yet not "unnatural" to time the placement of the sperm so that it does not fertilize the ovum. In either case, human intelligence is directing the process so that the ovum will not be fertilized. In the first case, a physical spatial object is inserted in the process; in the second case, an equally physical temporal gap is deliberately (and with such care!) inserted in the process. I do not understand why spatial objects are blameworthy, while temporal gaps are not. Both are equally "natural" (or "unnatural").[67]

In arguing as he does, Novak intends not to condemn the use of rhythm but rather to endorse the use of unnatural as well as natural contraceptives when a couple needs to limit the number of their children in order to care for them responsibly. He, as well as many contemporary Roman Catholics, believes that the theoretical assumptions of natural-law theory should be reinterpreted to better fit the practical realities of twentieth-century family life.

Contraception and Population Control

With the exception of strict natural-law ethicists, most ethicists support the use of contraceptives as a means of population control. Concern over the size of the human population is, of course, not peculiar to the twentieth century. As early as 1798, Thomas Malthus claimed that since population size "increases exponentially" whereas food supply "increases only arithmetically," the state would have to control the size of the population. Convinced that the lower socioeconomic classes lacked the restraint necessary to curb their "promiscuous breeding," Malthus urged the state to leave the poor to their fate—that is, to the vicissitudes of disease, epidemic, war, plague, and famine. To subsidize the poor, said Malthus, would be to interfere with nature's laws, harsh laws that must be obeyed in order to maintain an equilibrium between the human community's food supply and its population.[68]

Even though Malthus's views about population growth were largely discredited by the twentieth century, concerns about overpopulation were not thereby assuaged. During the 1960s and 1970s, a variety of thinkers argued strongly against unrestricted procreation. In *The Case for Compulsory Birth Control*, for example, Edgar Chasteen identified overpopulation as a leading cause of food shortages, crime, pollution, overcrowding in cities, apathy, alienation, high taxes, lagging development in the Third World, and especially the existence of "superfluous" people. Using emotional rhetoric, Chasteen wrote that:

Overpopulation is a child whose teeth decay, whose bones are malformed, whose eyesight goes uncorrected, and whose education is sporadic and totally inadequate for today's world. It is a body stunted by vitamin deficiency and beset by diseases unknown to the less crowded. It is a mind caged in a primitive world and dominated by the strong, where those ethics by which civilization maintains itself are irrelevant to the brutal demands of daily living.[69]

Frightened by the specter of this child, twentieth-century activists were even more inclined than their nineteenth-century counterparts to impose restrictions on individuals' right to procreate, recommending a wide variety of voluntary and involuntary means of contraception.

Voluntary Contraception and Population Control

Intent on safeguarding the right of individuals to procreate, some ethicists contend that even though overpopulation may be a serious problem, involuntary contraception (forcing people not to procreate) is no way to solve it. These ethicists assume that people are rational; that is, they do not desire to have more children than they or the world can support. The best way to solve the overpopulation problem, therefore, is simply to provide rational people with whatever medical, educational, and social services they need to produce only the number of children they want. In short, the real problem is not that people desire more children than they can support; rather, it is that they do not always have the means to prevent unwanted pregnancies.

Involuntary Contraception and Population Control

Advocates of involuntary contraception believe that voluntary contraception is an insufficient means to reduce population size. As they see it, not all people are rational; that is, some people do desire to have more children than is personally prudent or socially responsible. Such advocates use as examples families who refuse to use contraceptives for religious or cultural reasons and very young or otherwise immature people who refuse to use contraceptives simply because they regard them as aesthetically displeasing or a bother.

Under certain circumstances (extreme overpopulation would be one), advocates of involuntary contraception insist that the state may force such imprudent or irresponsible people to limit the size of their families. To the objection that the state may not interfere with an individual's right to procreate, these lobbyists reply that no right is absolute, especially one that, when exercised, permits already existent persons to bring into existence new person(s) who might, after all, not want the gift of life.

The advocates of involuntary contraception argue that procreating children who will lack adequate food, clothing, and shelter is a disservice not only to these children but also to the entire world population. Although the world's pie of natural resources can be cut more or less thinly, people cannot subsist on crumbs alone. Therefore, the state's duty is clear. To protect social values such as human survival and distributive justice, it not only may but must take one or more of the following forceful steps outlined by social ethicists Thomas Mappes and Jane Zembaty:

1. *Social structure adjustment*   For example, encouraging women to find employment outside the home or raising the minimum legal age for marriage, thus remotely affecting reproductive choices by affecting the context in which reproductive choices are made.

2. *Positive incentives*   Providing financial rewards for the practice of contraception, for not having children, etc.

3. *Negative incentives*   Inflicting financial penalties on those who have children or on those who have more than a certain number of children.

4. *Involuntary fertility controls*   For example, the compulsory sterilization of individuals after they have had a certain number of children, compulsory abortion in the case of mothers who already have had a certain number of children, or even the wide-scale control of fertility through the addition of a fertility-control agent to the water supply.[70]

The aim of each of these steps, ranging from the least coercive (social structure adjustment) to the most coercive (involuntary fertility controls) is to force people to conceive fewer children than they want.

The first one of these steps is probably the most effective way to limit people's desire to procreate. For example, one of the reasons that birth rates did not rise but actually fell in most industrialized Western countries during the 1970s and 1980s was that large numbers of women entered the work force. According to economist Gary Becker, a married woman living in an urban area and bringing home a good salary is likely to have fewer children than a nonemployed female homemaker living in a rural area.[71] Not only will the former woman not have the time and energy to care for a large family, she and her spouse actually *will not want* a large family. Becker explains that a relatively affluent couple's desire not to procreate makes sense because the demand for children depends on their relative cost—that is, on the money it takes to feed, clothe, and educate them minus the benefits they provide. Thus, the demand for children is relatively high in rural India where children are significant contributors to farm work by age 12 and relatively low in U.S. cities where children younger than 18 do only minor household chores (e.g., dish washing and lawn mowing).[72] Arguably, the easiest way for a couple to improve its standard of living is for each partner to work outside the home and for neither to pressure the other into having a big family. A small family means less stress, less expense, more time to spend with each child, more advantages for each child, and more time for career and personal interests.

Advocates of involuntary contraception concede that Becker's theory does not leave room for intangibles such as parental love. Nevertheless, they insist that the overpopulation problem requires everyone to become more realistic and less idealistic. If it is true that the population rate goes down when women enter the work force, then overpopulated countries should use legislation to achieve this salutary social structure adjustment.

Although opponents of involuntary contraception would object, for example, to a law requiring all women between the ages of 18 and 38 to enter the work force, India has considered legislation of this type. Contributing to India's over population problem is the fact that Hindus favor early marriage as a way to assure the groom and his family that his bride is indeed a virgin.[73] The earlier a girl marries, however, the more children she is likely to bear. For this reason, some Indian legislators have proposed that the legal age for marriage be raised. As they see it, even though this social structure adjustment would erode Hindu tradition, it may be the least coercive way to achieve the laudable goal of population reduction.

If adjustments in social structures are ethically problematic, so too are so-called incentive programs and involuntary fertility-control programs that tamper with people's motivational structures. By rewarding people for not procreating (or, as the case may be, for procreating), or by punishing them for one or the other of these acts, incentive programs can cause people to make reproductive decisions that they would not otherwise make. Depending on how irresistible the rewards or how dire the punishments are, critics regard incentive programs as more or less ethically suspect. So, for example, France's attempt to increase its population by offering to prolific couples tax breaks, day-care subsidies, parental leave, and so forth seems positively enlightened compared to Romania's now-failed attempt to increase its population by, among other things, banning all birth control and requiring fertile, married women to have a minimum of 5 children. Whereas the result of France's policy has been well-fed, well-clothed, well-loved children, the result of Romania's policy has been nearly 100,000 abandoned children living in "filth, degradation and misery."[74]

Contraception and Informed Consent

Unless a nation is either severely underpopulated or severely overpopulated, its government does not tend to interfere with its people's reproductive decisions. Thus, ethicists are far less worried about instances of involuntary contraception than they are about abuses of voluntary contraception. Certainly in the past, but even today, health care professionals have violated the doctrine of informed consent; that is, they have failed to give their patients the kind of information they require to choose voluntarily the contraceptive the patients judge to be in their own best interests. At times, these failures have been minor: The kind of information withheld has been of little consequence and the reasons for doing so have been benign. At other times, the failures have been major.

In the early 1970s, Dr. Joseph Goldzieher, for example, wanted to know whether some of the reported side effects of oral contraceptives were physiological or psychological. In a double-blind experiment on poor, Mexican-American women who had come to a clinic for contraceptives, 76 of the women got placebos whereas the rest received various kinds of oral contraceptives. None of the women were told that they were participating in a research experiment; and none of them were told that some of them would be receiving placebos. However, they all were told to use a vaginal cream just in case the "oral contraceptives" did not work. The results of the experiment were admittedly informative. The women on placebos experienced many of the same side effects as the women on the oral contraceptives. Unfortunately, 10 of the 76 women on placebos became pregnant. Clearly, the rights of all the women in this experiment, but especially of the 10 women who became pregnant, were violated. They had a right to be asked, as one critic suggested, whether they wanted to participate in the researcher's experiment, and they had a right "knowledgeably [to] refuse to participate" in what amounted to a game of Russian roulette. In sum, these poor, Mexican-American women had the right, as yet another critic suggested, to be treated in the same way that the researcher would have wanted his wife to be treated under similar circumstances.[75]

Clearly, then, the ethical implications of informed consent are several, especially because no one is certain how much information a person needs to make a truly informed decision about medical treatment. Ethicists as well as legal thinkers have proposed three possible standards to govern physicians' disclosure of information to patients. Physicians must disclose (1) what a responsible physician ordinarily tells a patient about various means of contraception; or (2) what a reasonable patient needs to know about various means of contraception; or (3) what an individual patient, however reasonable or unreasonable, wants to know, as well as needs to know, about various means of contraception.[76] We can better appreciate the differences among these three standards by focusing on a specific case, that of an allegedly unreasonable but nonetheless competent patient.

Imagine that an extremely well-educated woman with a history of hypochondria seeks out the services of an obstetrician-gynecologist (ob-gyn). Trained in a traditional and paternalistic school of medical thought, the ob-gyn evaluates the woman and decides she is an excellent candidate for oral contraceptives. She is young, healthy, and in a sexually active, monogamous relationship. Aware of the woman's tendency to make mountains out of molehills, the ob-gyn, who happens to be male, totally downplays the risks of oral contraceptives, emphasizing only their benefits. He sees no need to alarm the woman for fear that she will insist on using a less risky, but also less effective, means of contraception such as the cervical cap. Meanwhile, the woman senses that the ob-gyn is withholding information from her, including information about the harmful side effects of oral contraceptives. She demands that the ob-gyn tell her about all of the pill's harmful side effects, however rare. After all, she *knows* that her physical condition is such that what is a minuscule risk for most women is a colossal risk for her. The ob-gyn refuses to engage in a protracted discussion with her, insisting that any respectable ob-gyn would tell her the same thing—namely, that for young, healthy, sexually active patients such as herself, the benefits of oral contraceptives far outweigh their risks.

According to prevailing legal and ethical opinion, the ob-gyn in our case wronged the woman by failing to discuss with her the most typical negative side effects of oral contraceptives. Just because he had the reasonable medical belief that oral contraceptives were in the best medical interests of his patient did not justify his stonewalling her. Still, ethics and law do not require an ob-gyn to cater to an patient's excessive demands for information. Given her history of hypochondria, the ob-gyn in our case would have had enormous difficulty persuading his patient to use even the safest oral contraceptive on the market. All that ethics and law can comfortably require this ob-gyn to do, therefore, is to give his unreasonable patient the kind of information that would satisfy a reasonable patient.

Of course, it is difficult to determine just how much information even reasonable patients need in order to make informed decisions. Certainly, they need the kind of information, advice, and assurances that Dr. Robert Hatcher, author of *Contraceptive Technology*, urges ob-gyns to provide to patients. As he sees it, ob-gyns should (1) discuss the risks as well as the benefits of any recommended contraceptive; (2) explain how the recommended contraceptive works, urging the patient to ask questions and taking the time to answer them; (3) present alternatives to the recommended contraceptive (including abstinence from sexual relations and using no contraceptive whatsoever); (4) encourage the patient to report any problems she has with the recommended contraceptive and to discontinue its use if she finds it does not suit her specific needs; and (5) ascertain that the patient has understood items, through 4, requesting her to repeat in her own words, if necessary, the gist of the communicated information.[77] Although ob-gyns sometimes complain that there is no perfect way to meet these five requirements, most ethicists believe that there are better and worse ways. Grady Memorial Hospital, for example, has already developed an excellent consent form for its patients (figure 4.7).[78]

Provided that she is competent, a patient should be permitted to sign the consent form depicted in figure 4.7 if she claims to have understood it. Unfortunately, her signature will not constitute proof that she has really understood the risks and benefits associated with a myriad of contraceptives. Physicians' time is limited; there are only so many hours in the day, and they must be divided among many patients. A physician may be able to communicate effectively the risks and benefits of an IUD, for example, to a self-confident patient with an educational, racial, or socio-economic background similar to his or her own. But he or she may not be able to communicate effectively this same information to a patient who speaks poor English, who is afraid of physicians, or who does not think of questions to ask until she is on her way home from the physician's office. As regrettable as this state of affairs is, physicians can only do so much to inform their patients about their medical options. If a patient is competent, if she claims to have read and understood the informed consent form, and if her physician has used an office hour to discuss it with her, then the presumption must be that her signing on the dotted line is more than an act of blind faith.

Not all patients who need contraceptives fit the description of a competent patient, however. Some of them are incompetent—that is, simply *unable* to make their own decisions because of one or more physical or psychological impediments. Most mentally retarded persons and most normal children younger than 12 years, for example, would be bewildered by Grady Memorial Hospital's consent form, either because they could not read it or because they could not understand its terms fully. If she or he wishes to prescribe contraceptives for a mentally retarded person or a normal child, an ob-gyn will need to secure permission from the patient's guardian unless the patient is competent enough to make his or her own procreative decisions. If a person is only mildly mentally retarded, or if a young child is extremely precocious, for example, she or he may be able to understand basic facts about human reproduction, the salient risks and benefits associated with various contraceptive methods, and the personal

ORAL CONTRACEPTIVE CONSENT FORM
Grady Memorial Hospital
Atlanta, Georgia
Revised May 1985

I hereby acknowledge that I am voluntarily receiving birth-control pills. Pills are the method of family planning which I have chosen from the methods that have been explained to me. The advantages and disadvantages of the other methods of contraception have been explained to me.

BENEFITS: I am aware that oral contraceptives are *not* guaranteed to be 100% effective. It is my understanding that combined birth-control pills can be close to 99% effective if I take them consistently and correctly. It is my understanding that progestin-only pills (minipills) are slightly less effective even if taken consistently. I have been told that in addition to their benefits as a method of birth control, some women experience the following benefits from using birth-control pills:

- **Decreased menstrual cramps**
- **Decreased menstrual bleeding**
- **More regular menstrual bleeding**
- **Decreased pain at the time of ovulation**
- **Less risk of acute gonococcal pelvic inflammatory disease**
- **Improvement in acne**
- **Less risk of developing ovarian or endometrial cancer**
- **Less risk of developing benign breast tumors or ovarian cysts**

RISKS: I have been told to watch out for the following pill danger signals and return to the clinic or make contact with my clinician at once of I develop one of these problems. These could be warnings of serious or even life-threatening illness.

EAPLY PILL DANGER SIGNS

CAUTION

A • Abdominal pain (severe)
C • Chest pain (severe), cough, shortness of breath
H • Headache (severe), dizziness, weakness, numbness
E • Eye problems (vision loss or blurring), speech problems
S • Severe leg pain (calf or thigh)

See your clinician of you have any of these problems or if you develop depression, yellow jaundice, or a breast lump.

I am aware that while using oral contraceptives, I could experience the following side effects, many of which can be temporary:

Major Problems
- **Blood clots of the legs or the lungs**
- **Strokes or heart attacks**
- **Gallbladder disease**
- **One type of liver tumor**
- **Death**

Minor Problems
- **Nausea**
- **Spotting between periods**
- **Less menstrual bleeding**
- **Breast tenderness**
- **Weight gain**
- **Headache**
- **Depression**
- **High blood pressure**
- **Darkening of the skin on my face**
- **Worsening of acne**
- **Infections in the vagina**

I have been informed that a majority of the serious complications in pill users occur in women older than 30 who are heavy smokers (15 or more cigarettes per day).

Stopping Pills: I have been told that I may stop using the pills at any time. I have been told I should use another means of birth control until I have had three regular periods before attempting to become pregnant. I have also been informed that if my periods were very irregular, very heavy, or very painful before taking pills, they may return to this pattern when I stop taking birth-control pills.

Instructions for the use of birth-control pills have been given to me, and I have been given a patient package insert for my specific type of pill.

Questions: I have been given the opportunity to ask questions about all forms of birth control and about the pill in particular. My questions have been answered to my satisfaction.

Figure 4.7 Grady Memorial Hospital's oral contraceptive consent form. (Reprinted with permission)

ramifications of pregnancy. If this is the case, proxy consent may not be warranted and may even constitute a grave violation of the individual's rights.

Legal Aspects of Contraception

In the United States, early contraceptive legislation received its major impetus from a Protestant moral reformer, Anthony Comstock (1844–1915). Motivated by his efforts, Congress passed in 1873 a comprehensive federal statute titled, An Act for the Suppression of Trade in and Circulation of Obscene Literature and Articles of Immoral Use. This federal law imposed up to 10 years' imprisonment for sending through the mail any drug, medicine, or article able to prevent conception. It also imposed lesser penalties for advertising contraceptive articles, importing them into the United States, or manufacturing, selling, or even possessing them in the District of Columbia and federal territories.[79] Since state legislators were largely against contraception during the first quarter of the twentieth century, some 30 states followed the lead of the federal government, passing their own so-called Comstock laws. However, when public sentiment in favor of contraception began to swell later in the century, these state laws, like the federal law on which they were modeled, were no longer vigorously enforced. Nevertheless, bothered by the mere fact that these laws were still on the books, advocates of reproductive freedom began to challenge them in the courts.

Legal Challenges to Comstock Laws

Among the first laws to be challenged was a late-nineteenth-century Connecticut statute making it illegal either to use contraceptives or to "assist," "abet," "counsel," "hire," or "command" someone else to use them. In 1942, a physician sought a definitive ruling to determine whether he was truly violating the law by providing contraceptives to women, especially to women for whom pregnancy posed serious health risks. To his surprise and dismay, the Connecticut Supreme Court ruled that physicians were, in fact, forbidden to provide contraceptives even to such women. The court reasoned that if a woman knows that pregnancy is very risky for her, she should simply abstain from sexual intercourse.[80]

By the late 1950s, many physicians and patients had become so angered by this ruling that they pushed to have it declared unconstitutional. But because the law was largely unenforced, the state supreme court refused to hear cases against it, observing that it did not have the time to "umpire" debates on "harmless, empty shadows." In an effort to prove just how real their problems could be, Dr. Charles Lee Buxton, a physician-activist, and Mrs. Estelle T. Griswold, a community leader, opened a birth-control clinic in New Haven in 1961. Within a week, the police had closed the clinic and arrested Griswold and Buxton for passing out "immoral literature." Subsequently, Griswold and Buxton were found guilty and fined $100 each.[81]

After two unsuccessful appeals in Connecticut state courts, Griswold's and Buxton's case finally reached the U.S. Supreme Court in 1965. In the precedent-setting case, *Griswold* v. *Connecticut*, the majority of the Court articulated a fundamental right to marital privacy. No state may infringe on a married couple's procreative decisions unless infringing on them is the only, or the least coercive, way for it to further one of its "compelling interests"—for example, its interest in deterring premarital sex.[82]

Shortly after the *Griswold* decision was handed down in 1965, the Massachusetts legislature voted to give registered physicians and pharmacists special permission to dispense and exhibit contraceptives to *married* persons only. In 1967, William Baird, neither a registered physician nor a registered pharmacist, decided to test the constitutionality of this statute. Baird addressed a group consisting mostly of unmarried Boston University students on the topic of contraception. After his lecture, he invited the students to help themselves to the contraceptives he had displayed during the lecture. Baird deliberately handed a female student a package of vaginal foam, at which point he was arrested and charged with exhibiting and delivering contraceptive articles.[83]

After his trial and conviction on both counts, Baird spent years testing the constitutionality of Massachusetts' statute in several higher courts. He did not meet final success, however, until Massachusetts lost its 1972 case, *Eisenstadt* v. *Baird*, in front of the U.S. Supreme Court. The State of Massachusetts argued that its anticontraception statute was constitutional since it was the only, or least coercive, way to further two of its valid state purposes—the discouragement of premarital sex and the regulation of public health. However, the U.S. Supreme Court was not persuaded by Massachusetts' arguments.

To the first point, that depriving unmarried people of contraceptives discourages premarital sex, the Supreme Court replied that (1) fornicators are unlikely to be deterred by the unavailability of contraceptives; (2) no reasonable (i.e., humane) state should prescribe "pregnancy and the birth of an unwanted child as the punishment for fornication"; and (3) a statute that punishes with a 5-year prison term those who exhibit and deliver contraceptives to unmarried people is an oddly disproportional means to achieve the end of *possibly* deterring premarital sex, a crime that merits no more than a 90-day prison term.[84]

To the second argument, that depriving people of contraceptives saves them from health hazards, the Supreme Court replied that if a given form of birth control does not harm married people, then it will not harm unmarried people. Far from being concerned about its unmarried citizens' *health*, the Court suggested that what really concerned Massachusetts was its unmarried citizens' *morality*.

It is plain that Massachusetts had no such purpose in mind before the enactment of ... the statute.... Consistent with the fact that the statute was continued in a chapter dealing with "Crimes against Chastity, Morality, Decency and Good Order," it was cast only in terms of morals. A physician was forbidden to prescribe contraceptives even when needed for the protection of health.... Nor ... do we believe that the legislature suddenly reversed its field and developed an interest in health.[85]

In striking down Massachusetts' anticontraception statute as an unconstitutional exercise in thinly veiled legal moralism, the Supreme Court ruled that if the right of privacy means anything, it means that single as well as married adults have a right to decide whether to bear or beget a child.

Reproductive Rights for Adolescents

After *Eisenstadt*, unmarried as well as married adults had little difficulty securing contraceptives. Because of public debates about parents' purported rights to monitor their children's sexual conduct, however, health care professionals hesitated to prescribe or sell contraceptives to minors. The landmark case extending some measure of reproductive freedom to adolescents came in 1977. In *Carey* v. *Population Services International*, the U.S. Supreme Court held that personal autonomy over contraceptive choice applied to minors as well as to adults. Invoking the right to privacy, the Supreme Court held that contrary to Massachusetts' belief, nonprescription contraceptives do not pose significant health hazards to minors (or adults); in fact, most nonprescription contraceptives such as condoms, jellies, creams, and foams are virtually risk free. Likewise, contrary to Massachusetts' belief, displays of nonprescription contraceptives do not offend most minors' sensibilities. Minors may feel embarrassed to purchase condoms or other nonprescription contraceptives, but their discomfort is caused not by the sight of these devices but by the fact that they wish to keep their sex lives a secret. Although a state may have a compelling interest to protect its young (and old) citizens from harmful contraceptives, it does not have a compelling interest to protect them from harmless contraceptives, especially if they are displayed discreetly.[86]

In reaction to the Supreme Court's decision, many conservative groups objected that, in ruling as it had, the Court was depriving parents of an important opportunity to be involved in their children's lives. In an effort to strengthen the parent-child relationship, these groups lobbied for parental consent or parental notification requirements. Whereas the former requirements make a minor child's receipt of contraceptive services conditional on parental agreement, the latter require only that parents be informed that their children are receiving services.

Since they limit the privacy rights of minors very seriously, parental consent laws are subject to more constitutional scrutiny than are parental notification laws. For this reason, politically savvy conservative groups often play it safe, lobbying for notification rather than consent laws. Among the first government agencies to formulate a parental notification law was the U.S. Department of Health and Human Services (DHHS). In 1982, it proposed a regulation requiring publicly funded family-planning clinics to notify parents or guardians no later than 10 days after their children had received prescription drugs or devices from them. Exceptions to this rule could be made, but only in those cases where parents or guardians might physically harm a minor on account of her use of contraceptives. The DHHS defended its proposed regulation as one that would (1) break down "Berlin Walls" between parents and children; (2) permit parents to protect their children from the harmful side effects of some contraceptives; and (3) deter teenagers from having sex.[87]

Reaction to this and other parental notification rules has varied enormously. On the one hand, many conservative groups have praised them as a step in the right direction, hoping that future parental notification rules will require family-planning clinics to inform parents *before* they dispense contraceptives to their children. On the other hand, many liberal groups have condemned these same rules as a misguided government strategy, noting that contrary to common misconceptions, these rules do not improve parent-child communication. Nor do they necessarily decrease the premarital sex rate. In fact, the major result of parental notification laws seems to be a drop in teen clinic attendance and even a rise in teen pregnancy rates because sexually active, unprotected teens are at considerable risk for pregnancy.[87]

Currently, the United States has the highest teenage pregnancy rate (96 per 1000) among industrialized countries.[89] Many of these pregnancies are terminated before they ever come to term; 39 percent end in abortions and approximately 13 percent end with miscarriages.[90] The ones that do come to term often come to term poorly. Teenagers typically give birth to malnourished, low-birth-weight, or premature babies, approximately 20 percent of whom will die before their first birthday. The high rate of infant mortality among teenage mothers is due primarily to the lack of prenatal care for these young girls. Many pregnant teenagers cannot afford or do not know where to get proper prenatal care, and many more simply do not want to admit that they are pregnant. Given these stark realities, liberal groups urge their conservative counterparts to ask themselves whether parental notification laws tend to produce more in the way of evil than good consequences. That parents have a right and responsibility to communicate their moral beliefs to their children is clear; but if their children reject their parents' moral beliefs, then parents may need to consider that like adults, children have their own rights and responsibilities. By the time a child reaches the teenage years, he or she is probably autonomous enough to make his or her own decisions about being sexually active or bearing and begetting a child. If it is unconstitutional to impede competent adults' access to contraceptives, it is probably unconstitutional to impede competent adolescents' access to them.

Social Dimensions of Contraception

Although the individual's right to make his or her own reproductive decisions has been legally established, as we have just noted, not all citizens believe that contraception is necessarily in the best interest of sexually active persons, especially if they are minors. Whereas some adults believe that sex education in the public schools and access to contraceptives at family-planning clinics benefit minors, other adults believe they do not. Many ethnic minorities and women have also expressed concerns about the racist and sexist implications of birth-control policy.

Sex Education and Contraceptive Access for Minors

In the United States, the debate over contraceptive education is part of a larger debate over sex education in the public schools. For the most part, teachers instruct students about human sexuality in one of three ways: (1) narrowly, as a purely mechanical "nuts-and-bolts" lesson in physiology; (2) more broadly, as a psychological and sociological as well as physiological account of the entire spectrum of sexual activity and its ramifications;

or (3) most broadly, as a moral evaluation of human sexuality. Although parents tend to agree that a merely physiological approach to sex education leaves young people with the impression that a course on human reproduction is no different from a course on auto mechanics, they tend to disagree about the contents of an appropriate sex education course. Reliable and recent polls show that a majority of parents in the United States (upwards of 70 percent) believe that sex education courses should teach 12-year-olds not only about the dangers of AIDS, STDs, birth control, premarital sex, how men and women have sexual intercourse, homosexuality, and abortion, but also about moral values, what students should or should not do sexually.[91] Significantly, the very same majority that wants sex educators to teach moral values does not seem to agree on what these moral values are. As the following *Time* magazine poll suggests, a sex educator could not possibly please all the parents all the time.[92]

Should sex education courses:	**Yes**	**No**
Teach students that sex at too early an age is harmful?	79%	15%
Urge students not to have sexual intercourse?	67%	25%
Urge students to practice birth control when having casual sex?	84%	11%
Tell students that abortion is an option when pregnancy occurs?	56%	35%
Tell students that abortion is immoral?	44%	44%
Tell students that homosexuality is just an alternative sexual activity?	24%	64%
Tell students that homosexuality is immoral?	56%	36%

Despite the fact that Americans do not appear to share the same moral values, there may be ways to mediate between them. Some school districts are offering a variety of sex education courses. In Lindenhurst, NY, for example, 60 percent of the students attend a liberal "family life" course; 25 percent take a conservative "sexuality, commitment, and family" course; and 15 percent take a health course without sex education to suit the minority of American parents who object to any type of sex education that occurs outside the home.[93]

As heated as the battles over sex education curricula are, even more heated are the battles over school clinics, most of which are located in poor neighborhoods in big cities. Supporters of school clinics argue that they substantially reduce pregnancy rates for their students and, in some cases, even reduce sexual activity. They also point out that these clinics are not "sex clinics" imposed on students and parents against their wills. On the contrary, most school clinics encourage parents to oversee policy development and clinic quality, assuring parents that no services will be provided to students without parental knowledge and approval.[94] Opponents of school clinics argue that for every statistical study that supports the thesis that school clinics reduce sexual activity and pregnancy rates, there is another study that supports the counter thesis. They also argue that, no matter what school officials state publicly about the parents' right to shape their childrens' sexual mores, privately these officials advise teens to enjoy sex but guard against unwanted pregnancies and STDs, especially AIDS.[95]

Whether the opponents or the supporters of school clinics win the day may be irrelevant, however. Many teenagers tend to engage in premarital sex, get pregnant, and contract STDs not because they lack information or birth-control devices but because of social and psychological facts—for example, low self-esteem, impulsiveness, a sense that "it can't happen to me," and a bleak economic future. If parents really care about their children, they should find the words that will persuade their sons and daughters not to engage in behavior that is likely to harm them. And if society really cares about children, it should provide them with the kind of educational and occupational opportunities they need to *want* to make good lives for themselves.

Contraceptive Concerns: Issues of Race, Class, and Gender

Contraception is a matter for debate between various liberal and conservative groups, but it is a matter for even greater debate among women. Because contraception makes sex without procreation possible, it has supposedly led to new sexual responsibilities and rights for both men and women. As many women see it, however, these new responsibilities and rights are being distributed asymmetrically between them and men. Women are receiving more in the way of sexual responsibilities and less in the way of rights, whereas men are receiving more in the way of sexual rights and less in the way of responsibilities. When it comes to sexual responsibilities, women note that they are still the ones expected to protect themselves from an unwanted pregnancy and asked to bear the risks associated with contraceptive use. As most women view it, this state of affairs is an iniquitous one that needs to be remedied. Men, no less than women, are morally obligated to protect themselves from unwanted pregnancies (the baby is not only the "woman's problem") and, "if there are to be definite health risks associated with adequate contraception, these risks should be shared between the male and female partners."[96] Likewise, when it comes to sexual rights, women wonder whether contraception has really increased their ability to make uncoerced choices about when to have sex, with whom, and under what circumstances. With the widespread use of contraceptives has come the presumption that women are supposed to be more available for sexual intercourse than ever before. No longer can a woman discourage a man from making sexual advances with the chilling caveat, "I might get pregnant."

Stages of the American Birth-Control Movement

Given the asymmetry just cited, it is no wonder that many women regard contraceptive technology as a double-edged sword. Often women have chosen to use contraceptives to free themselves from the burden of unwanted pregnancies; but sometimes individual men as well as the state have forced women to use contraceptives to serve not women's interests but their own interests. Indeed, as social historian Linda Gordon sees it, the American campaign for contraceptive use has gone through three distinct stages, each of which has affected the reproductive rights and responsibilities of women, men, and the state differently.

The first stage of the birth-control campaign (1876–1910) is associated with the phrase *voluntary motherhood*. A diverse group of nineteenth-century suffragists, moral reformers, and free-love advocates insisted that women should be able to choose when and how many children to bear. Although this group of activists worked to correct the myth that women have no sexual drives, they also claimed that no self-respecting, sexually active woman should seek to control her reproductive functions "unnaturally"—by using a cervical cap, for example. Rather, a self-respecting, sexually active woman should seek to control her reproductive functions "naturally," by using either her powers of persuasion or her powers of refusal. Ideally, when a wife does not want to reproduce, she and her husband should be able to come to a mutually satisfactory agreement— for example, a decision to meet their sexual needs through the rhythm method, coitus interruptus, or dianaism (nonprocreative love). Less ideally, when a husband insists on having sexual relations with his wife no matter the consequences, she is entitled to refuse his overtures to avoid an unwanted pregnancy.[97]

Given that saying no to one's husband is not always, if ever, the best way to protect a wife from marital rape, Gordon wonders why proponents of voluntary motherhood opposed so-called unnatural contraceptives such as the cervical cap. After all, in the event of marital rape, it seems better to be safe (protected by an unnatural contraceptive) than sorry (pregnant with an unwanted baby). Gordon speculates that what really bothered "self-respecting" wives about contraceptives was not their unnaturalness but the fact that their widespread use would have enabled their husbands to have extramarital sexual relations with "good women" —that is, the women in their own social group—as well as with "bad women"—prostitutes and the like.[98] As humiliating and threatening as it is for one's husband to have sex with an anonymous prostitute, it is even worse for him to have sex with a neighbor.

The second stage of the birth-control movement (1910–1920) is the one primarily associated with the phrase *birth control*. The ideas of this stage of the movement were politically radical, focusing on the lot of all powerless people but especially on that of child-burdened, working-class women. The necessity of birth control for the poor was becoming much more evident, and attitudes toward birth control, and sex in general, were becoming much more permissive. The shift was dramatic. No longer was sexuality a taboo topic. Advertisements, movies, and magazines increasingly portrayed sexual images, and information about the availability of birth control became much more widespread.

The term *birth control* was coined around this time by Margaret Sanger (1883–1966), the U.S. woman whose name is most often linked with birth-control advocacy. A Socialist during the early years of her career, Sanger initially saw birth control as a way to make society more egalitarian as well as to increase women's autonomy. When party leaders began to describe birth control as a "dangerous distraction from class struggle," however, Sanger severed her Socialist connections.[99] After she left the Socialist camp, Sanger, in a gradual repudiation of her egalitarian beliefs, joined the eugenics movement.

Eugenic programs generally have two ultimately interrelated aims: (1) reduction of the frequency of presumably "deleterious" genes, and (2) improvement of the genetic status of the population. Such programs tend to be politically unpopular for a variety of reasons. Many nineteenth-century and early twentieth-century eugenists believed, for example, that certain races and certain classes (that is, the poor) were genetically inferior, and so they sought ways to control the size of their populations. Apparently, Margaret Sanger adopted this perspective later in her life. This woman who, as a Socialist, had attributed the impoverished condition of working-class women to capitalist economics eventually adopted a distressing blame-the-victim rhetoric, arguing that working-class women were "indiscriminate breeders." As she turned to upper- and middle-class women for financial support, "more children from the fit, less from the unfit" became Sanger's unfortunate motto.[100]

The third stage of the birth-control movement is associated with the phrase *planned parenthood*. Unlike the first two stages of the American birth-control movement, planned parenthood did not have among its goals such revolutionary ideals as equality between the sexes or the classes. It was, instead, a reformist movement seeking simply to strengthen the family unit by decreasing its size and increasing its quality. Under the auspices of the Planned Parenthood Federation of America, established in 1942, reformers organized clinics that offered birth-control information, birth-control devices, and counseling for sexual problems. Because segments of the public feared that Planned Parenthood was a free-sex movement, officials of Planned Parenthood initially stressed a hygienic, businesslike approach to sex and birth control.[101] Unfortunately, as political analyst Thomas Shapiro points out, Planned Parenthood's attempt "to decontaminate and depoliticize" the "sex issue" from any hint of promiscuity forced it to limit its services to married people only.[102] Single people were routinely turned away from Planned Parenthood clinics until the 1960s, when American society's sexual mores began to shift in more permissive directions.

The late 1960s and 1970s witnessed not so much the further liberalization of the American birth-control movement as its diversification. Whether these developments, which have spilled into the 1980s and 1990s, represent a fourth stage in the movement is not yet clear. Certainly no single term has been coined to capture the spirit of the various pro-choice and pro-life groups that have made the headlines in recent years. In an effort to establish firmly people's reproductive rights, many men and women have joined the pro-choice movement. In some cases, this has meant actively fighting laws limiting men's but especially women's access to contraceptives; in other cases, it has simply meant working toward the development of safer, more effective contraceptives. Largely in opposition to the pro-choice movement, other men and women have joined the right-to-life (or pro-life) movement, aimed primarily at the prevention of abortion but also, if only secondarily, at the restriction of contraception, especially those forms of contraceptives that act as abortifacients (for example, the IUD and RU 486). Although neither of these two groups is entirely satisfied with the status quo, they have reached an accommodation of sorts in that most people are able either to procreate or not to procreate as they see fit.

Concerns About Contraceptives

Although lack of access to contraceptives remains a problem for many people, especially young poor women, the fact that some contraceptives may pose serious health risks is the issue that presently attracts public attention. For example, in an interview with Rita Arditti and Shelley Minden, Martha Quintanales, a member of the Third World Women's Archives, outlines some of her complaints about current contraceptives. An immigrant from Cuba, Quintanales began to use contraceptives in college. She started with a series of birth-control pills that made her feel very ill and that her physician stopped prescribing to her, without explanation, after she developed infectious hepatitis, a disease she later discovered was associated with the particular kind of birth-control pill she had been taking. Having given up on the pill, she next tried an IUD, the now-banned Dalkon Shield. No one told her about its harmful side effects (including possible PID), and no one told her that should she become pregnant, an abortion would be indicated. Quintanales did indeed become pregnant and had to have an abortion. Later, during a second pregnancy, a physician prescribed a new kind of birth-control pill to prevent her from miscarrying. The prescription turned out to be the wrong one; instead of preventing a miscarriage, it caused one. After this traumatic experience, Quintanales tried another kind of IUD, the Copper-7, but she found it too painful to wear and had to have it removed. Finally, she discovered the safer, even if less effective and aesthetically pleasing, diaphragm and decided to take control of her body, vowing never again to hand it over to ob-gyns.[103]

To be sure, Quintanales's story reads like a nightmare. Many women who use contraceptives have experienced none of the problems that she experienced. On the contrary, they have been very satisfied with them, viewing them as one of the most significant contributions to twentieth-century women's liberation. Nevertheless, many other women have experienced at least some of the problems of which Quintanales speaks, and few women have been spared the anxiety that typically accompanies a close reading of the list of health risks routinely included in the material packaged together with most contraceptives. It is not surprising that some women believe once they begin taking contraceptives their bodies will be subjected to a series of unknown as well as known risks. And indeed, the history of several kinds of contraceptives, especially oral contraceptives, is not very reassuring. In 1990, the pill was 30 years old, and several mainstream newspapers chronicled its development, as shown in figure 4.8.[104]

The Birth of Control

The Pill, which turns 30 this year, was welcomed by many Americans, but others found it hard to swallow.

by Jeri Fischer

"This old maternity dress I've got is goin' in the garbage.
The clothes I'm wearin' from now on won't take up so much yardage!
Miniskirts and hot pants with a few little fancy frills,
Yeah, I'm makin' up for all those years since I've got the Pill."
—"The Pill," sung by Loretta Lynn in 1975

It was considered the ideal answer.

Effective. Simple.

Within two years on the market, more than 1 million U.S. women had prescriptions.

The Pill—the most popular birth control method in the United States, after sterilization—caused one of the biggest waves of moral turbulence in modern history.

This year, the Pill turns 30. Today it is less potent, but just as effective—and as controversial—as its predecessor.

When the Pill was approved for sale in 1960, women could at least experience sexual freedom without fearing pregnancy. For really the first time, they could control when they had babies. Higher failure rates of other contraceptives had made it impossible for them to be truly free from worry....

But while taking oral contraceptives was a liberating act for many, it threatened others. Some groups saw contraception as opening the door to sex outside marriage, or as interfering with God's plan for sex as a means of procreation....

Looking back, many people equate the Pill with the so-called sexual revolution of the 1960s.

"Birth control in the '60s and abortion in the '70s were primary causes of the sexual revolution because they took the consequences out of illicit sexual relations," says Charlotte lawyer Carl Horn, founder and president of the N.C. Policy Council, a conservative education coalition.

"They have substantially contributed to the breakdown of the family."

Others say a sexual revolution was inevitable, with or without the advent of oral contraceptives.

"A lot of people prophesied the Pill would do terrible things to society," says Dr. Elizabeth Corkey, 86, a former official of the Mecklenburg County Health Department. "But those people were usually the ones who didn't believe in birth control anyway.

Figure 4.8 On the occasion of the birth-control pill's thirtieth birthday, American newspapers chronicled its development. (Reprinted with permission of *The Charlotte Observer*)

"I don't think people would have been less sexually active without the Pill. I think they would have had more babies."

While some worried the Pill was a license to promiscuity, family planners sold it as the way to shrink the world's runaway population. But oral contraceptives turned out not to hold all the answers.

"People thought the way to solve overpopulation was by science," says Dr. Peter Hess, a Davidson College economist who studies population. "There was great enthusiasm for family planning programs in the 1960s, but there was a lack of appreciation of the cultural barriers to accepting those programs."

In some cultures, children are an economic asset, for example. "We found it wasn't a technical problem, but a behavioral challenge."...

By the 1970s, it seemed every other month a new study came out about the Pill's possible risks. Early research said oral contraceptives could cause blood clots, heart attacks and even strokes.

Today's Pill, used by 13 million U.S. women, is plugged as much safer than before, containing lower doses of estrogen and progestin.

In fact, it may have good side effects other than preventing pregnancy and childbirth, which is a health risk in itself. The female hormones in birth control pills appear to lower the risk of cancer of the ovaries and the endometrium (the lining of the uterus). The hormones also cut the risk of some forms of pelvic inflammatory disease, an infection in the uterus and the fallopian tubes that can cause infertility....

In the 1990s, the Pill hasn't lost its flair for breeding controversy....

The heated political climate has already helped discourage contraceptive research. In 1970s, nine U.S. pharmaceutical firms were researching and developing new forms of contraception. Now there's one.

"The Catholic Church sustained the anti-abortion movement from Roe vs. Wade in 1973 until about 1980, when it was swelled by conservative Protestants, Orthodox Jews and others," says the N.C. Policy Council's Horn.

"It may be that the Catholic Church's unchanging teaching on birth control may win similar support from other groups in the future."

Still, new ideas are on the horizon....

The History of the Pill

1960—The Food and Drug Administration approves oral contraceptives for sale.

1964—John Rock, the Pill's co-developer, writes the book *The Time Has Come*, in which he argues that oral contraceptives aren't evil.

1965—The U.S. Supreme Court throws out as unconstitutional an 86-year-old Connecticut law that forbids using contraceptives.

January 1976—Researchers link the Pill to increased dangers of gallbladder disease.

February 1976—A study says women older than 40 who take oral contraceptives face a risk of death much greater than the risk associated with any other method of birth control, including abortion.

February 1976—Researchers say oral contraceptives may cause liver tumors.

October 1976—Researchers dispute reports that say women who use the Pill are more apt to have girls.

1977—Dr. Robert Kistner, who helped develop the Pill, declares he's having second thoughts about the sexual freedom he helped bring to women. He says the Pill and the IUD (intrauterine device) have resulted in a gonorrhea outbreak.

1978—A study links fatal skin cancer to the Pill.

October 1980—Barbara Seaman, hailed as the Ralph Nadar of the women's health movement, writes *The Doctor's Case Against the Pill.*

October 1980—A study says the risk of taking oral contraceptives appear negligible. Increased risks in Pill users for heart disease, lung cancer, skin cancer and cervical cancer appear related more to lifestyle than Pill use.

January 1981—A Duke University scientist finds that exercise can lessen the Pill's dangers.

July 1981—A specialist says women who have delayed having children by taking birth control pills for some time are more likely to give birth to twins the first time they get pregnant.

1986—A study indicates that longtime Pill use does not increase a woman's risk of breast cancer.

1988—A preliminary report suggests that oral contraceptives may facilitate infection by the AIDS virus in women.

June 1989—A study says women with a family history of breast cancer do not appear to increase their risk of the disease by taking the Pill. Experts with the American College of Obstetricians and Gynecologists say they're confident that oral contraceptives are safe.

September 1989—The largest study on the effect of birth control pills eases fears of a breast cancer–birth control pill link by suggesting there is no unusual risk of the cancer for women who didn't start taking the Pill until their mid-20s.

October 1989—An FDA advisory panel agrees that the advantages of birth control pills outweigh the possible risks of heart attack and stroke for healthy women older than 40 who don't smoke.

Figure 4.8 (cont.)

Though science has established that the health risks of most contemporary contraceptives are small indeed, some women continue to be suspicious of them, especially the contraceptives they view as interfering with their bodies' normal functioning. For this reason, there is renewed interest among some women in barrier methods of contraception. Although less effective than the IUD and oral contraceptives, many women endorse barrier methods simply because they provide women with another option.[105] Despite its relative unreliability, a woman may choose to use a barrier method because she prefers risking an unwanted pregnancy to some of the more serious side effects that have been associated in the past with oral contraceptives and IUDs.

Other women, however, are content to let bygones be bygones. As they see it, whatever the health risks of past contraceptives may have been, these risks no longer apply. Nonetheless, many of these women do want to see contraceptives that are not only more effective than oral contraceptives but also more convenient and long-lasting. Predictably, these women have reacted very positively to the implant, Norplant. In large measure, this reaction is attributable to Norplant's clean bill of health, which stands in marked contrast to the poor bill of health that until recently was delivered to the relatively long-lasting injectable, Depo-Provera.

Although both Depo-Provera and Norplant are indeed long-lasting (3 months and 6 years, respectively), they are by no means perfect contraceptives. Neither agent is without side effects (very similar to those of oral contraceptives), and both raise significant issues of reproductive control for women. Should a woman decide that these contraceptives' side effects are too much for her to handle, she cannot remove the effects of a 3-month Depo-Provera injection from her blood stream or extract a Norplant implant safely and painlessly from her arm without a physician's assistance. For this reason alone, women who opt for Depo-Provera or Norplant should understand fully the implications of using these contraceptives.

Regrettably, conditions of informed consent were not always met in the early days of Depo-Provera's development, particularly in some Third World countries. In their eagerness to help control certain nations' overpopulation problems, some health care professionals injected women with Depo-Provera without warning them about its possible side-effects and possible links to certain forms of cancer.[106] Because of this type of abuse in the Third World countries, critics arised concerns about marketing not only the injectable Depo-Provera but also the implant Norplant in the United States. They note, for example, that the need for informed consent does not seem to be a major concern for those persons who recommend the imposition of Norplant on young, sexually active women whose failure to use effective contraceptives supposedly leads to 1 million accidental pregnancies each year.[107]

But just because some persons recommend using implants such as Norplant and injectables such as Depo-Provera coercively, this does not mean that these kinds of contraceptives should not be marketed in the United States. Is it fair to deprive women who want to use these long-lasting contraceptives of them so that they cannot be forced on women who do not want to use them? One can only hope that our society will find ways to promote, in equal measure, the freedom and well-being of all women whether or not they choose to use effective contraceptives.

Contraceptive Responsibilities and Rights: Closing the Gender Gap

Whatever concerns they currently have about contraceptives, women are not likely to discontinue using them. Most sexually active women have decided that the risks to their health posed by most contraceptives are worth the benefits—namely, the opportunity to be sexually active without becoming pregnant. This decision, together with the fact that almost all contraceptives are female contraceptives, has tended to place the responsibility for contraception on women.

As a result of a variety of factors, including the AIDS epidemic, however, society is reassessing its views on procreative responsibility. Condom use is definitely increasing. Men who were unwilling to use allegedly pleasure-limiting latex condoms as contraceptives are now apparently willing to use them as health-protecting devices. Women regard men's new willingness to use condoms as an opportunity for them to challenge men about matters of reproductive responsibility. It is not uncommon for a woman to question a man as follows: If you are willing to use a condom to protect yourself (us) from AIDS, then why weren't you willing to use it to protect me (us) from an unwanted pregnancy? You know that I was distressed about the side effects of an intrauterine device and oral contraceptives, and that I wanted us to use a somewhat less effective contraceptive—namely, the condom—to minimize the risks to my body. But you said that sex with a condom wasn't fun enough, romantic enough, for your tastes. Why, then, is it fun enough, romantic enough now that you (we) are worried about AIDS?

To be sure, not all men respond well to this type of challenge, but many do. Indeed, an increasing number of men maintain that were some of the male contraceptives we discussed earlier developed, they would be willing to use them. Were men as well as women to use contraceptives, women, especially young women, would be spared not only some of the risks associated with contraceptive use but also some of the social embarrassments associated with it. According to feminist writer Anne Woodhouse, our society continues to associate birth control with promiscuity to such a degree that young, unmarried women often refuse to use contraceptives for fear that men will get the wrong idea about their sexual availability.[108] Were men as responsible for contraception as are women, chances are that society's attitudes about the relationship between birth control and promiscuity would change. Indeed, use of birth control could come to signal not sexual promiscuity but sexual responsibility, a willingness for men and women to consider the full meaning and consequences of sexual intercourse before they engage in it.

The time is ripe for researchers to focus more attention on the development of male contraceptives. Even though men cannot get pregnant and experience the pleasures and pains of those 9 months, they can play a more active role in preventing pregnancy in a partnership. Perhaps it is time for society to shift the major burden of responsibility for contraception off of women and onto both men and women, particularly if researchers can develop safe and effective contraceptives for people of either gender. If contraceptive technology continues to develop in the current directions, pregnancy will no longer be a woman's "problem." Instead, it will be the concern of a man and a woman equally responsible for, as well as equally free to bear and beget (or not to bear and beget), children in a way that serves the best interests of themselves and society.

5   Sterilization

Over the past 30 years, attitudes toward sterilization as well as the techniques used to achieve sterilization have changed. Until the 1950s, many physicians were less willing to sterilize patients they judged fit than those they judged unfit—the poor, the uneducated, minority members, the retarded or insane. They used the *rule of 120* to determine eligibility for sterilization: A woman's age times the number of her living children had to equal 120 (for example, 30 years × 4 children) before a physician would recommend that a woman, especially a so-called fit woman, be sterilized. Since then, laws articulating the reproductive rights of all citizens have made it increasingly clear that all competent adults—irrespective of their race, socioeconomic class, gender, age, and health status—have the right to decide whether sterilization is an option for them.[1]

Sterilization is the most common form of birth control used by married couples, and its popularity is growing every year. In 1970, 20 million people worldwide had chosen voluntary sterilization as a means of birth control; by 1980, that number had increased to 100 million.[2] Each year, in the United States alone, more than 700,000 women and 400,000 men choose to be sterilized.[3] Vasectomy for the man and tubal ligation for the woman are the most common types of sterilization.

The Technology of Sterilization

Male Sterilization: Vasectomy

The Process

Vasectomy is a fairly simple surgical procedure that has changed very little over time. After giving the patient a local anesthetic, the surgeon makes a small incision on the upper part of each side of the scrotum

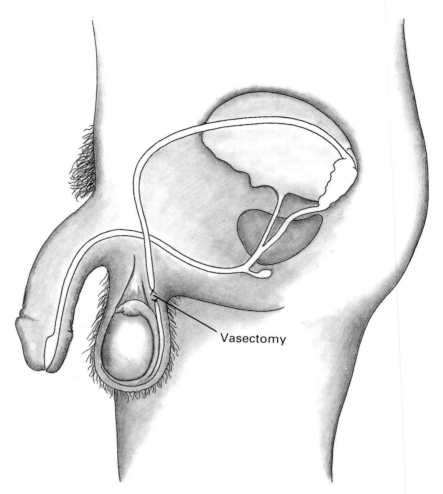

Vasectomy

Figure 5.1 The male reproductive system showing how a vasectomy severs the vas deferens through an incision in the scrotum. Of course, the vas on both sides are severed.

to expose the vas deferens, the tube that channels the sperm from the testicles to the penis (figure 5.1.) Having made this incision, the surgeon removes a section of the tube on each side to prevent it from joining together and carefully ligates each end to shut it completely but not so tightly that the suture cuts the vas. After the vasectomy, the patient continues to produce sperm in the testicles, where they are trapped for reabsorption into the body.[4]

In 1974, researchers perfected a new no-scalpel technique in China where it has become the standard vasectomy technique. Using this procedure, the vas is reached through a puncture in the scrotum rather than through a scalpel incision. Not only does this procedure lower the complication rates associated with some other modes of sterilization, but it also seems to reduce patient anxiety rates.[5]

Currently, researchers are debating whether both ends of the vas should be tied or whether the testicular end should be left opened. The latter option has two obvious advantages: (1) It avoids a troublesome pressure buildup that sometimes dilates and ruptures the tied testicular end of the vas, and (2) it facilitates the reversal of the sterilization process should a man so desire.

In the past, researchers were largely convinced that the risks of leaving one end of the vas untied—namely, the formation of large, painful spermatic granulomas or the spontaneous rejoining of the vas's two ends—outweighed its benefits.[6] They have recently changed their minds, however. Evidence shows that if they are small enough not to be painful, spermatic granulomas can actually be beneficial. Not only do they alleviate pressure buildups in the vas's testicular end; they also play a helpful role in reversing the sterilization process. Evidence also indicates that some of the new surgical techniques are able to decrease, and even to eliminate, spontaneous rejoining of the vas's two ends. Thus, an increasing number of researchers and surgeons believe that it is best to tie only one end of the vas and to place a sheath over the other.[7]

The entire sterilization procedure takes between 15 and 20 minutes and is relatively painless. Although the patient usually can resume sexual activities after approximately 1 week, he and his partner are advised to use contraceptives until he has ejaculated all the active sperm remaining in his body, a process that takes between 7 and 12 ejaculations. Usually, physicians ask their patients to submit sperm samples to a clinical laboratory until there have been two consecutive counts that show no sperm present. Ninety-five percent of all patients are completely sterile after 10 weeks;[8] the rest take a little longer.

Complications

Male sterilization is usually very safe and easy, with few complications. There may be some swelling and discomfort with any vasectomy, but this is generally short-lived and slight.[9] In 1 of every 100 cases, a man will develop cellulitis or scrotal abscesses. Occasionally, a man will develop painful spermatic granulomas but, as mentioned earlier, most spermatic granulomas are painless and may be beneficial. The most serious problem would be spontaneous recanalization (the rejoining of the vas), making the vasectomy useless. However, provided that a vasectomy is done carefully, this is an uncommon occurrence and one that need not concern the patient unduly.

Vasectomy Reversal

The main drawback to vasectomy is its permanence. As the demand for vasectomy has increased, so too has the demand for vasovasostomy, a resectioning of the vas tube after it has been occluded by vasectomy. Although there are no guarantees, the development of microscopic techniques in vasovasostomy procedures has dramatically increased the odds of a successful sterilization reversal. Whereas in 1948 the success rate for the presence of sperm in an ejaculation after a vasovasostomy was between 35 and 40 percent, microsurgery has increased this success rate to 90 percent, which has resulted in a pregnancy rate of 50 percent.[10]

Surgeons use either traditional macrosurgical techniques or contemporary microsurgical techniques when they perform a vasovasostomy. The *macrosurgeon* anesthetizes the patient, locates the vasectomy scar on the scrotum, and makes an incision to uncover the two ligated ends of the vas. He or she then removes the scarred tissue and rejoins the ends of the vas so that the sperm can once again move from the testicles to the penis.

In contrast to the macrosurgeon, the microsurgeon does not remove the scarred tissue and rejoin the ends of the vas at this stage of the operation. Instead, she or he cuts the proximal end of the vas until fluid is seen. Then the microsurgeon removes a sample of fluid to test it for sperm, the presence or absence of which predicts the overall chances of a successful operation. Next, the microsurgeon cuts back the distal end of the vas to a healthy, undamaged section and dilates it. Finally, she or he brings the two ends of the vas together in a vas deferens approximator clip, which holds them in place during the suturing process.

Both types of vasovasostomies are considered minor outpatient surgery. After being released, the patient is advised to avoid ejaculating or lifting anything heavy for 2 weeks. No matter how successful the surgery is, it takes time for a man to regain fertility. Three months after a successful operation, the sperm count is still low and sperm motility remains poor. After 6 months, however, the sperm count is usually higher and sperm motility should be almost normal.

A vasovasostomy is more likely to be successful if the surgeon uses microsurgical techniques and if she or he performs it no more than 10 years after the vasectomy (this factor alone can change the success rate from 35 percent to 91 percent). Two other factors that bode well for a vasovasostomy's success are the presence of spermatic granulomas and the presence of sperm in the fluid tested from the proximal end of the vas.[11]

Currently, researchers are trying to build the vasovasostomy procedure into the vasectomy procedure. One way to make a vasectomy easily reversible is to clamp the vas deferens with a clip that can be unclamped at any future time. Although this method is very easily reversed, it is not nearly as effective a contraceptive as is the standard vasectomy, and it is still being perfected.[12]

Conclusions

Vasectomies are the most effective form of male contraception currently available. Indeed, failure rates are a scant 0.15 per 100 persons, with most failures due to one of four infrequent causes: (1) the vas deferens spontaneously rejoined and healed by itself; (2) the patient had a third undetected tube; (3) the physician mistakenly left one of the vas deferens unsevered; or (4) the patient failed to use proper contraception directly after the operation.[13] Although a vasectomy is safe and effective, some men nevertheless fear that it may in some way reduce their manhood or their sexual performance. As understandable as this fear may be, it is completely unfounded. A vasectomy is not the same as castration. Indeed, most men have reported positive rather than negative changes in sexual performance after their vasectomies.

Female Sterilization: Tubal Ligation

The Process

The principle behind female sterilization is similar to that behind male sterilization. The surgeon occludes the fallopian tubes leading from the ovaries to the uterus so that the woman's eggs remain trapped in the tubes for reabsorption into the body (figure 5.2). But even if the principle behind tubal ligation is akin to that behind vasectomy, the method is not. A tubal ligation is more complex than a vasectomy because access to the fallopian tubes in the female is more complex than access to the male vas deferens. Until recently, a tubal ligation was a matter of major, not minor, surgery. In the past, the surgeon typically put the patient under general anesthesia, made a 3- to 4- inch incision across her abdomen, and then "tied" her tubes. As difficult as it was for the woman to recuperate after this invasive procedure, her trials and tribulations were small compared to those of the woman whose surgeon instead performed a hysterectomy. Unlike a tubal ligation, a hysterectomy involves removal of the entire uterus and involved a significant time of postoperative bed rest.

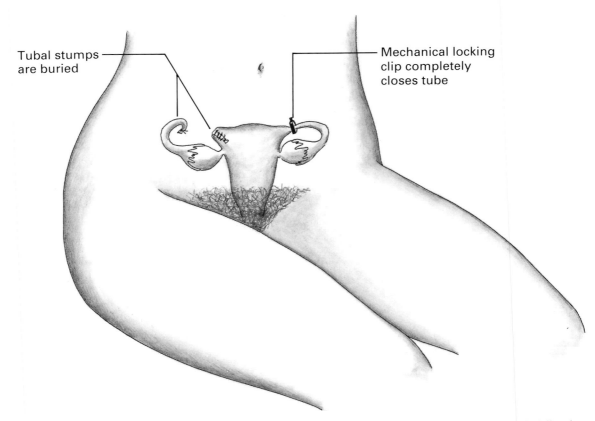

Tubal stumps
are buried

Mechanical locking
clip completely
closes tube

Figure 5.2 Various methods for achieving female sterilization. A tubal ligation severs the fallopian tubes through an incision in the abdomen. A clip may be used to occlude the fallopian tubes.

Fortunately, surgeons no longer regard hysterectomy as a desirable female sterilization technique.[14]

Although tubal ligations remain more painful and complex than vasectomies, fiberoptic procedures are gradually eliminating the need for major surgery. Such procedures require the use of a laparoscope, an instrument that consists of a fiberoptic bundle in a tube of stainless steel. After injecting gas to expand the woman's abdomen, the surgeon makes a small incision and then inserts the laparoscope through it. There the laparoscope illuminates a small abdominal section, reflecting the image outward through a lens. At this stage of the procedure, the surgeon makes a second, small incision. Using the image projected by the laparoscope, she or he locates and occludes the two fallopian tubes. In another, even simpler procedure, the surgeon inserts the cutting or cauterizing tool through a special tube in the laparoscope so that only one incision is needed. Both versions of this operation take approximately 20 minutes and require a couple of adhesive strip bandages afterward. Although it is commonly referred to as Band-Aid sterilization in the United States, the painfulness and seriousness of this operation should not be underestimated. Many women have a great deal of pain from the injected gas as it moves to the chest, affects the joints, and is slowly absorbed by the body. As with any operation, the significance of the procedure cannot be judged by the size of the incision.[15]

Whether they use contemporary laparoscopic techniques or traditional surgical techniques, surgeons can select any one of several occlusion methods but, given the increasing interest in sterilization reversal, surgeons prefer to use an occlusion method that is minimally damaging to the patient's tubes.

Some surgeons favor the Pomeroy technique (developed in 1930), whereas others favor the Uchida technique (developed in 1945). Surgeons who use the Pomeroy technique double up the tube and tie it with a dissolvable suture. They then cut the doubled-up tube without crushing it. As a result, the two ends of the doubled-up tube grow apart, usually eliminating the problem of spontaneous rejoining.[16] In contrast, surgeons who use the Uchida technique inject a saline solution into the tube. Because this solution separates the serosa layer of the tubes from the muscle layer, surgeons find it easier to cut and tie the tube. Rather than removing any part of the tube, surgeons bury each of the tube's two ends into the serosa where they are unlikely to rejoin spontaneously. The popularity of this technique lies in the fact that it is still one of the easiest both to perform and to reverse successfully.[17]

Other surgeons favor electrocoagulation and electrocautery techniques. In electrocoagulation, surgeons use either a unipolar or a bipolar method to run an electrical current through the tubes to cauterize them. Unfortunately, complications attend both of these methods. When surgeons use the unipolar method, the electrical current sometimes strays from its destination (the fallopian tubes), burning the bowels instead of the tubes; and even when they use the more controllable bipolar method, surgeons are not always able to manage the electrical current in such a way that it burns only the tissue they want it to burn.[18] In electrocautery, surgeons occlude the tubes by applying a heated hook directly onto them and pulling them against an insulated backing.[19] Although surgeons are able to localize both the electrical current and its burning effect in this procedure, it is not clear how the failure rates of this method compare with those of others.[20]

Finally, some surgeons favor transcervical sterilization and the colpotomy. During transcervical sterilization, the surgeon inserts a laparoscope and a cauterizing tool through the vagina and dilated cervix into the uterus. There the physician uses the cauterizing tool to seal the areas where the fallopian tubes meet the uterus. Although this fiberoptic procedure eliminates the need for incisions, takes only 15 minutes to perform, and necessitates merely a 2- to 4- hour recovery period, researchers believe it is still relatively unreliable and are working to perfect it.[21] Slightly more reliable than transcervical sterilization is the colpotomy, often referred to as *a stitch in the vagina*. After administering a general anesthetic to the woman, the surgeon makes a small incision in the vagina and severs the fallopian tubes by inserting a tool up through the cervix. Although the colpotomy leaves no visible scarring, it is a bit more complex than the fiberoptic procedures we have discussed and usually requires a couple of days in the hospital.[22]

In response to the increasing demand for reversible sterilizations, researchers have been developing two kinds of sterilization techniques—clips and rings—that completely eliminate the necessity of cutting or cauterizing the tubes. Surgeons who choose to use clips fit them over the tubes to block the egg's passage by pressing the walls of the tube together. Although clips met with less than complete success in the past, a new titanium clip lined with Silastic, the Filshie clip, promises to be highly effective.[23] Surgeons who choose to use rings, most often the so-called Falope ring, insert them tightly over a doubled-up loop of the fallopian tubes. Over time, the tubes atrophy. The occlusion process with the Falope ring is very simple, but its effectiveness as a complete form of sterilization is uncertain.[24]

Many researchers believe that other techniques are even more promising than clips and rings when sterilization reversal is a desirable goal. Some researchers are experimenting with highly controlled electrical currents that would burn only the insides of the fallopian tubes, thereby decreasing the chance of the currents straying and burning other organs. Other researchers are experimenting with caustic chemicals that would burn or scar the insides of the fallopian tubes to seal them. Because the burning or scarring would be confined to such a localized, limited piece of tissue, these researchers believe that reversal would be fairly simple and likely to succeed, but they worry about the possibly harmful side effects of injecting even a small amount of caustic chemicals into a woman's body.[25] Finally, other researchers are experimenting with flexible silicone plugs that the surgeon would insert into a woman's tubes. Although no confirmatory studies have been undertaken yet, these researchers hypothesize that to reverse a woman's sterilization, a surgeon would simply remove these tube plugs.[26]

Complications

Although tubal ligation is much safer today than it was in the 1950s, it is by no means risk free. Female sterilization in the United States results in 3.6 deaths per 100,000 women. Sterilization through a hysterectomy offers the greatest risk both in terms of morbidity and complications. Compared to a very low complication rate for laparoscopy, abdominal hysterectomies have a relatively high complication rate. Other procedures with high complication rates include the colpotomy, associated with a high risk of cellulitis, pelvic abscesses, and hemorrhaging, and the electrocoagulation methods, associated with bowel burns.[27]

Problems common to all tubal ligation techniques are infection and hemorrhaging. Infection depends greatly on the type of sterilization procedure performed. Colpotomy is the worst culprit, with problems ranging from minor irritations to abscesses to pelvic inflammatory disease. Hemorrhaging usually results from incorrect procedure by the surgeon: incomplete coagulation of the tubes, a clumsy resectioning of the tubes, or a poor attempt to resect burned bowels (after an incorrect attempt at electrocoagulation). Although risk of hemorrhaging is also dependent on the type of sterilization procedure, the use of laparoscopic operations has reduced this risk to less than 0.5 percent.[28]

Another problem common to female sterilization is post–tubal ligation syndrome, a condition that consists of a variety of postoperative problems including cramps, headaches, nausea, or spotting. Whether or not these postoperative problems develop depends on several different factors such as the patient's age, the method of sterilization used, the kind and extent of postoperative care given, and the contraceptive and medical history of the patient.[29]

Sterilization Reversal

As the popularity of sterilization has increased, so too has the desire to have the process reversed. Some women seek a reversal operation because they have had a major change in life-style since their sterilization: a divorce, a remarriage, the death of a child. Others seek a reversal operation because they were relatively young when their sterilizations were performed—too young, perhaps, to have made a fully informed decision about not having any, or more, children. Still others seek a reversal operation because they were pressured into their sterilizations by spouses, parents, or welfare administrators. For these and other reasons, approximately 10 percent of sterilized women later desire a reversal.[30]

Techniques for reversal are still very new and, depending on the type of sterilization procedure used and the condition of the fallopian tubes, the operation can range from difficult to impossible. An ideal candidate for a reversal is a healthy woman who went through sterilization less than 5 years earlier, and whose operation left the tubes fairly well intact (it seems that the Pomeroy technique, the clip, or the ring cause the least destruction, whereas techniques such as electrocoagulation cause the most). However, even if a woman is an ideal candidate for a reversal, the operation may not succeed. In fact, only 58 percent of attempted reversals now succeed. As techniques for reversible sterilizations improve, and as more physicians begin to master and use them on a routine basis, the rate of successful sterilization reversals will undoubtedly increase.[31]

Conclusions

Sterilization is a very effective form of birth control for women. The failure rate is between 0.04 and 0.08 per 100 women per year, and most of these failures are not actual failures in the operation but are attributable to the fact that the patient was already pregnant before the sterilization procedure. When the operation actually fails—a rare event indeed—it is usually the result of incomplete cauterization or spontaneous healing of the fallopian tubes.[32] Moreover, like a vasectomy, a tubal ligation does not lessen a woman's sexuality. Sterilized women are no less sexually desirous or active than nonsterilized women. In fact, many sterilized women report that their sexual desire or activity increased subsequent to their sterilizations because they no longer had to worry about unwanted pregnancies.

The Ethics of Sterilization

To determine when sterilization is morally permitted, required, or forbidden, we must distinguish voluntary sterilization, in which the person who is sterilized has given informed consent to the appropriate medical operation, from both involuntary and nonvoluntary sterilization. If a person actively objects to being sterilized, or if a person decides to be sterilized only, or primarily, because of serious ignorance or severe coercion, then she or he is sterilized *involuntarily*. However, if a person is literally unable to give or withhold informed consent to his or her sterilization because he or she is incompetent (for example, an infant or a severally mentally disabled adult), then that person is being sterilized *nonvoluntarily*.

Voluntary Sterilization

The only ethical tradition that seriously opposes voluntary sterilization is the natural-law tradition. According to natural-law theorists, human beings have a duty to cooperate with their supposedly innate human drives toward life, procreation, knowledge, and community. When a woman or man chooses to be sterilized, she or he chooses deliberately to frustrate her or his drive to procreate. In so doing, that person defies the natural law, acts immorally, and reveals herself or himself as less than fully human.

Critics of the natural-law tradition object that *if* human beings do have innate drives, there is no reason to believe that the drive to procreate is somehow preeminent. To survive, a couple may have to limit the size of its family so that the already existing children can be fed, clothed, and sheltered; and to educate their children properly and express their love for them adequately, a couple may have to forego more than 1, 2, or 3 children. However natural procreation is, insist the critics, what makes it *human* rather than *animal* procreation is the ability to control it through a variety of means.

Whether the natural-law theorist can prove that to be fully human a person has to remain fertile is doubtful. What is certain is that most ethicists outside the natural-law tradition are persuaded that voluntary sterilization is morally justified. Utilitarians believe that voluntary sterilization tends to maximize the group's good because it is an excellent means of birth control; and rights-oriented thinkers believe that it maximizes autonomy because it provides the individual with a sure means to serve his or her goal of not procreating. If individuals have the right and, conceivably, the duty not to procreate, then voluntary sterilization is a permissible, even required, course of action for them.

Involuntary Sterilization

Involuntary sterilization, performed against the wishes of an autonomous person, is the kind of sterilization that concerns ethicists most. One of the factors that complicates any moral evaluation of involuntary sterilization, however, is the fact that very few human decisions are fully voluntary.

Persons make fully voluntary decisions only when they are totally aware of all relevant facts and known contingencies and entirely free of all external pressures and internal compulsions. But given that virtually all people lack something in the way of knowledge or power—that is, that their decisions are affected by factors such as "neurotic compulsion, misinformation, excitement or impetuousness, clouded judgment (as, for example, from alcohol), or immature or defective faculties of reasoning"[33]—it seems that few human decisions are fully voluntary. However, just because a decision is less than fully voluntary does not mean that it is fully involuntary and, therefore, utterly suspect from a moral point of view. Few sterilizations are fully voluntary, but a sterilization that is less than fully voluntary is not necessarily fully involuntary.

The distinction between fully involuntary and less than fully voluntary sterilizations is similar to the one between so-called blatant and subtle sterilizations. Adele Clarke writes that blatant sterilization "includes forced sterilization against a person's will, sterilization without telling the person [he or she] will be sterilized, and sterilization (in the United States) without the patient's informed consent to the procedure."[34] Under such conditions, a person's knowledge or power is so constricted that it is scarcely conceivable that it is the individual's autonomous choice to be sterilized.

A clear example of a blatant sterilization on the microlevel (involving a specific individual) is the 1964 case of Nial Ruth Cox. Cox, who was living with her 8 siblings and her mother (a welfare recipient), gave birth to a child. When she turned 18 a year later, Cox was no longer entitled to receive welfare benefits. Nevertheless, a welfare caseworker told her that because of her "immorality," she would have to be sterilized "temporarily" or else her mother and siblings would all be stricken from the welfare rolls. Also told that the "temporary" sterilization procedure was reversible, Cox underwent the procedure. Afterward, she was reassured that she would be able to have children in the future.[35] If any case of sterilization is a case of fully involuntary sterilization, this would seem to be it. Cox was deprived of anything resembling the kind of knowledge necessary for informed consent. In fact, she observed, "Nobody explained anything. They treated us as though we were animals."[36] Thus, rights-oriented ethicists will condemn Cox's sterilization as a clear instance of using a person as a mere means to secure a desired social end. In its eagerness to shrink its welfare rolls, the state played "footloose and fancy-free" with a young woman's hopes for the future, caring nothing about her personal goals and everything about its own purposes—presumably, a balanced budget.

In contrast to blatant (or fully involuntary) sterilization, says Clarke, subtle (or less than fully voluntary) sterilization includes situations in which a woman or man legally consents to sterilization, but the social conditions in which she or he does so are such that they limit her or his capacity to exercise genuine reproductive choice and autonomy.[37] Among the conditions likely to eventuate in a subtle sterilization are the following ten: (1) lack of abortion options, (2) unnecessary hysterectomy, (3) economic constraints on reproductive choice, (4) lack of awareness of the permanence of sterilization, (5) lack of knowledge of, or access to, other means of contraception, (6) simultaneous sterilization and childbirth or abortion, (7) iatrogenic (medically caused) sterility or infertility, (8) disproportionate sterilization of welfare women, (9) ideologies of "appropriate" family size and structure, and (10) lack of counseling to cope with sterilization.[38] Depending on how many of these conditions are present and depending on the degree to which any of these conditions are manifest, a subtle sterilization may or may not be morally objectionable.

An example of a morally objectionable subtle sterilization at the microlevel (involving individuals) is that of one 24-year-old, unmarried, black mother of 4. Prior to her last delivery, her attending physician informed her that unless she submitted to sterilization, he would (1) "refuse to attend her or her child during or after labor," (2) deny her access to the hospital with which he was associated, and (3) see to it that her welfare payments were terminated.[39] Because of these threats, the young woman consented to be sterilized despite her desire to have more children.

At the macrolevel, the People's Republic of China recently organized a sterilization campaign that combines disincentives with incentives to motivate people to "choose" a course of action that is, at best, the lesser of two evils for them. Couples who agree to be sterilized after the birth of a first child are rewarded with pay bonuses, special privileges for their child, job promotions, and government approval.[40] Couples who refuse to be sterilized and then have a second and even a third child are penalized with pay cuts, no privileges for their additional child(ren), job demotions, and government disapproval.

Clearly, negative incentive systems are far more coercive than positive incentive systems. To forsake an added benefit to have a large family is one matter; to suffer an added burden is quite another. Although this program has curbed China's population growth, it has also led to a high rate of infanticide. Because the ancient Chinese preference for male children has not disappeared under modern Socialist rule, some couples who cannot afford the penalties associated with having more than 1 child kill their firstborn child if it happens to be female. Nevertheless, despite the severe ethical problems that negative incentive programs pose, such programs may be justified if communal survival is at substantial risk, but only if penalties for noncompliance are not too great and are applied in such a way that the children of overpopulating parents do not suffer serious harm as a result of their parents' decision to bear and beget them.

In addition to blatant and subtle sterilizations, there are those involuntary sterilizations that fall somewhere between these two extremes. A good example of these amorphous cases is Indian sterilization policy during Indira Ghandi's years as prime minister. Largely as a result of offering material goods to poor, illiterate men, India set the world record for vasectomies at 10 million in 1977. Not only did the government fail to obtain the informed consent of many of these men prior to their sterilizations; it also often neglected to give them the promised material goods subsequent to their sterilizations.[41] When these facts became known, the general public lost confidence in Indira Ghandi's regime. That some of the men who were sterilized knew what sterilization was and nonetheless agreed to be sterilized to receive "prizes" such as money, food, clothes, and transistor radios bothered the public almost as much as the fact that some men who were sterilized did not understand how enduring the consequences of sterilization usually are.[42]

Clearly, involuntary sterilization is a moral problem both at the individual and social level. However, the fact that many individuals are somewhat ambivalent about their decision to be sterilized does not necessarily mean their decision constitutes involuntary sterilization, even a subtle sterilization. A couple may *want* 10 children but nonetheless realize that they are equipped to handle only 2 or 3. Should one or the other partner choose to be sterilized on account of this realization, her or his decision will not be any more involuntary than most decisions human beings routinely make. Limits are an essential component of the human condition. They are suspect only when they are imposed arbitrarily on some individuals and segments of society but not on others. Then, and only then, do we need to worry about people being sterilized against their own best interests.

Nonvoluntary Sterilization

Provided that a competent adult's decision to be sterilized is made with a good measure of his or her own knowledge and power, it will probably escape moral condemnation.[43] But competent adults are not the only people who get sterilized. Many incompetent adults and adolescents— usually, but not always, mentally retarded—are also sterilized. Given that incompetent people are unable to make their own sterilization decisions, what morally justifies their surrogates to make these decisions for them?

In the attempt to answer this question, we need to look at some specific cases. Consider the case of Fred, a mentally retarded young man. Fred is largely unable to take care of anything more than his simplest needs. He lives at home with his widowed father, who loves him very much. Although Fred enjoys physical intimacy, including sexual intimacy with women, his father tells him repeatedly that "sex is bad," fearing that Fred will impregnate one of the mentally retarded young women with whom he associates. Besides confusing and possibly traumatizing the young woman, such a pregnancy would produce a child whose biological parents could not care for it without a great deal of assistance. As a result of these considerations, Fred's father concludes that it is in Fred's best interests to be sterilized so that Fred can enjoy consensual acts of sexual intimacy with women without impregnating them. Because Fred would probably come to a similar conclusion if he could reason as well as his father, this may be a case where nonvoluntary sterilization is morally justified. Fred is sterilized not so much against his will as in accord with a will that, due to various mental impediments, he cannot express.

In the case of an incompetent such as Fred, then, rights-oriented ethicists hold that Fred's father may make decisions for his son provided that he takes the ends, aims, or goals of Fred as primary. Whereas it would be wrong for Fred's father to have him sterilized simply because it would then be easier to care for Fred, the father may have Fred sterilized if (1) anyone in Fred's place would want to be sterilized and (2) the procedure enhances Fred's position in the moral community.

According to philosopher Robert Neville, membership in the moral community means that a person is held morally responsible for those actions she or he is able to perform knowingly and willingly.[44] Because Fred is unable to understand the repercussions of begetting a child, the community cannot hold him morally responsible if he impregnates one of his female friends. In contrast, because Fred is able to understand that sexual intercourse is a way of being nice to someone who likes you, the community can hold him morally responsible if, for example, he rapes one of his female friends. Thus, if the community wants to treat Fred as a person—as someone who is morally responsible for at least some of his actions—it should permit him to engage in sexual activity, even if it requires him to be sterilized. Less violence is done to Fred by sterilizing him and allowing him to enjoy sex than by not sterilizing him but depriving him of the opportunity for personal growth through physical intimacy.

One final point is in order here. Many mentally retarded people are able to make informed decisions about whether to be sterilized. There are, after all, varying degrees of mental retardation and, therefore, varying degrees of incompetency. Consider the case of Mary, a 23-year old, mildly retarded woman, who lives with her parents in comfortable surroundings. She would like to have a child, and her parents believe she could adequately care for a child with some help from them. However, mental health officials have asked the court to order Mary's sterilization. Mary begs not to be sterilized, and her parents concur with her that sterilization is not necessary in her case. Should the court order her sterilization anyway, Mary's sterilization must be considered more involuntary than nonvoluntary because sterilization is against not only her own expressed will but also the expressed will of her parents. In contrast to Fred's situation, it is doubtful that everyone in Mary's situation would want to be sterilized. Moreover, Mary will not gain stature in the moral community if she is sterilized. On the contrary, she will lose stature because she will no longer be able to make the procreative choices she was capable of making before the operation and because she will no longer have the opportunity to develop her skills as a nurturing person.

Legal Aspects of Sterilization

Voluntary Sterilization

As we noted earlier, voluntary sterilization is any medical procedure performed on a consenting, competent adult that renders him or her permanently sterile. Although voluntary sterilization is now legal in all 50 states in the United States, it has not always been readily available, particularly for women. Until 1969, women requesting sterilizations were routinely checked against the so-called rule of 120 mentioned earlier. This formula enabled members of the American College of Obstetricians and Gynecologists (ACOG) to refuse sterilization requests under otherwise compelling circumstances.[45] As late as 1970, the ACOG also required the permission of 2 doctors and a psychiatrist before a married woman's sterilization request could be honored. Like the notorious rule of 120, however, this rule was often selectively enforced. Apparently, some physicians were more reluctant to sterilize rich, healthy, white, and educated women who, they believed, would produce "solid stock" than they were to sterilize poor, sickly, black, or illiterate women who, they believed, would produce yet more mouths for the state to feed at the taxpayers' expense. As more upper- and middle-class women began to demand a foolproof means of birth control, however, the ACOG largely abandoned its double standard for voluntary sterilizations.

Though some states continued to enact legislation to control voluntary sterilization, in *Hathaway* v. *Worcester City Hospital* the U.S. First Circuit Court of Appeals clearly stated that individuals have the right to both therapeutic and elective sterilization.[46] The court grounded its opinion, in part, on the conviction that Worcester City Hospital's prohibition on voluntary sterilization violated the equal protection clause of the Fourteenth Amendment. No other elective procedures or therapeutic procedures of equal risk were prohibited. The opinion recognized the legitimacy of the state's interest in protecting a viable fetus but noted that this interest was far less compelling in the context of sterilization than in that of abortion. To protect an actual fetus is one thing; to protect a potential fetus is quite another.

Because voluntary sterilization is now a legally protected procedure, an increasing number of sterilizations are performed annually. Because blatant and subtle sterilization abuse is always a possibility, some organizations such as the Committee to End Sterilization Abuse (CESA) prompted the then Department of Health, Education and Welfare (DHEW) to mandate uniform guidelines for voluntary sterilization, including a minimum waiting period of 72 hours between the decision to be sterilized and the actual operation, a minimum age of 21 years, and valid informed consent.[47]

Unfortunately, sterilization abuse did not disappear with the 1974 publication of the DHEW's guidelines. In 1975, an ad hoc committee on sterilization guidelines found that, in the 20 New York City hospitals they investigated, the DHEW's guidelines were neither consistently known nor consistently followed. Subsequent to their investigation, this committee revised the DHEW's guidelines so that they could no longer be easily circumvented. The new requirements included a 30-day waiting period, no sterilization of people younger than 21 years, full counseling on all methods of birth control, informed consent with comprehension *proved*, and a prohibition against securing consent during childbirth or abortion procedures.[48] Significantly, hospitals, Planned Parenthood, the Association for Voluntary Sterilization, and feminist organizations such as the National Organization for Women opposed these guidelines. These groups feared that the strict guidelines for voluntary sterilization would not so much prevent sterilization abuse as block or make difficult some women's bona fide decisions to be voluntarily sterilized. Although the opposition's arguments were strong, the revised regulations were adopted, first in New York City, then in New York State, and finally nationwide. Currently, these regulations continue to protect against sterilization abuse in the United States, although it remains unclear how effective the regulations are and whether they do, in fact, have the unfortunate side effect of impeding some sterilizations that are wanted.

Involuntary Sterilization

Most involuntary sterilizations in the United States have occurred under eugenic sterilization laws. The early advocates of eugenics (from the Greek, meaning "well-born")[49] were so zealous that there were hundreds of eugenic sterilizations even before there was any legislative authority for the procedure. During the 1880s and 1890s, a strong movement built up in favor of eliminating the "unfit" by means of discouraging the reproduction of inferior stock. A combination of social Darwinism and the belief that idiocy and mental illness were strictly hereditary resulted in the involuntary sterilization of hundreds of allegedly feebleminded persons in Kansas, Pennsylvania, and Indiana, the first state to pass a Eugenic Sterilization Law (1907).[50]

Although eugenic sterilization met with the Indiana State Legislature's approval, it did not secure the state supreme court's stamp of approval. In 1921, Indiana's Eugenic Sterilization Law was declared unconstitutional, a precedent that caused several similar state laws to topple.[51] However, this domino effect was slowed in 1927 when *Buck* v. *Bell* reached the U.S. Supreme Court.[52] In 1924, Virginia had passed a law that included among its provisions the following:

> ... *that the health of the patient and the welfare of society may be promoted in certain cases by the sterilization of mental defectives ... that the sterilization may be effected ... without serious pain or substantial danger of life; that the Commonwealth is supporting in various institutions many defective persons who if now discharged would be a menace but if incapable of procreating might be discharged with safety and become self-supporting with benefit to themselves and to society; and that experience has shown that heredity plays an important part in the transmission of insanity, imbecility.*[53]

Invoking the provisions of this law, Virginia wished to sterilize an 18-year-old, supposedly feebleminded welfare recipient named Carrie Buck on the grounds that every Virginian's best interests, including those of Carrie Buck herself, would be served by her sterilization. Though Carrie Buck and her attorneys did not believe her sterilization was in *her* best interests, they were not able to convince the U.S. Supreme Court that Virginia's involuntary sterilization statute was unconstitutional. Speaking for the Court, Justice Oliver Wendell Holmes held that it was within the police power of the state to force certain persons to be sterilized. Referring to the arguable fact that, like Carrie, Carrie's mother and daughter were also "feebleminded," Holmes proclaimed that "three generations of imbeciles are enough"[54] and that society had the right to protect itself against "defective" progeny.

Since 1927, the scientific community has become increasingly dubious of the empirical claim on which the *Buck* decision was based—namely, that mental illness, mental retardation, and criminality are hereditary conditions. Contemporary geneticists point out that even if Carrie Buck, her mother, and her daughter had been as feebleminded as the Court said they were—a questionable finding given that a health professional had classified Buck's 1-month-old daughter as an "imbecile" merely by looking at her—feeblemindedness is not hereditary in any straightforward sense. Although specific types of retardation may have a genetic component, how that component is expressed depends on both genes and environment, with the environment sometimes playing a more influential role than the genes themselves. In the case of Carrie Buck, a disadvantaged member of society, there is reason to believe that better nourishment and a better education could have strengthened her "feeble" mind as well as her mother's and daughter's.[55]

Another shortcoming of the *Buck* decision is its contention that retarded persons are necessarily unfit parents and that they have no business procreating. In opposition to this contention, Dr. Leo Kannen has written:

> *In my twenty years of psychiatric work with thousands of children and their parents, I have seen percentually [sic] at least as many "intelligent" adults unfit to rear their offspring as I have seen such "feeble-minded" adults. I have—and many others have—come to the conclusion that, to a large extent independent of the I.Q., fitness for parenthood is determined by emotional involvements and relationships.[56]*

Kannen's statistical evidence challenges the reasoning behind the *Buck* decision and, although the issue of involuntary sterilization for eugenic reasons has yet to be resolved completely, recent U.S. Supreme Court decisions have made it increasingly clear that there is a right to procreate that cannot easily be violated.

Next to *Buck*, *Skinner* is the most instructive involuntary sterilization case of the twentieth century. *Oklahoma State* v. *Skinner* (1941) involved an Oklahoma law that provided for the sterilization of "habitual criminals" —that is, persons who had been convicted three times of felonies involving moral turpitude. Deliberately excluded from the list of targeted felonies were several so-called white-collar crimes (for example, offenses arising from the violation of prohibitory laws, revenue acts, embezzlement, or political offenses).[57] Jack Skinner was convicted of stealing chickens (more than $20.00 worth therefore constituting grand larceny) and, subsequently, of two counts of robbery with firearms. Each of these felonies involved moral turpitude, and so the state ordered Skinner's sterilization for eugenic reasons.

To establish the validity of this statute, Oklahoma needed to produce evidence to support its belief that children born to habitual criminals inherit their parent(s)' criminal tendencies. Although Oklahoma never produced this evidence, the majority of the Oklahoma Supreme Court nonetheless ruled that such evidence had to exist. After all, said the court, Oklahoma would not have enacted its involuntary sterilization if such evidence did not exist. States can be trusted to tell the truth!

Despite the Oklahoma Supreme Court's decision to take Oklahoma's word at face value, the U.S. Supreme Court struck down Oklahoma's law in *Skinner* v. *Oklahoma* (1942).[58] The Court held that, in crafting its statute, Oklahoma had laid "an unequal hand"[59] on its population of criminals, subjecting for involuntary sterilization people who had committed repeated acts of grand larceny but not people who had committed repeated acts of embezzlement. After emphasizing the necessity of strict scrutiny in sterilization cases, Justice Douglas asserted that distinguishing between repeated acts of grand larceny and repeated acts of embezzlement constitutes invidious discrimination. If "he who commits larceny by trespass or trick or fraud has biologically inheritable traits,"[60] then he who commits embezzlement has similar traits, reasoned Douglas. In its desire to come down hard on those it perceived as low-life types but to treat upper-crust types with kid gloves, Oklahoma had constructed a bogus distinction between larceny and embezzlement, a distinction so forced and strained that the U.S. Supreme Court recognized the classist mentality behind it. The importance of *Skinner*, then, is that it exposes the class bias that sometimes underlies involuntary sterilization proposals, including a very recent proposal to sterilize welfare recipients to end a cycle of poverty that seems intractable.[61]

Nonvoluntary Sterilization

If a person is incapable of giving informed consent to sterilization, it is incorrect to call the proposed operation either *voluntary* or *involuntary*. Rather, as we noted previously, the sterilization of such a person is best termed *nonvoluntary*. Of course, it is just as difficult for a lawyer as it is for an ethicist to determine whether a person is able to understand the interrelationships between sexual intercourse, pregnancy, having a child, and being a parent. In 1980, for example, the parents and physician of a 19-year-old woman with Down's syndrome sought to have her sterilized at their local hospital. The hospital refused to sterilize the young woman, Lee Ann, without court approval. In the process of seeking the court's approval, lawyers for Lee Ann's parents and physician described her condition as follows:

She is the oldest of three children, lives at home with them and her parents, and has never been institutionalized. Her IQ is in the "upper 20's to upper 30's range." She can converse, count to some extent, and recognize letters of the alphabet. She can dress and bathe herself. Her life expectancy and physical maturation are normal; however, her mental deficiency has prevented the normal emotional and social development of sexuality. If she becomes pregnant, she will not understand her condition, and she will not be capable of caring for a baby alone.[62]

Reasoning that it would be in Lee Ann's best interest for her to live in a group home for mentally retarded adults, her parents also reasoned that it would be in her best interest to be sterilized before this move. In this way, they could be assured that their daughter would not face a frightening pregnancy, or worse, an entirely burdensome motherhood.

Lee Ann's case led to the landmark decision, *In re Grady* (1981).[63] In deciding this case, the court had three options. First, it could hold that only persons legally capable of giving or withholding consent can exercise the right not to procreate and, therefore, that persons lacking legal capability—persons such as Lee Ann—may not be sterilized under any circumstances. Second, it could hold that only parents or a court-appointed guardian has the right to make such a momentous decision for persons such as Lee Ann. Third, it could hold that only the court itself has the right to decide for persons such as Lee Ann whether sterilization is in their best interest.[64]

The court quickly rejected its first option, reasoning that if sterilization is sometimes in the best interest of a competent person, then it is sometimes in the best interest of an incompetent person. After some debate, the court also rejected its second option. Recalling that the *Quinlan* court had permitted Karen Ann's parents to turn off their comatose daughter's respirator, the *Grady* court initially reasoned that if the Quinlans had the right to make a life-or-death decision on behalf of Karen Ann, then the Gradys had the right to make a sterilization decision on behalf of Lee Ann. As the *Grady* court reflected more on the case before it, however, it realized that there was a major distinction between it and the *Quinlan* case. Whereas there was no history of abuse in Quinlan-type decisions— that is, of parents deciding to turn off their children's life-support systems prematurely—there was a history of abuse in Grady-type decisions—that is, of parents deciding to have children sterilized needlessly. Given this crucial difference between *Grady* and *Quinlan* the court ruled that parents or guardians may not make unilateral sterilization decisions on behalf of their charges. Fearing that those closest to a mentally retarded child are not always ready, willing, or able to decide what is in that child's best interest, the court took its third option, reserving for itself the right to determine finally whether sterilization is in a mentally retarded child's best interest.

Certainly, *In re Grady* is a controversial decision. Many people believe that parents or guardians are better judges of their children's best interests than are the courts. But even if this is ordinarily the case, a court's motives in ruling for or against a sterilization procedure may be less conflicted or complex than those of parents who love their child either too much or too little to see his or her best interests clearly.

Social Dimensions of Sterilization

In our discussion of the ethical and legal problems surrounding abortion (see chapter 2), we alluded to several of the social problems as well. With respect to involuntary sterilizations, we have focused on issues surrounding the forced sterilization of so-called unfit people. Lest we give the mistaken impression that involuntary sterilization is no longer a problem or that people no longer espouse policies that fit under the rubric of eugenics, we discuss these issues in more detail here. In addition, we focus on men's and women's attitudes toward sterilization, particularly some of the fears men and women have expressed about the procedure and some of the reasons that people choose sterilization over contraception.

Minority and Majority Attitudes Toward Eugenics

Over the years, a number of social commentators have expressed the view that people should not be permitted to procreate severely defective or seriously diseased children. Arguing from a variety of perspectives, most of these commentators classify themselves as (1) eugenicists, (2) utilitarians, or (3) rights-oriented thinkers. As the eugenicists see it, people act irresponsibly when they choose to procreate knowing full well that the statistical odds are such that they are likely to produce either (1) a child who is burdened with mental or physical defects or disease or (2) a child who is a carrier of the defects and diseases she or he escaped. If the human race is to progress—that is, to become physically and mentally better—then, say the eugenicists, people with harmful genes must not procreate. Hence, for example, people who are carriers of sickle-cell anemia (a disease for which there is no known cure and that severely debilitates its victims, shortening their life span considerably),[65] or Tay-Sachs disease (a deadly nervous system disorder), or hemophilia (a hereditary condition in which one of the normal blood-clotting agents is missing, causing prolonged bleeding from minor injuries) should be voluntarily sterilized. Other forms of birth control are simply not as effective. And in the event that these people refuse to be voluntarily sterilized, insist the eugenicists, they should be involuntarily sterilized. Their individual right to procreate is simply not as important as humankind's interest in progressing.

Although utilitarian thinkers agree with the thrust of the eugenicists' arguments, their approach to irresponsible procreation (by which they mean procreation that fails to maximize the aggregate's well-being) is less directly motivated by scientific considerations. As they see it, even if a person is not a carrier of a harmful gene, he or she should not be permitted deliberately to produce a child that is doomed to lead a very short and painful life or a somewhat longer and less painful, but still tragically limited, life. So, for example, all people (but especially women) who are addicted to drugs, including alcohol, or who have the acquired immunodeficiency syndrome (AIDS) should practice voluntary contraception and, to the degree that their addiction or disease cannot be overcome, should consider voluntary sterilization just to be "on the safe side." To produce a cocaine-addicted baby, a baby suffering from fetal alcohol syndrome, or a baby afflicted with AIDS is not to serve aggregate utility, insists the utilitarian. Therefore, in the event that a woman with AIDS, for example, refuses to practice birth control but insists on engaging in sexual intercourse, utilitarians believe that the state may consider sterilizing her against her will should some purportedly less restrictive option, such as threatening her with imprisonment, fail.

Ordinarily, rights-oriented thinkers recoil from the suggestion that a person's right to procreate be limited but, as we noted in chapter 4, the right to procreate is not absolute. Even rights-oriented thinkers are prepared to justify involuntary sterilization if it is the *only* way to prevent a child from being born who would beg not to be born. These thinkers claim that a child has a right not to come into existence if its existence will amount to severe, unmitigated physical pain, for example.

Unimpressed by most of the arguments favoring involuntary sterilization, opponents of it note that rights-oriented thinkers, utilitarians, and eugenicists all go astray when they presume to distinguish between lives worth living and lives not worth living. They single out eugenicists for particular criticism. Not only is it not certain that a life with sickle cell anemia or even Tay-Sachs disease is one not worth living, for example; it also is not certain that a policy of eliminating deleterious genes will truly serve humankind's long-term best interest. A gene that is bad in some ways may be good in other ways. For example, the gene that causes sickle cell anemia also protects the carrier from contracting malaria, and the gene that causes Tay-Sachs disease also provides the carrier with a resistance to tuberculosis. Depending on the course of human events, an ability to resist malaria or tuberculosis may become humankind's saving grace should, for example, one or the other of these diseases suddenly become more widespread and life-threatening than it currently is. Moreover, note the opponents of involuntary sterilization, when it comes to eugenics, politics and genetics inevitably become mixed. At first, there is a push to prevent genetically defective people from procreating, but rapidly there is a push to prevent allegedly dangerous or undesirable people from procreating. Regrettably, the people who are labeled "dangerous" may simply be the people who threaten the established powers—high-spirited revolutionaries and social reformers. Similarly, those who are labeled "undesirable" may be the people who disgust the powers that be—aliens, weirdos, the shiftless, the homeless. After a while, the public forgets that dangerousness and undesirability are not genetic traits but social labels and that today's desirable person could easily become tomorrow's undesirable person depending on how the prevailing political winds shift.

Although most people concede that the right to procreate is not absolute, few of them wish to limit this right unless it is absolutely necessary to do so.[66] Through his or her act of procreating, an individual helps weave the tapestry of humankind, a tapestry that simultaneously reaches into the past and projects into the future. To prevent an individual from participating in this project is to deprive him or her of what may be the most meaningful task that any human can perform. Thus, involuntary sterilization seems justified only if there is no other way to prevent clear, present, and very serious harm from befalling the human community in general. Nonetheless, the loss of freedom and self-respect associated with forcibly invading an individual's body to sterilize him or her—a form of involuntary sterilization that is rare—may be too great a price to pay even for communal survival. People who prize their freedom are not likely to forsake it for the privilege of continued existence in a "safe" society that cares too little about the individual's rights in its relentless drive to achieve the collectivity's good.

Men's Attitudes Toward Sterilization

An interesting social aspect of sterilization is men's growing comfort with the idea of voluntary sterilization. At one time, many men feared having a vasectomy because they mistakenly believed that sterility and impotence were causally linked. Over time, however, an increasing number of men have become convinced of what was always true—namely, that sterility and impotence are not causally linked. For example, in a study of more than 1000 couples in which the man had chosen sterilization, 73.1 percent of the men reported an increased satisfaction in their sexual lives, whereas only 1.5 percent reported deterioration.[67] Thus, the major reason for a man not to use vasectomy as a reliable form of contraception is that he still has an interest in procreating children who are genetically related to him. If a man is indecisive about having a vasectomy for this very reason, he may want to consider the possibility of storing some of his sperm in a sperm bank (see chapter 8). Should he wish to father a child later, and should a surgeon be unable to reverse his sterilization, the woman with whom he wishes to have a child could be artificially inseminated with some of his banked sperm.

As men become increasingly convinced that they ought to bear their fair share of the responsibility for contraception, the demand for voluntary sterilization is increasing among them. Nevertheless, couples continue to resort to female sterilization (17.6 percent) more often than male sterilization (7 percent).[68] Given that a tubal ligation is a more invasive procedure than a vasectomy, and given that it remains approximately 20 percent more difficult to reverse female sterilization, there is good reason for a couple to choose male over female sterilization.[69] Should long-lasting male as well as female contraceptives be developed that have no more complications or side effects than male and female sterilization, sterilization's popularity may wane.

Women's Attitudes Toward Sterilization

Before the days of effective contraceptives such as the birth-control pill and the intrauterine device, many women turned to sterilization as their best birth-control option. Admittedly, some of these women were ambivalent about being sterilized. They feared that they would no longer be "real women" once they lacked the power to procreate; they also feared that sterilization would somehow "desex" them. Fears about being desexed were the first ones to be mitigated. Studies on women who had chosen sterilization routinely showed that the large majority were satisfied that the operation had not diminished their sexual desire.[70] Fears about no longer being a "real woman," however, were harder to mitigate. To the degree that our society associates womanhood with motherhood, and because many women judge their self-worth in terms of their fecundity, some women reason that, for all practical purposes, a sterilized woman is a defective woman.

Not surprisingly, educationally and economically privileged white women were among the first women in the United States to seek voluntary sterilization. Convinced that sterilization was safer, more effective, and less bothersome than any contraceptive on the market, these women were angered when, as we noted earlier, medical, legal, and clerical authorities put obstacles in their path. In an effort to establish women's right to bodily control, these women joined with groups such as Zero-Population Growth, Inc., the American Civil Liberties Union, and the Association for Voluntary Sterilization in the 1970s to force hospitals to provide voluntary sterilizations "free from sectarian influence and antiquated pro-natalist policies."[71] As a result of such campaigns as Operation Lawsuit, these groups were able to obtain sterilizations for women previously denied the procedure and to liberalize hospital regulations to make the operation freely available. They were particularly relieved that hospitals would no longer routinely counsel women seeking sterilizations to seek psychiatric help on the grounds that women who do not want children are asking for unhappiness.[72]

The organizers of Operation Lawsuit certainly had good intentions; they hoped to make it as easy as possible for a woman to be voluntarily sterilized by reducing the time gap between her decision to be sterilized and the actual operation. What they did not anticipate was that some physicians would use this shortened waiting period to rush certain women, especially women of color or poor women, into sterilizations not so much for their own good as for that of society.

Whereas one type of sterilization abuse consists, then, of the effort to deprive a woman of a *wanted* sterilization, the more common type of sterilization abuse consists of the effort to impose an *unwanted* sterilization on a woman. Such impositions generally take one of the following forms:

1. A person is sterilized without informed and voluntary consent.

2. A person "chooses" sterilization because lack of access to contraception and abortion makes it the only alternative to having more children.

3. A person "chooses" sterilization because poverty and lack of social services make it an alternative to increased misery.[73]

Clearly, legal restraints or economic constraints shape people's reproductive decisions and, depending on how restrictive or burdensome these restraints and constraints are, they can constitute an unjustified limitation on a woman's or, for that matter, a man's reproductive choices.

That existing sterilization policies tend to shape poor women's reproductive options in ways that they do not shape affluent women's options is clear. As of 1975, Medicaid assumed 90 percent of the cost of sterilization for all indigent people. In contrast, as of 1977, Medicaid stopped funding all medically unnecessary abortions for indigent people. Funding at the state level is also slanted in favor of sterilization, some states reimbursing 90 percent of the costs of a sterilization but only 50 percent of the costs of an abortion. Lest there be serious doubt that this asymmetrical funding pattern has an effect on women's behavior, data from Illinois shows that as the cost of abortions went up there, the number of sterilizations increased, rising from 3625 in 1979 to 6219 in 1980.[74]

In what seems like an attempt to discourage reproduction among the poor or to reduce the number of abortions, the state makes sterilization the most attractive, and most available, method of birth control for them. Women who depend on public funding for contraceptives and abortion as well as sterilization do not have as much reproductive freedom as women who do not depend on public funding. Thus, the only way to give *all* women control over their procreative choices is not only to provide adequate funding for alternatives to sterilization (i.e., contraception and abortion) but also to provide women with the material requirements, including jobs, necessary to support a family.

Of course, making contraception and abortion somewhat expensive or, alternatively, making sterilization somewhat inexpensive are relatively noncoercive ways for the state to influence women—at least, certain classes of women—to make the reproductive choices it wants them to make. As noted previously, various nations have used sterilization laws to control the size of their populations or the physical and mental quality of their citizens. Indeed, some nations have manipulated sterilization policy in an effort to consolidate their power. Adolf Hitler, for example, believed he could strengthen Germany by simultaneously replenishing desirable Aryan stock and preventing undesirable non-Aryan stock from reproducing. In the 1930s, he outlawed voluntary sterilization for Aryan women and created the *Mutter Krueze* (Mother's Cross) for patriotic German women who had borne 4 or more children. At the same time, he legalized and ordered the sterilization of non-Aryan or otherwise undesirable (that is, Jewish, Gypsy, lesbian) women.[75]

Although the United States has never legislated a wholesale program of involuntary sterilization for large segments of the population, enough people, especially women, have been sterilized against their own best interests to attract the public's concern. A host of citizens' groups and women's organizations have suggested various ways to protect people from involuntary sterilization, but there is a growing consensus among them that, in terms of the formal protection of citizens' rights, the current Health, Education and Welfare guidelines are as good as any proposed alternative. These guidelines require the following:

1. Informed consent in the language spoken or read by the person

2. Extensive counseling, which will include information about alternatives

3. A prohibition on consent at times of delivery or at any other time of stress, and on overt or veiled pressures on welfare patients

4. The right to choose a patient advocate throughout the counseling, as in any other aspect of the process

5. A 30-day waiting period between consent and procedure

6. No sterilization of people younger than 21 years of age.[76]

Nonetheless, as good as these guidelines are in theory, in practice they are only as good as the people who enforce them.

Sterilization abuse is likely to be far less of a problem in the future if the means for sterilization reversal are perfected. Should this happen, there will no longer be meaningful distinctions between sterilization and contraception. Of course, new opportunities for abuse may arise. For instance, some people worry that the state will seek to plug the tubes of all female adolescents in an effort to reduce teenage pregnancy rates. Because this would be gender discrimination at its worst, the vasa of all male adolescents would have to be clamped as well. Concerns such as these are somewhat alarmist. In the United States, parents are not likely to sit idly by as their children are hauled off to be plugged or clamped. Nevertheless, should plugging or clamping become perfected birth-control options, a development in technology will have erased a whole set of moral problems related to sterilization. No longer a final or ultimate decision about relinquishing one's procreative powers, sterilization will lose the most fearsome of its stings. It will become, instead, a sure way to protect oneself from pregnancy without having to live with the kind of risks many contraceptives impose.

6   Abortion

As one of the most complex ethical, legal, and social issues of our time, abortion has generated debates that threaten the integrity of a pluralistic system intended to tolerate differences. No doubt these debates make it difficult for people to discuss abortion, including abortion techniques, dispassionately. But unless we understand what abortion is—namely, the premature expulsion of a fetus from the uterus in either a natural (spontaneous) or unnatural (induced) manner—and how one is performed, we will be unable to understand the ways in which technology is actually changing the parameters of the abortion debate.

The Technology of Abortion

Spontaneous Abortion

A spontaneous abortion, or miscarriage, is the body's natural rejection of the fetus. Estimates of the occurrence of spontaneous abortion range from 10 to 50 percent of all pregnancies.[1] During the first trimester (3 months) of pregnancy, fetal deformities are the usual cause of a spontaneous abortion; abortions occurring after this are primarily due to other complications—for example, an incompatibility in the Rh factors of the mother and the fetus. If a mother with Rh-negative blood is exposed to the red blood cells of an Rh-positive baby at the time of birth, she will develop antibodies against the Rh factor, which acts as a foreign substance in her body. These antibodies may be fatal to a subsequent fetus with Rh-positive blood since they will remove the red blood cells from the fetus's circulation. Fortunately, such fatalities are less likely today than they were even a decade ago. Researchers have now devised ways to protect an Rh-positive fetus from its Rh-negative mother. This procedure involves giving Rh-negative mothers an injection of Rh antibodies a few days after the birth of an Rh-positive baby. These antibodies interact with the Rh-positive antigens on the surface of the fetal red blood cells and prevent the mother from producing her own Rh antibodies. Since her system is never stimulated to produce them, Rh antibodies will not be present to harm a subsequent Rh-positive fetus. Other complications include allergies, uterine deformities, and toxemia of pregnancy. Like Rh incompatibility, all these conditions were once extremely problematic during pregnancy, but prenatal care has developed to such an extent that physicians can detect, monitor, and sometimes treat these conditions throughout pregnancy, thereby lessening the risk to both the mother and the fetus.

Induced Abortion

Although induced abortion is a topic that has always generated heated controversy, its practice can be traced back to ancient times. Among the methods women have used to induce abortions are inserting abortifacients such as the herbs rue and ergot into the cervix (still used in some Third World countries), wearing tight corsets, falling down intentionally, physically abusing the abdominal region, and ingesting chemicals such as lead, arsenic, phosphorous, quinine, and apiol.[2] In the years just before the decriminalization of abortion in the United States, physicians saw numerous women who needed emergency treatment as a result of self-induced or otherwise illegal abortions. Abortionists and pregnant women used coat hangers, knitting needles, and knives, potassium permanganate tablets, and other dangerous vaginal and uterine soaps and pastes to extract the fetus from the womb.[3] Sometimes these abortion techniques were effective, but sometimes they were not. Whether or not they managed to abort, the women were often harmed in the attempt. With the physical methods came the danger of uterine perforation, uterine rupture, or hemorrhaging. With the chemical methods came the danger of poisoning or drug overdoses. Nevertheless, women continued to choose dangerous, illegal abortions as an alternative to having an unwanted child.

Partly in reaction to this state of affairs, the U.S. Supreme Court ruled in the 1973 case *Roe* v. *Wade* that citizens' right to privacy includes their procreative freedom. However, the Court also declared some interest in unborn human life and therefore dictated that the decision to have an abortion is completely up to the woman and her physician in the first trimester; that the state has the option to regulate abortions in the second trimester in order to preserve maternal health; and that the state has the option to regulate or ban abortions in the third trimester to protect potential human life, except in cases where the pregnancy seriously threatens the life or health of the woman.

Whether an abortion is performed in the first, second, or third trimester, however, the attending physician must collect as much medical information and history about the patient as possible. To determine the age of the fetus, the physician not only asks the woman about the date of her last menstrual period but also gives her a complete physical and pelvic examination. To identify problems in the pregnancy that might complicate the abortion, the physician analyzes the blood and urine of his or her patient to determine blood type, Rh type, and the presence of infection or communicable diseases. Finally, the physician asks questions about the patient's use of contraceptives—past, present, and possibly future—and the use of other medications.[4]

After the physician has collected all the relevant information, she or he is in a position to decide what abortion technique to use. In the past, abortion was a relatively dangerous procedure, but this is no longer true. Whether induced by surgical or chemical means, abortion (especially when performed in the first trimester) is actually less risky than a normal pregnancy.[5]

Surgical Techniques

Surgical abortions range from the fairly simple and safe to the very extreme procedures that are performed only to save the life of the woman. Among the surgical techniques are vacuum aspiration, dilation and curettage, dilation and evacuation, hysterotomy, and hysterectomy (figure 6.1). In general, the farther along a woman is in her pregnancy, the more risky the abortion becomes.

Vacuum aspiration

Vacuum aspiration is the most common form of surgical abortion and has been used since 1967. The procedure has been perfected so that it requires only local anesthesia, 20 minutes on the operating table, and a short time in the recovery room. The physician dilates the cervix gradually with laminaria or, more rapidly, with a dilator. *Laminaria* are slender rods made of seaweed that have been processed and sterilized for medical use. As shown in figure 6.2, they are inserted into the cervical canal and, over several hours, absorb moisture, swell, and gently widen the canal.[6] As soon as the canal is widened, the physician judges the size and the angle of the uterus, inserts a vacuum tube into the uterus, and removes the fetus quickly, sometimes using curettage to make sure that all the

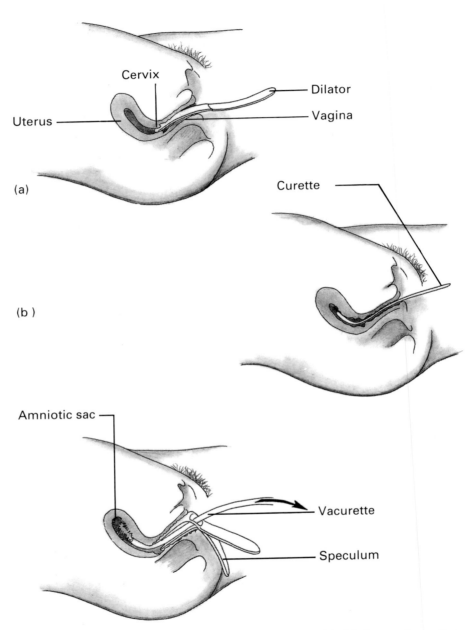

Figure 6.1 The two common methods of abortion, (a) dilation and curettage and (b) vacuum aspiration.

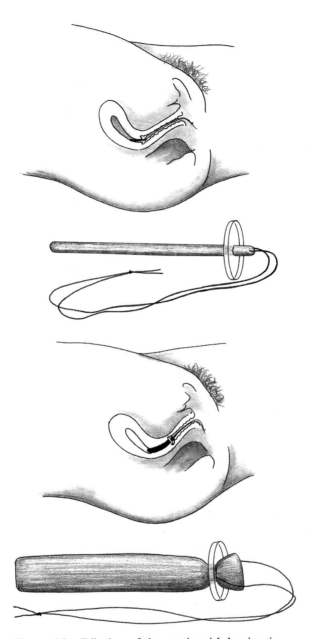

Figure 6.2 Dilation of the cervix with laminaria.

material has been removed. The material is then examined for any problems, and the woman can go home after a brief recovery period.[7]

Dilation and curettage

Although the procedure for dilation and curettage (D & C) is more painful and more complicated than that of vacuum aspiration, it is still used in many clinics. The D & C requires general rather than local anesthesia, and the patient usually stays in the hospital overnight. The cervix needs to be dilated more than with vacuum aspiration, and a steel curette needs to be inserted to scrape out the inside of the uterus. Once again, the procedure takes only approximately 20 minutes.

Dilation and evacuation

Both the vacuum aspiration and the D & C are ideal for first-trimester abortions, up to 13 weeks after the last menstrual period. However, after this time, they are no longer the best choices. For a pregnancy between 13 and 16 weeks, and sometimes even up to 20 weeks, dilation and evacuation is the preferred technique. Once again, the cervical dilation needs to be more extensive. The procedure is performed with a large vacuum curette and an instrument for crushing and dismembering the fetus to remove the pieces. Sometimes a drug called *oxytocin* is used to induce labor contractions (RU 486 is also effective) to ease removal and lessen blood loss. One of the common dangers is that the fetal skull might get trapped in the cervix.

Hysterotomy and hysterectomy

Although both the hysterotomy and the hysterectomy can be used as second-trimester abortion methods, they involve major surgery and are performed only when the woman's life is endangered by the continuation of the pregnancy. A hysterotomy is a minor cesarean section that removes only the fetus. In contrast, a hysterectomy is a major operation that removes the entire uterus along with the fetus. It leaves the woman permanently sterilized. Obviously, neither of these methods of abortion is quick, easy, or without risk, and both require an exceptional reason to even be considered as the best abortion procedure.

Chemical techniques

RU 486 is an abortifacient that was first made available to women in France to terminate a pregnancy within the first 7 weeks. While avoiding the risks of surgery and anesthesia, its only complication appears to be a 4 to 5 percent chance of hemorrhaging. As we mentioned in chapter 4, RU 486 is not yet on the U.S. market. This does not mean, however, that other sorts of chemicals are not used to induce abortions in the United States. In fact, the common methods of second-trimester abortions in the United States—an abortion of the fetus from 14 to 24 weeks after the last menstrual period—all involve the introduction of chemical substances into the woman's body to induce premature labor, to kill the fetus, or both. The three regularly used substances are prostaglandins, hypertonic saline, and urea.

Prostaglandins

The prostaglandins are a family of hormones present in semen, in the uterine lining, and in many body tissues. Although their role is not yet fully understood, they are the cause of ordinary menstrual cramps and are suspected of playing a role in initiating labor at the end of pregnancy. In semen, they may facilitate sperm transport or in some way enable the sperm to unite with the egg. Their only approved medical use is for termination of pregnancy.[8] Currently, physicians favor two types of prostaglandins, both of which are effective in inducing uterine contractions during the second trimester. One requires an intraamniotic injection, and the other requires a vaginal suppository. With either administration, labor begins fairly rapidly. The negative side effects of both methods include gastrointestinal symptoms and cervical lacerations. Neither treatment is inexpensive, and both leave open the possibility for birth of a live fetus, a problem that is becoming more common and more complex to handle with the increasing sophistication of premature infant care.

Hypertonic saline

Another option for a second-trimester abortion, used between the seventeenth and twentieth week of pregnancy, is an injection of hypertonic saline (a solution more concentrated in salts than normal cellular fluid). The physician withdraws a small amount of amniotic fluid and replaces it with a 20 to 25 percent saline solution that effectively kills the fetus within the uterus. Labor is induced, and the dead fetus is usually delivered in 24 to 72 hours. A saline abortion is simpler and less expensive than a prostaglandin abortion. However, it too has its negative side effects. It may cause intravascular clotting, myometrial necrosis, a cerebral edema, or other problems if the saline enters the blood stream. All in all, the method presents many more complications and risks than an early (first-trimester) abortion.[9]

Urea

The third option for a second-trimester abortion is the injection of urea (a concentrated solution of a nitrogen compound that is normally produced by the kidneys) into the amniotic sac in a method similar to the one used in the saline abortion. Like the saline abortion, this type of abortion aims to end the life of the fetus within the womb and induce premature labor, but it is not always effective alone and is therefore usually used in combination with another abortifacient. Among the advantages of a urea abortion are its relative simplicity, inexpensiveness, and safety.[10]

Abortion Complications

Before the decriminalization of abortion in the United States, when desperate pregnant women were seeking unlicensed, untrained, and unsanitary abortionists, there was a fairly high rate of complications and even death from botched abortions. Now, with sanitary clinics and trained physicians, abortion is no longer a particularly dangerous procedure, especially when performed in the first trimester. Indeed Dr. Christopher Tietze has pointed out that abortion's attendant risks are no greater than the pill's attendant risks:

Under the conditions of mortality prevailing in developed countries, the known risk of life due to thromboembolic diseases resulting from the use of currently available oral contraceptives over a given period of time is estimated to be on the same order of magnitude as the risk incurred by preventing births exclusively by abortions in hospital, not making any contraceptive efforts over the same period.[11]

Nevertheless, the relatively small risks associated with abortion are sometimes exacerbated by three factors: length of pregnancy, the method of abortion used, and the postoperative care given.

The shorter the pregnancy, the less fetal tissue there is to be removed and the less danger there is to the woman. For this reason, abortion counsellors urge their clients to have their abortions early in their pregnancies when simpler methods can be used, general anesthesia is not always needed, and the whole operation is much shorter.[12]

Although the method of abortion depends on the length of the pregnancy, physicians agree that, as a rule, the vacuum aspiration abortion is safest for early pregnancy and the saline abortion is safest for later pregnancies. A first-trimester vacuum aspiration is quick, fairly simple, and requires the least possible dilation of the cervix. Safer than a hysterotomy, hysterectomy, or prostaglandin abortion, a second- or third-trimester saline abortion is still more problematic than a first-trimester vacuum aspiration, especially in terms of its psychological impact on the woman. It is one thing to undergo a D & C, and quite another to go through the labor and delivery process with the intent of expelling a dead fetus.[13]

To determine what kind of postoperative care a woman needs, physicians must be familiar with the symptoms of abortion complications, the length of time it takes each symptom to develop, and the best treatment for each symptom. For example, trained physicians will suspect an infection, quickly prescribing antibiotics, should their patient develop a fever and a tender abdomen 48 to 72 hours after her abortion. Similarly, the trained physician will suspect hemorrhaging, quickly prescribing a blood transfusion or shock treatment, should his or her patient begin to bleed heavily, externally or internally, 12 to 24 hours after her abortion. If physicians are not attuned to these kinds of complications, the risks of abortion will be much greater for the patient than they would otherwise be.[14]

After any abortion, the recovering woman should avoid certain activities to safeguard against infections. She should refrain from sexual intercourse, use of tampons, and douching for a week or so, carefully monitoring her temperature to be aware of any irregularities. The recovering woman should also watch for problems such as severe pain, hives or rashes, intense bleeding, the continuation of the symptoms of pregnancy, or the failure to begin menstruation within 6 weeks after the abortion. If she notes any of these symptoms, or anything else that is troublesome or unusual, the recovering woman should immediately consult her physician instead of waiting for her 2-week postabortion office visit.[15]

Medical Problems that May Lead to Abortion

The moral arguments for and against abortion are very complex, as we will discuss later in this chapter. Although some groups deny that there is any justification for abortion, other groups accept several justifications for it, including a wide variety of medical reasons that range from emotional stress on the woman to a life-threatening pregnancy. Whatever disagreements they may have among themselves, however, these latter groups concur that if any abortion is justified, it is one that will terminate a pregnancy whose complications (either fetal infections or genetic abnormalities) will result in a severely imperiled newborn.

Fetal Infection

Usually the fetus is protected from infection by the placenta but, when the mother becomes sick, the infection sometimes travels into the placenta and infects the fetus. Minor infections such as a cold or influenza virus do not usually affect the fetus, but other more serious infections can leave the fetus with problems such as blindness, deafness, congenital diseases, hydrocephalus, microcephalus, or severe retardation. Fortunately, two of the worst culprits, polio and rubella, have virtually disappeared in the United States owing to vaccination.[16] However, other types of infection, such as toxoplasmosis (parasite *Toxoplasma gondii* transmitted most commonly by eating poorly cooked meat containing cysts of the parasites or through contact with the feces of infected cats), are still present and, although rare, they are relatively untreatable. More than 50 percent of the pregnant women infected with toxoplasmosis have healthy children, but since there is no way for a particular woman to know whether the fetus *she* is carrying has been harmed, she may desire an abortion to be on the safe side.[17]

Genetic Abnormalities

More serious and more common than fetal infections are fetal genetic abnormalities. Researchers estimate that there are 15 million Americans with birth defects, 80 percent of which are genetic. In 50 percent of the mentally disabled infants born each year, the root of their problems can be traced back to genetic abnormalities, as it can be in 40 percent of the infants who die each year.[18]

Although medical technology in the United States is still not advanced enough to protect fetuses from most genetic defects, it is advanced enough to detect many different kinds of genetic and chromosomal problems. An increasing number of disorders are being diagnosed by techniques such as amniocentesis (developed in the 1960s), ultrasonography, and chorionic villi samplings. Although critics charge that the women who use these techniques almost invariably have an abortion if the test results reveal fetal defects, in fact this is not the case. Ninety-five percent of the time, these diagnostic tests reveal a genetically normal fetus and, when the tests do reveal a genetically abnormal fetus, abortion is not always the course of action chosen by the couple. On the contrary, many couples use the knowledge they have obtained through these tests to prepare to rear a child who will be burdened with an extraordinary number of physical or mental challenges throughout life.[19] Additionally, an increasing number of physicians are using this knowledge to treat some of these fetal defects in utero. As these treatment options grow, more couples will feel free to bring their fetuses to term, confident that they will be born healthy.

The Ethics of Abortion

Depending on which religious beliefs, philosophical assumptions, sensory impressions, aesthetic images, and personal recollections dominate a person's psyche, she or he will tend to adopt either a so-called pro-choice position or a so-called pro-life position on abortion.[20] What is particularly disturbing about this polarizing state of affairs is that many of the differences that separate pro-choice and pro-life advocates seem non-negotiable. When people cannot make progress on a moral issue, when they seem no closer to achieving consensus at the beginning than at the end of a conversation, their temptation is to throw their hands up and declare that their opponents are morally befuddled and benighted. Such defeatism is regrettable, however. No society that wishes to live in relative harmony can permit its members to stop conversing with one another about the matters that will otherwise tear them apart.

In the first 8 years after *Roe* v. *Wade*, the annual abortion figure rose from 744,600 to 1.5 million, terminating approximately one-third of all pregnancies in the United States. Undoubtedly, the circumstances surrounding these difficult decisions varied widely. Given our general attitudes about life and death, and our predisposition to treasure a human life no matter how fragile or tenuous, the decision to terminate a pregnancy is almost always made with some feelings of regret or guilt. Thus, it is not surprising that the ethics of abortion preoccupies people especially insofar as (1) the status of the fetus and (2) the needs, interests, and rights of all affected parties are concerned.

Status of the Fetus

The status of the fetus raises a fundamental question: When does *truly* human life begin? According to theologian Charles Curran, we must emphasize the qualifier *truly* in the phrase *truly human life* in order to distinguish adequately between mere *human life* and a full *human person*.[21] Reinforcing Curran's point, philosopher Frederick Jaffe notes that the outcome of the abortion debate depends on how its central questions are framed. If we ask the question, "When during gestation does *human life* begin?" our conclusions about abortion are likely to be different than if we ask instead "When does a fetus become a *person* who merits protection equal to or greater than the woman in whose body it is located and without whose body it would cease to exist?"[22] Jaffe insists that the choice between these two ways of posing the abortion question is value-laden. Most people will be much more concerned about killing a human person than about ending a human life that is not yet personal.

Most theorists admit that there is a distinction between having human life and being a human person. The empirical claim that a conceptus, zygote, embryo, or fetus has human life can be established scientifically. In contrast, the conceptual claim that a conceptus, zygote, embryo, or fetus is a person cannot be established scientifically without begging the question whether what makes a human life *truly* human is simply membership in the biological species *Homo sapiens*. If a theorist believes that membership in the biological species *Homo sapiens* is not a sufficient condition for personhood, she or he must be able to name those extra characteristics that transform a member of the biological species *Homo sapiens* into a full human person. As Charles Curran sees it, these characteristics are (1) individual-biological, (2) social-relational, (3) conferred-rights, or (4) multiple. So complete is Curran's classification scheme that we will follow its general contours with some noticeable detours.

Individual-Biological Approach

Some theorists believe that what transforms a fetus into a person is some biological moment such as (1) birth, (2) viability, (3) the formation of the senses, the nervous system, and brain, (4) the formation of the cortex of the brain, or (5) conception. As intuitively plausible as this approach to the status of the fetus may be, there are problems with identifying any one of these five biological moments as *the* moment when personhood, or truly human life, begins.

Birth does not seem to mark the beginning of personhood since there is little difference between a fetus the day before it is born and the day after it is born. The fact that the fetus is in the womb one day and outside of it the other should not transform its moral value.

Viability is also a poor criterion for the passage to personhood. Currently, *viability* is understood as the point at which a fetus can survive outside its mother's womb. As a result of certain technological advances, very premature infants are now able to be sustained ex utero. Since advances such as the artificial placenta may one day enable blastocysts, zygotes, embryos, and fetuses to survive ex utero, will everyone then agree that these entities are human persons simply because they are not dependent on a natural womb for life? Or will some people simply reject viability as a criterion for personhood, reasoning that if ventilator dependence, for example, does not rob a grandmother of her personhood, then ventilator independence should not confer personhood on her newly born granddaughter.

Because neither birth nor viability seem to qualify as the biological moment of personhood, several proponents of the individual-biological approach have speculated that fetuses become persons at earlier developmental moments than those of either birth or viability. Some of these theorists claim that the fetus becomes a person when it assumes a characteristically human morphology—that is, a human shape with basic human organs. Working with St. Thomas Aquinas's (1227–1274) idea that there is a fit between the material and formal aspects of being, theologian Joseph Donceel has argued that the fertilized ovum, the morula, the blastula, and the early embryo cannot become persons because they are not materially organized enough to receive the truly human form, or soul. The form of the soul cannot animate the matter of the body, he says, until the fetus's senses, nervous system, and brain have emerged, a point of development that occurs only after several weeks of pregnancy have elapsed.[23]

Articulating another version of Donceel's theory, philosopher Wilfried Ruff pinpoints the moment of "ensoulment" (his term for personhood) at the formation of the brain's cortex during the eighth week of pregnancy. Since most people associate personal life with consciousness and self-reflection, and since consciousness and self-reflection have their indispensable substratum in the cerebral cortex, Ruff is confident that persons—truly human lives—cannot exist before the eighth week of pregnancy.[24] After all, if the cessation of brain waves is evidence that a person has ended, then the inception of brain waves may be evidence that a person has begun. But even if Ruff's line of reasoning makes sense, the fact remains that both brain birth and brain death are debatable indexes for the presence or absence of personhood, respectively.

Given that it is difficult to identify any moment in the continual progressive development of the fetus as *the* crucial moment when it becomes a human person, many proponents of the individual-biological approach have retreated to the moment of conception. John T. Noonan, Jr., for example, argues that "at conception the new being receives the genetic code. It is this genetic information that determines his characteristics, which is the biological carrier of the possibility of human wisdom, which makes him a self-evolving being. A being with a human genetic code is man."[25]

To the objection that the *possibility* of human wisdom is not equivalent to the *actuality* of human wisdom, Noonan points out that the fetus is best thought of as the *probability* of human wisdom. To clarify his point, he contrasts a sperm's potentiality for personhood with that of a fetus's probability for personhood:

If a spermatozoon is destroyed, one destroys a being which had a chance of far less than 1 in 200 million of developing into a reasoning being, possessed of the genetic code, a heart and other organs, and capable of pain. If a fetus is destroyed, one destroys a being already possessed of the genetic code, organs, and sensitivity to pain, and one which had an 80 percent chance of developing further into a baby outside the womb who, in time, would reason.[26]

The fact that the conceptus will probably, and not just possibly, become a person is reason enough for Noonan to treat that conceptus as if it were already a person. Of course, theorists who believe that only actual persons, and not also possible or even probable persons, should be treated as persons will not find Noonan's line of reasoning cogent.

Social-Relational Approach

Unlike those who stress individual-biological criteria for personhood, those who emphasize social-relational criteria insist that what makes human life truly human life is some set of cultural responses (being socially accepted as a person to whom one can relate, for example). However, object the critics, if an individual's personhood depends on whether other people accept him or her as someone to whom they can relate, then these people have the power to drum him or her out of the corps of personhood at will. Indeed, if the social-relational test for personhood is taken too seriously, say the critics, a mother may be morally justified to kill her always wailing 1-month-old son on the grounds that she does not view him as a person to whom she can relate.[27] Likewise, if this test for personhood is adequate, a son may be morally justified to kill his Alzheimer's-afflicted mother on the grounds that he does not view her as a person to whom he can relate.

As most relational thinkers oppose both infanticide and parricide, they specify the relational criteria for personhood in such a way that only fetuses and not also infants, for example, count as nonpersons. With respect to infants, H. T. Engelhardt argues that what distinguishes them from fetuses is that the mother-infant relationship is a "social and willed structure of interaction and a cultural enterprise," whereas the mother-fetus relationship is merely a "biological and imposed structure and a physiological enterprise."[28] A fetus starts to become an infant, says Engelhardt, at the point of viability after which mothers supposedly relate to their fetuses as if they were persons. The main problem with Engelhardt's distinction between a biological mother-fetus relationship on the one hand and a personal mother-infant relationship on the other is that relational capacities vary greatly from person to person. For every woman who claims that she was unable to relate to her fetus as a person at the point of viability or even later, there will be a woman who claims that she related to her fetus as a person from the moment it was conceived.

Conferred-Rights Approach

Unlike proponents of the individual-biological and social-relational approaches, proponents of the conferred-rights approach resolve the issue of personhood in a legalistic manner: An entity becomes a person when a society formally confers on it the rights of a person. According to philosopher R. B. Brandt, rational and impartial agents who do not know whether they will exist as fetuses or as adult persons under a proposed moral code will reason that it is prima facie wrong to kill any sentient being that wants to live. Since a fetus is probably not the kind of creature that is able to formulate any kind of wants, including the "want to live," Brandt concludes that it is probably not prima facie wrong to kill it.[29]

At the root of Brandt's line of reasoning, then, is the conviction that fetuses, especially very early fetuses, are not sentient—that is, capable of feeling pleasure and pain and, therefore, of formulating wants. As Brandt's critics see it, however, it is not clear that fetuses are nonsentient and, even if fetuses are nonsentient, presence or lack of sentience is not necessarily the ultimate criterion for personhood. Indeed, those who deny that fetuses have rights usually stake their claim not on the fetus's lack of sentience but on its inability to reason, to engage in self-motivated activity, to communicate, or to formulate a self-concept. Of course, if what makes an entity a person is, for example, its ability to formulate a self-concept, then the class of nonpersons probably includes infants and severely mentally impaired adults as well as fetuses.[30] Be this as it may, Brandt cannot simply *assume* that society confers rights on entities if and only if they have wants. He has to prove that having wants, rather than some other higher-order capacity, is the basis for rights.

Over the past few years, many theorists have retreated from the conferred-rights approach. Not only is it inordinately difficult to define *rights*; it is, as we have just noted, equally difficult to decide what rights should be assigned to which entities and on what basis. Given the fact that rights frequently conflict, Larry R. Churchill and José Jorge Simón have argued that, when it comes to abortion, the rhetoric of rights has been misused to the point of creating an ethical cul-de-sac. Both sides of the abortion debate have appealed to the notion of rights—the fetus's right to life, on the one hand, and the woman's right to privacy and control over her body, on the other. As Churchill and Simón see it, these rights "have taken on an absolutist flavor" that threatens to leave ethics "dead in the water."[31] To resurrect ethics, parties to the abortion debate must, at the very least, remind themselves that no right is absolute. Better yet, parties to the abortion debate must recognize that moral deliberation includes more than a proper assessment of competing rights claims. To decide whether a given abortion decision is morally justified, people must be attentive not only to the fetus's and woman's respective rights but also to the motives and intentions of the involved agents; the origins and consequences of the decision; the loyalties, traditions, and customs at risk; and the economic conditions under which the decision is made.[32]

Multiple Approach

Since the individual-biological, social-relational, and conferred-rights approaches are inadequate taken separately, some theorists have developed a multiple, or integrated, approach to determine the point at which truly human life begins. Among these theorists is Edward Langerak, who combines all three of the standard approaches to abortion in order to provide a comprehensive framework for evaluating the status of the fetus. Langerak claims that the fetus is a potential person, "a being, not yet a person, that will become an actual person in the normal course of its development."[33] Because we often rely on high probabilities to make judgments in an uncertain world, and because there is a high probability that the fetus will become a person, the potentiality principle helps explain the belief that something about the fetus itself makes abortion morally questionable. Nevertheless, because the potentiality principle does not explain another belief many people have—namely, that late abortions are somehow morally worse than early abortions—we must rely on some insights present in the social-relational and conferred-rights approaches to account for this belief.

Reflecting on the developing fetus with the potentiality principle in mind, Langerak observes that implantation, quickening, viability, and birth are the usual candidates for *the* moment when the developing fetus becomes a truly human person. The difficulty is to provide nonarbitrary reasons for conferring the rights of personhood at one of these moments but not another. Because Langerak believes that postquickening abortions (abortions after the mother feels the fetus move in her womb) as well as postviability abortions and acts of infanticide erode people's already limited capacity for sympathy, he suggests that society should confer a claim to life on the fetus at the beginning of the second trimester—a claim that can, however, be trumped by other serious claims such as that of a mother to mental or physical well-being.[34] Whether Langerak's answer to the question of the status of the fetus is satisfactory depends on how able and willing we are to live with conceptual as well as moral ambiguity. Perhaps we need to think of persons, no matter their age, less as products and more as processes, who gradually weave themselves into the fabric of society's moral network of relationships. Langerak advises us that we may be doing violence to ourselves as well as to fetuses whenever we *unnecessarily* rip vulnerable entities in process out of the cloth of our shared existence.

Utilitarian and Rights-Oriented Approaches to the Needs, Interests, and Rights of Those Affected by the Abortion Decision

The abortion debate is not only about the status of the fetus. Is it or is it not a person? Does it or does it not have needs, interests, and rights? It is also about the status as well as the needs, interests, and rights of *all* the people who, directly or indirectly, will decide the fetus's fate. Therefore, whether they emphasize the aggregate's well-being (the utilitarian approach) or the individual's rights (the rights-oriented approach), ethicists approach the issue of abortion fully aware that more is at stake than the personhood of the fetus.

Utilitarian Approaches to Abortion

For utilitarians, the abortion decision is a decision about which course of action (abortion or continuing the pregnancy) is most likely to maximize the aggregate's utility (pleasure, happiness, well-being). Since utilitarians consider the interests and needs of all the sentient creatures who will be affected positively or negatively by the abortion decision, philosopher Baruch Brody wonders if and when the fetus's interests and needs should be factored into their calculations. On reflection, Brody concludes that utilitarians should include the fetus in their calculations only when a woman *does not want* to abort it. He reasons as follows: Since utilitarians are bound to consider the desires of all the persons who will be affected by an action, a woman who does not want to abort her fetus must consider not only her own desires and those of her friends and family but also those of the fetus which, if it is born, will exist as a person with desires. She must ask herself questions such as, Would I want to exist if I were going to be born to a drug-addicted, unwed, poverty-stricken teenaged woman? or Would I want to exist if I knew I were going to be born with a severe and painful physical defect? In contrast, a woman who *does want* to abort her fetus needs to consider only her own desires and those of her friends and family. The fetus drops out of the picture "because if the fetus is destroyed it will not have had desires, and nothing will have been satisfied or frustrated."[35]

    Although Brody's argument makes sense if fetuses do not, as he assumes, have desires, it loses force if fetuses do have desires. Nevertheless, even if a fetus has desires, depending on how important those desires are relative to the desires of the people who will be affected by its continued existence, a woman's decision to abort it may still be justified. For example, even if a fetus is healthy and desires to live, its desire to live may be outweighed by its mother's desire to live.[36]

This line of reasoning suggests I that from a utilitarian perspective, the morality of an abortion depends on complex predictions about whether aborting a fetus will maximize aggregate utility. What saves a fetus from being aborted is not proof of its personhood but an argument that the aggregate in which it is included as one, but no more than one, will be worse off if it is not born. But because situation-by-situation determinations of aggregate utility are so difficult to make, many utilitarians refuse to take a situational approach to abortion. Instead, they search for a rule that either usually permits or usually forbids abortion. The main problem with this rule-oriented approach to the morality of abortion is that it is unclear what the long-term effects of regarding fetal life as less than truly human life (personhood) will be, even if it is somewhat clear what the long-term effects of disregarding women's bodily integrity will be and already are.

Rights-Oriented Approaches to Abortion

Rights-oriented thinkers do not believe that an abortion is justified simply because aggregate utility is thereby maximized. Rather, they believe that even if an abortion maximizes aggregate utility, it may still be wrong if one or more individuals' rights have been violated. So, for example, if a fetus has a right to life, it is wrong to abort it even if its procreators (two college students who do not want to interrupt their career plans to get married and have a baby) will be much happier if it is never born. There is a problem with this line of reasoning, however. It leads us back to the question of the status of the fetus: Is, or is not, a fetus the sort of entity that has rights?

Because the status of the fetus is such a debatable issue, some theorists have suggested that we simply assume that the fetus is a person and that every person has a prima facie right to life. Even so, says philosopher Judith Jarvis Thomson, it may not always be wrong to abort a fetus. As Thomson sees it, "Having a right to life does not guarantee having either a right to be given the use of or a right to be allowed continued use of another person's body—even if one needs it for life itself."[37]

Given her understanding of what the right to life does and does not include, Thomson has little difficulty justifying abortion in those cases in which a woman will die unless she aborts the fetus. Because the right to self-defense is a right that virtually every ethical system accepts, Thomson wonders why the natural-law tradition forbids abortion even in those cases where the mother's life is at stake. What she forgets is that natural-law theorists invoke the principle of self-defense only against noninnocent aggressors. Because a fetus is innocent—it did not, after all, deliberately invade a woman to gestate in her womb—and because every person's right to life is equal, natural-law theorists reason that there is no way to choose between the fetus's life and that of the woman. Nature must simply be permitted to take its course when only 1 of 2 people can live.[38]

Although Thomson agrees that the fetus is innocent, and although she concedes that both the fetus and the woman who is gestating it have a right to life, she insists that when the fetus's life comes into conflict with that of the woman in whom it is gestating, the woman's right to life overrides that of the fetus. Thomson bases her judgment on the observation "that the mother and the unborn child are not like two tenants in a small house which has, by an unfortunate mistake, been rented to both: The mother *owns* the house."[39] In other words, the mother has a prior moral claim—her right to bodily integrity—that tips the scales of justice in her favor despite the desperate plight of the innocent fetus that depends on her for existence.

Thomson goes even further in her defense of abortion, however. She argues that possessing the right to life does not automatically give one person the right to use another person's body in order to keep on living. A person who needs to use a set of healthy kidneys cannot justifiably kidnap a woman and plug himself or herself into that woman's kidneys for even a short period of time. Analogously, the fetus has no right to use the body of the woman who is gestating it even if it cannot live outside of that woman's body.[40]

Thomson admits that her analogy is imperfect, that it applies better to cases of unwanted pregnancy after rape or failed contraceptives than to cases of unwanted pregnancy after voluntary intercourse. If a woman invites a person to use her kidneys for a specified number of months, if she enters into a caring relationship with him or her, she may owe that dependent person access to her body even if that dependent person has no right to such access. For her suddenly to break the caring relationship she initiated is prima facie wrong, even if such a rupture does not constitute a violation of the dependent person's rights. Analogously, if a woman becomes pregnant because she wants to have a child, it is probably wrong for her to break her relationship with the fetus simply because she has an urge to fit into a slinky designer gown.[41]

Despite the flaws in her argument, Thomson correctly argues that the mother, regarded as a person who is being pursued, has the right to take the life of the fetus who is pursuing her. But, says Baruch Brody, the whole matter of pursuit needs to be carefully analyzed before we decide that it is morally permissible for a woman to abort the fetus to save herself. According to Brody, if we look at a normal case of pursuit—for example, a case in which B is about to shoot A—three conditions are involved:

1. *The condition of danger* The continued existence of B poses a threat to the life of A, a threat that can be met only by the taking of B's life.

2. *The condition of attempt* B is unjustly attempting to take A's life.

3. *The condition of guilt* B is responsible for his or her attempt to take A's life.[42]

Although it is always morally forbidden to kill B if no condition of danger exists, it is sometimes morally permissible to kill B even if no condition of guilt exists. For example, a police officer does no wrong when, in pursuit of an armed suspect, she or he shoots the suspect in self-defense, even if it is later revealed that the suspect was a crazed psychotic who mistook the officer for the Loch Ness monster.

There are also cases—for example, the following one described by Brody—when it is morally permissible to kill B even if no condition of attempt exists:

B is about to press a button that turns on a light, and there is no reason for him to suspect that his doing so will also explode a bomb that will destroy A. Moreover, the only way in which we can stop B and save A's life is by taking B's life, for there is no opportunity to warn B of the actual consequences of his act. In such a case, B is not attempting to take A's life and, thus, he is neither responsible for nor guilty of such an attempt. Nevertheless, this may still be a case in which there is justification for taking B's life in order to save A's life.[43]

To those who would protest that it is morally forbidden to kill B to save A, Brody replies that in cases of self-defense the only condition that always needs to be met over and beyond the condition of danger is something he calls "the condition of action": B is doing some action that will lead to A's death and that action is such that if B were a responsible person who did it voluntarily, knowing the consequences, B would be responsible for the loss of A's life.[44]

Brody's conditions (condition of danger plus condition of action) may or may not bolster Thomson's view that if any abortions are morally permissible, it is those that are performed to save the mother's life. Certainly, the condition of danger is met since the continued existence of the fetus poses a threat to the life of the mother, a threat that can be defused only by killing the fetus.

Far less certain is whether the condition of action is met. Some ethicists claim that merely by existing, the fetus is doing some action that will lead to its mother's death and that action is such that if the fetus were a responsible person who did it voluntarily, knowing the consequences, the fetus would be responsible for the loss of the mother's life. Other ethicists instead claim that existing does not count as an action; it is simply a state of being.

In any event, even if the fetus is not, by existing, engaging in the action of "pursuing" its mother, its life may still not count as much as its mother's. What determines the rightness and wrongness of an abortion decision is not only who has the most rights but also who has the most responsibilities and to whom. If a woman who already has 4 children will die or become seriously debilitated unless she has an abortion, then the fact that she is already enmeshed in a web of prior personal responsibilities should be taken into account. In some ways, her life belongs not only to her but also to the children who are dependent on her.

A final ethical matter to address as an addendum is the distinction between fetal extraction and fetal extinction. As many people see it, when a woman asks to have an abortion, she is requesting only that the fetus be removed from the body. Although she foresees that the fetus will die as a result of this procedure, her intention is to restore her bodily integrity and not to kill her fetus. The problems with this distinction, however, are twofold.

First, fetuses that would have died naturally on extraction 15 years ago (so called nonviable fetuses) are now able to survive owing to the ever-improving state of neonatal technology. When the Supreme Court decided *Roe* v. *Wade*, viability (the age at which fetuses can be expected to live outside the womb) was set at between 24 and 28 weeks. Today physicians are able to save fetuses as young as 22 weeks and weighing 500 grams (1.1 lb).[45] Thus, if killing the fetus is not the true intent behind a woman's decision to abort, other things being equal, we would expect her to request an abortion technique least likely to harm her *possibly* salvageable fetus.

Second, even if the point of viability were not being pushed back into the fifth month of pregnancy, the fact is that most women who seek abortions desire not only that the fetus be extracted but that it be killed. A pregnant woman who is a victim of rape or incest usually wants every reminder of the rape or incest to be destroyed, including the most conspicuous reminder, the fetus. Similarly, a pregnant woman who is not a victim of a violent sexual assault usually wants her fetus to be killed simply because she wants that chapter of her life to be expunged. The question, then, is whether a woman has a right not only to bodily integrity but also to kill her fetus. If it becomes possible to extract fetuses from the womb without extinguishing them, will women have the right to choose between life and death for their fetuses? Just how far does the right to privacy extend?

Legal Aspects of Abortion

General Legal Background

Because abortion is so hotly debated, it has presented legislators and judges with the formidable challenge of separating legal exigencies from ethical and social considerations. Recent technological advances in medical science have made this unenviable task even more difficult. Nevertheless, legislators and judges have worked toward the resolution of the abortion debate, specifically by developing three different paradigms for abortion legislation and adjudication.

The first paradigm forbids a woman to have an abortion unless her physical life is clearly and presently at risk. This antiabortion approach is usually justified in terms of a need to protect the interests of the unborn child, but it also has been justified in terms of a need to support population growth or, in the past, to reduce medical risk to pregnant women.[46]

The second paradigm permits a woman to have an abortion provided that at least 2 physicians and psychiatrists agree with her decision. The problem with this approach to abortion is that it invites the medical establishment to do one of two things: (1) to set up its own institutional principles and policies to guide physicians and psychiatrists through the abortion decision systematically and uniformly, or (2) to leave the abortion decision to the idiosyncratic judgments of individual physicians and psychiatrists. On the one hand, if the medical establishment devises its own rules to govern abortion decisions, we must question the appropriateness of delegating quasi-legislative and quasi-judicial authority to a group of experts none of whom are legislators or judges. Why should the American Medical Association (AMA) and the American Psychiatric Association (APA) determine abortion policy? Is this not a matter for the legislatures and courts? On the other hand, if the AMA and APA do not devise institutional positions on abortion, this second paradigm leaves the abortion decision to the idiosyncratic judgments of 2 or more physicians and psychiatrists who may be biased by their own value preferences. Though it avoids the problem of adding to the AMA's and APA's institutional power, this version of the second paradigm gives physicians and psychiatrists too much individual power. In either event, however, the medical establishment usurps not only the authority of the legislatures and the courts but also the autonomy of the women seeking abortions. If the abortion decision is anyone's to make, it seems that it should be the woman's.

The third paradigm, which is the reigning one, permits a woman to abort any *previable* fetus provided that the abortion is performed in a way that accords with the state's compelling interests in preserving maternal health. This approach to abortion permits a woman to make her own procreative choices without securing anyone's imprimatur, including that of the medical establishment, unless her fetus is viable.

Apparently, these modern abortion paradigms have medieval and even ancient points of reference. Although some early Christian thinkers insisted that *animation*, the moment when the soul supposedly enters the fetus's body, occurs at conception, most fourteenth- to sixteenth-century Christian thinkers set the point of animation at 40 days for male fetuses and at 80 days for female fetuses.[47] Later, English jurists reached the not unreasonable conclusion that animation occurs when the male or female fetus quickens, or moves in its mother's womb. From this belief arose the seventeenth- and eighteenth-century English common-law rule that since life begins at quickening (which usually takes place after the sixteenth week of pregnancy), abortion after quickening is a felony. But because it proved difficult, if not impossible, to determine whether a fetus had been aborted after or before its quickening, when English common law gave way to statutory law in the early nineteenth century, Parliament ruled that all abortions, prequickening as well as postquickening, were felonious.[48]

Until the middle of the nineteenth century, American abortion laws bore the clear imprint of their English counterparts. Distinctions were made between postquickening and prequickening abortions, and the penalties provided for the former were initially much higher than those provided for the latter. Of special interest, however, is the fact that pre–Civil War abortion legislation was aimed primarily at the practitioner, not the mother. Apparently, the number of "quacks" performing abortions was high, and something had to be done to prevent them from using dangerous "herbal abortifacients" on women.[49] The trend to punish the practitioner, not the mother, continued until approximately 1871 when the

AMA prompted no less than 36 states and territories to pass legislation aimed at the mother as well as the practitioner.[50] Having seen the sperm and the egg unite under their microscopes, many physicians concluded not only that truly human life begins at conception but also that the woman who has an abortion "overlooks the duties imposed on her by the marriage contract ... [yielding] to the pleasure, but [shrinking] from the pains and responsibilities of maternity."[51]

Although restrictive abortion laws were not uniformly enforced by the states, the sentiment in favor of them did not abate until the late 1960s. At that point, a series of events, including the refusal of some hospitals to abort thalidomide fetuses, an outbreak of fetus-deforming German measles, growing concerns about overpopulation, and the establishment of the National Organization for Women (NOW), convinced many people that some abortions were indeed morally justified. In 1962, the American Law Institute (ALI) proposed that all states decriminalize abortion performed (1) for therapeutic reasons such as the protection of the life or health of the mother; (2) for humane reasons such as the severely defective state of the fetus; and (3) for intensely personal reasons such as pregnancy due to rape or incest. Colorado, North Carolina, and California quickly enacted the ALI proposal into law. Shortly thereafter, New York passed a law permitting abortions on demand through the first and second trimesters of pregnancy.[52]

Not every state, however, moved in the direction of more permissive abortion laws. Some courts, legislatures, and citizens continued to insist that, no matter the circumstances, abortion is always wrong. As a result, some women had easy access to abortions, whereas others did not. The time had come to take the abortion issue out of the states hands and to determine whether the United States Constitution could force the states to achieve some parity in abortion legislation and adjudication.

Roe v. Wade (1973)

The case that determined the constitutionality or unconstitutionality of a variety of state abortion laws was *Roe* v. *Wade*. In a seven to two decision, the U.S. Supreme Court ruled that the right to privacy entails that:

1. During the first trimester of pregnancy, states may not enact laws to interfere with a woman's *and* physician's abortion decision.

2. During the second trimester of pregnancy, states may enact laws but only if such laws aim to preserve and protect maternal health.

3. During the third trimester of pregnancy, states may enact laws to protect the viable fetus, but only if such laws make exceptions for those instances in which the woman's life or health (physical or mental) are at risk.

4. States may not enact laws requiring all abortions to be performed in accredited hospitals, or to be approved by hospital committees or a second medical opinion, or to be performed only on state residents.[53]

Although many ethical, social, and legal commentators have praised the *Roe* v. *Wade* decision for giving women the kind of reproductive freedom they need to live life autonomously, others have criticized it for overemphasizing the right to privacy and for relying too heavily on viability as the point after which a fetus's life becomes more meaningful and worthy of preservation.

Lawyer John Hart Ely, for example, has objected that the *Roe* v. *Wade* Court came close to "using the word *privacy* to mean the freedom to live one's life without governmental interference."[54] As he sees it, the way to resolve the abortion dilemma is not by overemphasizing a woman's right to privacy, implying that she has the right to do as she pleases provided that she is able to keep it secret. Rather, it is to discover values that are situated not at the periphery but at the core of the Constitution, values that can help us balance a woman's interests against those of her fetus without playing a cruel zero-sum game in which either the mother wins or the fetus wins.[55]

The more crucial objection against *Roe* v. *Wade* is probably that viability is an increasingly useless criterion for distinguishing between fetuses who have a claim to life and those who do not. As neonatal medical technology and care have improved, the point of viability has shifted downward from approximately 28 weeks to 23 weeks. The primary obstacle to lowering the point of viability still more is that before 23 weeks or so the fetus's lungs are too immature to function even with respirator assistance.[56] Should scientists and technologists develop some sort of an artificial womb in the future, however, aborted fetuses could continue to develop their lungs ex utero. The abortion question would then be transformed into the question of whether a fetus, at a very early stage in development, has the right to be transferred from a natural to an artificial womb so that it can continue developing toward truly human life, or personhood.

Whatever the objections to *Roe* v. *Wade* and its companion case, *Doe* v. *Bolton*, may have been, these two cases ushered in an era that moved abortion from back alleys into hospitals and clinics. Indeed, it was *Doe* v. *Bolton* even more than *Roe* v. *Wade* that provided the momentum for this transition. In *Doe* v. *Bolton*, the plaintiffs challenged the constitutionality of a Georgia statute that required all abortions to be performed in hospitals. The Court struck down the statute by a vote of seven to two for several reasons, including the fact that Georgia had failed to demonstrate that the only safe place to perform an abortion, including a first-trimester abortion, was in a hospital.[57] The *Doe* decision is also significant because it permitted physicians to interpret the phrase *medically necessary abortion* broadly. In deciding whether their patients need an abortion, physicians may take into account *all* factors relevant to their patients' well-being, including age and familial circumstances as well as physical and psychological conditions.[58]

Post–*Roe* v. *Wade* Decisions

The two decades since *Roe* v. *Wade* and *Doe* v. *Bolton* have been marked by efforts to clarify the decisions' character and scope. Three issues have dominated legal debate during this period: funding restrictions, third-party consent or notification requirements, and procedural requirements.[59] Although *Roe* v. *Wade* and *Doe* v. *Bolton* initially withstood most of the challenges mounted against them, recent developments suggest that these landmark abortion decisions may yet be overturned.

Funding Restrictions

Immediately following the Court's decisions in *Roe* v. *Wade* and *Doe* v. *Bolton*, antiabortion groups began to exert pressure on all levels of the government, seeking restrictions on federal and state abortion fundings. By 1977, these efforts had met with some success. The Court's six to three decisions in *Maher* v. *Roe*[60] and *Beal* v. *Doe*[61] limited Medicaid benefits to include only those abortions that were "medically necessary" under the provisions outlined in *Doe* v. *Bolton*.

While *Maher* and *Beal* were being decided in the courts, a legislative battle was brewing over Representative Henry Hyde's (R-IL) proposed amendment to the Department of Health, Education, and Welfare's (DHEW's) Appropriations Act. Whereas the August 4, 1977, version of his amendment counted as medically necessary, and therefore Medicaid-fundable, only those abortions performed to save the life of the mother,[62] the modified August 26, 1978, version of his amendment also included as medically necessary those abortions "where severe and long-lasting physical health damage to the mother would result if the pregnancy were carried to term when so determined by the physician" and those performed on victims of rape or incest "when such rape or incest has been reported promptly to a law enforcement agency or public health service."[63]

Given that the Hyde Amendment was at odds with *Doe* v. *Bolton's* broad interpretation of what constitutes a medically necessary abortion, and given that the amendment was likely to affect not all pregnant women but only indigent women, critics immediately attacked it. One of the most provocative of these challenges was a New York suit, *McRae et al.* v. *Califano*, whose plaintiffs faulted the Hyde Amendment for four reasons.[64]

First, the *McRae* plaintiffs pointed out that Medicaid legislation mandates that all eligible patients receive an equal measure of medically necessary care. Whereas the *Maher* and *Beal* decisions allowed for all medically necessary abortions, the Hyde Amendment funded only certain kinds of medically necessary abortions—namely, those in which medical necessity jibes with a moral point of view according to which an abortion is necessary *only* when the pregnant woman's life is at stake, when her physical health will be permanently and severely damaged, or when the pregnancy is a result of rape or incest. Abortions motivated by a desire to limit family size or by a desire to abort a severely defective fetus lie outside this interpretation of medically necessary. The plaintiffs insisted that it is the task of physicians and not of moralists to decide what kinds of abortion are medically necessary; the Hyde Amendment transforms a medical determination into a legal one.[65]

Second, the *McRae* plaintiffs noted that, according to the Fifth and Fourteenth Amendments of the Constitution, the state may not single out for funding deletion a medically necessary procedure that only one group of people needs—in this case, pregnant, indigent women. People—be they male or female, rich or poor—who need medically necessary procedures are similarly situated with respect to their need for these procedures. To make funding deletions that have a variable impact on persons depending on their gender, race, or ethnic group is to fail to extend the equal protection of the law to all persons.[66]

Third, the *McRae* plaintiffs noted that the Hyde Amendment's vague wording made it difficult for physicians and pregnant women to determine when an abortion is, in fact, medically necessary. In the *McRae* suit, physicians testified that the Hyde Amendment's major criterion for medically necessary abortions was *life endangerment*, a term that is not "a common phrase" in "medical parlance."[67] By *medical necessity* physicians mean "all factors relevant to a person's well-being, not just physical facts predicting whether she will live or die."[68] In other words, as physicians see it, abortions may be medically necessary for any one of the following not necessarily life-endangering reasons: (1) physical reasons such as phlebitis, varicose veins, cancer, diabetes, myoma of the uterus, urinary tract infections, intrauterine device in utero, ulcerative colitis, previous cesarean sections, anemia, malnutrition, hyperemesis, and obesity; (2) psychological reasons such as stress; (3) humane reasons such as nonreported pregnancies due to rape or incest; (4) age reasons (teenage pregnancies); (5) familial reasons such as fetal abnormality; and (6) emotional reasons.[69] Moreover, even if physicians agreed to interpret the phrase *medically necessary abortion* to mean "life-threatening abortion," they would still find it extremely difficult to identify precisely which members of a high-risk group of patients will, in fact, succumb to the risk that threatens them. In other words, physicians cannot always predict when a pregnancy is actually going to be life-threatening for a particular woman who has diabetes or phlebitis, for example. Whereas one diabetic woman may nearly lose her life carrying a pregnancy to term, another may experience few difficulties.[70]

Fourth, and finally, the *McRae* plaintiffs argued that by depriving pregnant, indigent women of abortion funding, the Hyde Amendment served no secular purpose. Maternal health was not served by such a strategy, since carrying a pregnancy to term is actually more risky than having an abortion, especially a first-trimester abortion. Likewise, economic considerations were not served by such a strategy since abortions, especially first-trimester ones, are far less costly than carrying a pregnancy to term. Thus, if the Hyde Amendment was not serving a secular purpose, reasoned the *McRae* plaintiffs, it must be serving a nonsecular, even religious purpose, and because the First Amendment provides that "Congress shall make no law respecting the establishment of religion ...," the Hyde Amendment was very likely unconstitutional.[71]

Of all the attacks on the constitutionality of the Hyde Amendment, this last one was both the most novel and the most arguable. The fact that the Hyde Amendment served neither to safeguard maternal health nor to conserve state financial resources did not necessarily warrant the plaintiffs in *McRae* to conclude that it served *no* secular purposes whatsoever. Although many Catholics and other religious people supported the Hyde Amendment, so too did some non-Catholics and even some nonreligious people. Because debates about the status of the fetus are often as philosophical or political as they are theological, persons may have philosophical or political reasons rather than theological reasons for opposing the federal funding of Medicaid abortions. Be this as it may, during the 6-month debate before the Hyde Amendment's passage, the main arguments advanced for limiting federal funding of abortions were, as the *McRae* plaintiffs alleged, not philosophical or political but theological. For this reason, Judge H. Dooling, the presiding judge, chose to rule in favor of the plaintiffs. He observed that the mere fact that some nonreligious as well as some religious people believe that abortion is wrong does not automatically protect the Hyde Amendment from First Amendment challenges. If it did, no bill or amendment, except one obviously establishing a state church or one clearly eliminating freedom of worship, could be successfully challenged on First Amendment grounds.

Although the *McRae* plaintiffs convinced Judge Dooling that the Hyde Amendment was unconstitutional, the U.S. Supreme Court disagreed. In *Harris* v. *McRae* (1980), the Supreme Court ruled five to four that the Hyde Amendment was constitutional for four reasons. First, if the fact that some atheists lobbied for the Hyde Amendment does not make it a secular manifesto, then the fact that many religious persons also lobbied for it does not make it a religious manifesto. Otherwise, all bills and amendments would be subject to scrutiny depending on how many nonreligious or religious groups supported them in one way or another. Second, the fact that the Hyde Amendment does not fund abortions for poor women does not mean that it is violating the "due process" rights of these women. Although the state may decide to subsidize all medical procedures, it is not required to do so; and because "the Hyde Amendment leaves an indigent woman with at least the same range of choice in deciding whether to obtain a medically necessary abortion as she would have had if Congress had chosen to subsidize no health care costs at all,"[72] the Hyde Amendment does not deprive her of her constitutionally protected abortion rights. Third, although the "due process" clause ensures protection against state interference with freedom of choice, "it does not confer an entitlement to such funds as may be necessary to realize all the advantages of that freedom."[73] Only Congress has the power to decide whether a constitutionally recognized freedom warrants a federal subsidy. Fourth, and finally, the fact that the Hyde Amendment "makes childbirth a more attractive alternative than abortion for persons eligible for Medicaid"[74] is rationally related to the state's legitimate interest in protecting potential human life, an interest affirmed in *Roe* v. *Wade*.

Decidedly unimpressed by the Majority's reasoning in *Harris* v. *McRae*, the Minority of Justices (Brennan, Marshall, Stevens, and Blackmun) marshalled three arguments against it. First, both the intent and the effect of the Hyde Amendment is such as to "coerce indigent pregnant women to bear children that they would otherwise elect not to have."[75] Even if the state has no duty to ensure a woman access to an abortion, it has no right to make it all but impossible for her to secure one. Second, both the intent and the effect of the Hyde Amendment is to block not only all medically unnecessary abortions but also as many medically necessary abortions as possible. Third, and finally, if not in intent then in effect, the Hyde Amendment has a detrimental impact on only one segment of the female population—pregnant, indigent women, many of whom are also members of a minority race. Since the "discriminatory distribution of the benefits of government largess can discourage the exercise of fundamental liberties just as effectively as can outright denial of those rights through criminal and regulatory sanctions,"[76] the Hyde Amendment ought to be ruled unconstitutional.

Consent and Notification Provisions

In addition to public-funding restrictions on abortions—restrictions that are more the rule than the exception today—antiabortion activists have favored consent and notification provisions as a means to limit women's reproductive freedom. The benign intent of this kind of legislation is to involve interested third parties (parents and spouses) in a woman's abortion decision so that she will have the benefit of their wisdom; the less benign intent of this legislation is to open up the woman's psyche to the kind of pressures only family members and friends can exert. To date, this type of legislation has been ruled unconstitutional in one form only to be ruled constitutional in a slightly different form.

Planned Parenthood of Central Missouri v. Danforth (1976)
In a six to three vote, the Supreme Court invalidated a Missouri statute that gave husbands veto power over their pregnant wives' decision to abort their pregnancies and, in a five to three vote, it also invalidated a Missouri statute that said parents of minor, unwed girls could be given an absolute veto over abortions.[77] Apparently, the Court's reasoning was that neither a genetic father's interest in his wife's abortion decision nor a genetic grandparent's interest in his or her daughter's abortion decision is strong enough to override a woman's or girl's right to make her own decision about abortion during the first and second trimesters of her pregnancy. Among other matters, what the Court left open to question was whether a state could require physicians to notify spouses or parents about their wives' or daughters' plans to have an abortion and whether a state could require more than parental notification in the case of minor daughters who are not able to give informed consent to an abortion.

Belloti v. Baird, H. L. v. Matheson and the "Akron Ordinances"
Because the *Danforth* decision left open several matters about consent and notification legislation, antiabortionists found the requisite legal loopholes

through which to string new legislation that finally did limit the reproductive freedom of minor girls' though not of adult women. In the 1979 case, *Belloti* v. *Baird*, the Court voted eight to one that parental *consent* statutes are permissible provided that the state provides an alternative procedure, such as letting the minor girl seek judicial consent for her abortion.[78] Cheered by this decision, antiabortionists believed that they would have a relatively easy time securing court support for notification legislation. To their surprise, lower courts did not immediately endorse the view that notifying a parent, let alone a spouse, about an impending abortion is always an innocuous, and even potentially beneficial, communication of information.

As most lower courts saw it, a woman's moral duty to discuss an abortion decision with the fetus's genetic father is not a matter for legislation. After all, the woman may be a victim of rape or incest, in a very unhappy marriage, or an adulteress. Similarly, a child's moral duty to discuss an abortion decision with her parents is not a matter for legislation. Even if most parents have the best interests of their children at heart, some of them do not. Given that parent-child relationships vary from the blissful to the abysmal, "the ameliorative qualities of a third person's wisdom and experience" in a child's abortion decision is "uncertain."[79]

But even if the lower courts were unfavorably disposed to both spousal and parental notification statutes, the Supreme Court was not. In *H.L.* v. *Matheson* (1981), the Court ruled six to three that states may require parental notification if the minor girl seeking an abortion is still dependent on her parents and too "immature" to decide such a matter for herself.[80] But even in the kind of case the Court had in mind, say that of an 11-year-old pregnant girl, states must still provide a judicial alternative to parental notification and consent.

Even more recently, in *Hodgson* v. *Minnesota* (1990), the Court ruled five to four to uphold a Minnesota law requiring unwed teenagers to notify both parents before having an abortion, provided the law allows the teenager to go to a judge instead. The Court also upheld in a six to three vote an Ohio law that requires physicians to notify one parent of a pregnant minor of the girl's intent to have an abortion. This law also provides for judicial bypass.[81]

Whether it is correct for the Court to limit the reproductive freedom of very young girls in this way continues to be a matter of much debate. On the one hand, there is the argument that parents have a right to be involved in their children's decisions, especially momentous ones such as the abortion decision. Many parents plead to be notified about their daughters' impending abortion not because they want to make things difficult for their daughters but because they want to support them with every financial and emotional resource available. On the other hand, there is the argument that parents do not have a *right* to be involved in their children's decisions; at most, they have an *interest* in being involved, an interest that must be balanced against the children's right to make their own decisions. Only if it can be proved that a child is not autonomous should parents have a say in her abortion decision and then only if it can be proved that their parental interests coincide with their child's best interest.

However successful antiabortion legislation may have been with respect to parental notification or consent legislation, it has been decidedly unsuccessful with respect to spousal notification or consent legislation. In general, adult women are able to give informed consent to abortion; they do not need their husbands to make this momentous decision for them. Antiabortionists concede that, in principle, women are able to give informed consent, but they have argued that women are sometimes deprived of the information they need to give informed consent. In the early 1980s, for example, Akron, Ohio's municipal government enacted a set of ordinances, later referred to as the *Akron Ordinances*, that put physicians under the affirmative obligation to inform patients that truly human life, or personhood, begins at conception.[82] Inspired by Akron's actions, other municipal governments enacted their own Akron Ordinances, going so far as to require physicians to show their patients pictures of the about-to-be-aborted fetus.

Although informed consent is assuredly in the best interests of any patient, many courts came to the conclusion that the intent of so-called Akron Ordinances was not so much to provide women with factual information about fetal development and abortion as to interpret for women the significance of this information in order to convince them that abortion is murder. The obligation of physicians is to inform their pregnant patients about the major physical and psychological risks of carrying a fetus to term, on the one hand, and aborting a fetus, on the other. It is not also the obligation of physicians to convince their pregnant patients that fetuses are persons. Not only is it debatable whether a fetus is a person; it is also debatable whether a woman who is forced to focus on the most physically painful and psychologically distressing aspects of abortion will be in a position to give her informed consent to it.

Currently, the consensus of the courts is that physicians are under no legal obligation to instruct their pregnant patients as to the moral status of the fetus. Indeed, according to the 1986 Supreme Court decision *Thornburgh* v. *American College of Obstetricians and Gynecologists*, physicians are not even required to inform women seeking abortions about available benefits for prenatal care and childbirth.[83] However, this does not mean that pregnant women seeking abortions can demand some right to moral insulation; in other words, pregnant women seeking abortions may have to withstand orderly picketers and chanting, for example. Part of the price of living in a pluralistic society is having to listen to people with whom one disagrees.

Procedural Issues

In addition to focusing on consent and notification issues, antiabortionists have also focused on procedural issues, especially the state's interest in regulating the time, place, and method of abortion from the second trimester on, and the state's interest in protecting viable fetal life. At first, these procedural attacks on *Roe* v. *Wade* were unsuccessful. In three 1983 decisions, *City of Akron* v. *Akron Center for Reproductive Health*,[84] *Planned Parenthood Association of Kansas City* v. *Ashcroft*,[85] and *Simopolous* v. *Virginia*,[86] the Court said that states may not require that all second- or third-trimester abortions be performed in a hospital. The Court also struck down regulations that imposed not only a 24-hour waiting period between the signing of the abortion consent form and the abortion itself but also blanket restrictions on the method of abortion that could be performed after viability.

The fact that the Court ruled as unconstitutional blanket restrictions on certain abortion methods is of special significance. Antiabortionists wanted to ban the use of abortion methods that would certainly kill the viable fetus. What the Court decided was that such a ban could put physicians in the untenable position of failing to serve the best interests of their patients (i.e., the women seeking abortions). For example, the abortion method most likely to preserve the life of a viable fetus may be the prostaglandin method, whereas the abortion method most likely to preserve the life and health of the mother may be saline amniocentesis, which is fatal to the fetus. Given this state of affairs, it seems that the physician's duty is to use saline amniocentesis because she or he cannot serve 2 patients at once, and it is debatable whether the viable fetus is his or her patient at all.

But what if the physician realizes that in the case of a certain woman, saline amniocentesis or the prostaglandin method would be equally acceptable? Should there be laws to the effect that, provided the woman's health and life is in no way jeopardized, the physician should employ that method of abortion most likely to preserve the life and health of the viable fetus? At least two arguments were brought against such laws in the mid-1980s.

First, it is unclear who is to decide whether a given fetus has attained viability—the attending physician in the good-faith exercise of his or her medical judgment or a prosecutor and jury in the course of a criminal proceeding. Second, and more problematically, it is unclear how the medical profession, and the public at large, are to construe abortion. Is it simply a matter of wanting to remove the fetus from a woman's uterus, or is it actually a matter of wanting to destroy the fetus? If fetal extraction is the goal of abortion, then physicians should use whatever abortion technique maximizes the survival chances of a possibly viable fetus if that technique does not increase the risks to the mother. For example, physicians should use the prostaglandin method (as opposed to saline amniocentesis) for second-trimester and early third-trimester abortions since this method of abortion constitutes the least direct danger to the fetus. But if, as is far more likely, fetal extinction is the goal of the abortion, then physicians should, if at all possible, use an abortion technique that guarantees the death of the fetus. Using an abortion technique expressly calculated to save the fetus would certainly traumatize a woman who does not want to give birth to a live child.

What is likely to traumatize a woman seeking an abortion to an equal if not greater degree, however, is the fact that the Supreme Court ruled in *Webster* v. *Reproductive Health Services* (1989) that states may demand physicians to perform viability tests on any fetus at least 20 weeks old. If these tests indicate that the fetus is indeed viable, then the state's interest in protecting the life of that fetus is compelling enough to prevent its mother from aborting it unless her life is at risk.[87]

Another front on which antiabortionists have had some success is that of "institutional conscience." Antiabortionists argue that hospitals have a right to refuse to perform certain kinds of medical procedures and that reasons of conscience as well as fiscal reasons are adequate for such refusals. However, it is not clear that institutions can really have consciences. Opponents argue that it is one thing to say that no person should be coerced, held liable, or discriminated against in any manner because of a conscientious refusal to perform, accommodate, or assist in an abortion, and it is quite another thing to say that hospitals have the same right. Nevertheless, the courts have been sympathetic to the argument that private, sectarian hospitals (for example, Catholic hospitals) can have an institutional conscience that says no to abortion for religious reasons.

In the past, the fact that some private, sectarian hospitals refused to perform abortions did not seriously interfere with women's access to safe abortion facilities.[88] There were still plenty of public hospitals and clinics as well as private, nonsectarian hospitals, clinics, and individual physicians that offered abortion services. But this is changing. In *Webster* v. *Reproductive Health Services*, the Court ruled that states may require that (1) public health care facilities not be used for performing medically unnecessary postviability abortions and (2) public health care providers not perform or assist at medically unnecessary postviability abortions.[89] Conceivably, a woman who wants an abortion could still secure one at a private, nonsectarian hospital or clinic, but because many of these hospitals and clinics receive public money or have contractual arrangements with state or local governments, they might fall under the *Webster* ruling. Moreover, even if a private, nonsectarian clinic is not dependent on public monies, it operates under public health and safety regulations. *Turnock* v. *Ragsdale* challenged the Illinois statute that clinics must maintain the same standards as hospitals. If this statute were in effect, many clinics may have had to close, and since approximately 60 percent of abortions are performed in clinics, this could have severely limited the ability of women to secure abortions. The Supreme Court ruling upheld a lower court's injunction against the statute[90] and the feared closings did not take place.

A final procedural ploy to limit abortions consists of attempts to limit the dispersal of abortion information. In May 1991, the Supreme Court ruled that anyone who works in one of 4,000 federally funded family planning clinics must conceal from the women who use them any information about their right to abortion. Writing for the majority, Chief Justice William Rehnquist based his opinion on Section 1008 at Title X of the Public Health Service Act, which says that "none of the funds appropriated under this subchapter shall be used in programs where abortion is a method of family planning."[91] Critics of the Court's ruling observe that it is one matter to interpret Title X to mean that federally funded clinics must not perform or advocate abortions and another to interpret it to mean that clinic physicians, for example, may not explain the abortion option to their pregnant patients or refer them to physicians outside the clinic who perform abortions, even when their patients request such referrals. To "gag" clinic physicians and other clinic employees, they maintain, is to violate their First Amendment right to free speech. Defenders of the Court's ruling maintain that the new rules are not meant to inhibit any physician's point of view but to promote the government's "value judgment favoring childbirth over abortion."[92] If a clinic does not share this value judgment, it can refuse federal monies and provide as much abortion information as it chooses. The problem with this solution to a clinic's dilemma is that, if it needs federal monies to operate, it will collapse and the women it serves (usually indigent women) will be deprived of important health services.

Undoing *Roe* v. *Wade*

Webster v. *Reproductive Health Services*, alluded to earlier, represents the greatest erosion of *Roe* v. *Wade* to date. This 1989 Supreme Court decision upheld a Missouri law that restricted abortion in three ways. It said: (1) that public hospitals or other tax-supported facilities may not be used for performing abortions not necessary to save the mother's life; (2) that public employees may not assist an abortion not necessary to save the mother's life; and (3) that medical tests must be performed to determine the viability of any fetus believed to be at least 20 weeks old.[93]

Of all of those provisions, the third is probably the most significant. When *Roe* v. *Wade* was decided in 1973, fetal viability was believed to occur in the third trimester of pregnancy (sometime around the twenty-eighth week or so). States were not permitted to restrict abortions in any way except to preserve maternal health prior to fetal viability. Since 1973, however, fetal viability has been pushed back into the second trimester. Twenty-three weeks is now considered the point of fetal viability, and the Supreme Court apparently is no longer willing to uphold what Chief Justice Rehnquist has termed the *rigid trimester analysis* of *Roe* v. *Wade*.[94] Viability is what counts and not length of pregnancy. The significance of abandoning the trimester system in favor of viability is that it permits states the freedom to ban or restrict second-trimester as well as third-trimester abortions.

Since *Webster*, a number of states have either proposed or passed laws banning virtually all abortions, including those in the first and second trimesters as well as the third trimester. Idaho passed a bill that would have permitted an abortion only if a woman's life was imperiled, if an incest victim was younger than 18, or if a rape was reported to the police within 7 days (when the rape victim would not yet know whether she was pregnant), but Governor Cecil Andrus vetoed the bill largely because of its restrictions on abortions due to rape or incest.[95] More recently, Louisiana passed a bill much like the Idaho bill except that it goes further: A physician can be sentenced to a minimum of 1 year at hard labor and be fined $10,000 for performing an abortion, and a woman can be charged as an accessory to his crime. Governor Roemer's veto of this bill was overridden by a majority of the Louisiana State Legislature.

Although pro-choice forces believe that Louisiana's law will ultimately be declared unconstitutional, they are worried that less restrictive versions may still pass. Over the next few years or so, an increasing number of states might seek to limit women's access to abortion.

Social Dimensions of Abortion

As abortion has presented legal scholars and ethicists with many intractable problems, it has also led to interminable conflict among social forces. While pro-choice and pro-life forces continue to pit the rights to privacy and bodily integrity against the right to life, some concerned men's groups as well as women's organizations and minority caucuses are looking for new ways to reconceptualize these old arguments. Clearly, we need to rethink the abortion issue if we ever expect to free ourselves from its socially harmful consequences.

Liberals and Conservatives on Abortion

In general, people who identify themselves as pro-choice are liberals who espouse the principles of pluralism, a philosophy that "was formulated to enable individuals and groups to coexist in society despite deep-seated differences on fundamental matters of religion, morality, and conscience."[96] Convinced that the Constitution protects freedom of choice, pro-choice activists argue that society must accept people's individual choices, including women's abortion choices, even when these choices fail to reflect majoritarian views. People who identify themselves as pro-life argue that there are some individual choices that no decent society can accept and that the choice to kill innocent human life is among these unacceptable choices. In general, people who identify themselves as pro-life tend to be conservatives who believe that unless the state preserves majoritarian values, American society will disintegrate into chaos. As these pro-life activists see it, pro-choice activists use the rhetoric of freedom of choice to disguise the fact that great numbers of self-indulgent women are killing their babies.[97]

By closely attending to the rhetoric and structure of the abortion debate, we begin to see how deep the ideological chasm is between pro-life and pro-choice advocates. According to Randall Lake, whereas the anti-choice position favors deontological over teleological argumentation, the pro-choice position favors teleological over deontological argumentation.[98] In deontological ethics, persons are required to perform certain duties whether or not performing these duties brings happiness to them or anyone else. As pro-lifers see it, the unique advantage of deontological ethics is that it "counteract[s] the urge to place one's self-interest first."[99] Supposedly, when a woman is tempted to abort her fetus on the grounds that she is unready, unwilling, or unable to carry it to term, the imperatives of duty will help her see that her unreadiness, unwillingness, and inability might simply be convenient excuses for a very selfish act.

In contrast to the deontological approach to abortion, the teleological approach to abortion does stress personal or collective happiness. As pro-choice advocates see it, there are particular goals that persons seek for themselves or their families and friends. When a woman is about to make an abortion decision, she should ask herself whether aborting her fetus will bring her closer to or further from these particular goals. If a system of teleological ethics is egoist (focused exclusively on the individual's self-interest), then a pregnant woman seeking an abortion is permitted, even required, to place her own self-interest first; but if a system of teleological ethics is utilitarian (focused on the aggregate's collective interests), then a pregnant woman seeking an abortion is required to consider other people's interests as being as important as her own self-interest. In either event, however, the woman will be asking herself questions such as, "Will aborting this fetus bring about more *happiness* for me (alternatively, for all considered)?" She will not be asking herself whether she has a *duty* not to abort (alternatively, a duty to abort).

Were the abortion debate not as heated as it is, pro-life advocates might ask themselves whether the rules they are following are perhaps too rigid. If they adhere to the rule that life must be preserved at all costs, then this rule has as many implications for the end of life as for the beginning. Hence, for example, if a pro-life activist wants to save the life of an anencephalic fetus, then she or he must also want to save the life of an 80-year-old brain-dead woman. Admittedly, some pro-life advocates would insist that life is life and that it is wrong for human beings to make any judgments about the quality of any life. All life, even brain-dead and anencephalic life, must be preserved. Other pro-life advocates, however, are less absolutistic and are not eager to save the lives of human beings who are experiencing nothing at all or merely pain.

Similarly, if the abortion debate were not as heated as it is, pro-choice advocates might ask themselves whether the rights they are proclaiming are truly rights. Although a pro-choice activist might feel comfortable justifying a woman's decision to abort a fetus afflicted with Down's syndrome or spina bifida, she or he might have a difficult time justifying a woman's decision to abort a fetus solely on account of its gender. Indeed, confronted with this last possibility, the pro-choice person might simply deny that any uncoerced, reasonable woman would choose to abort a fetus solely on account of its gender. Comments Frances Kissling, president of Catholics for a Free Choice in Washington, DC:

... the notions that women would seek abortions in the mid to late second trimester because the nursery is painted blue or hubby's family has had firstborn boys for generations is ludicrous. It really deserves no response. It also deserves no defense. I would seek no laws to prevent that which does not happen, but I would not oppose such laws. This is an area for self-regulation, and one hopes that responsible providers of abortion would decline their services in such cases.[100]

In a similar vein, although a pro-choice advocate might ardently defend a cocaine-addicted teenager's choice to abort a first-trimester fetus that she cannot raise, she or he might refuse to endorse a wealthy woman's choice to abort a third-trimester fetus that she has come to view as an inconvenience.

Unfortunately, the abortion debate *is* as heated as it is, and because deep passions are flaring, the two sides of the abortion debate are unable to see just how confused they both are. In a recent poll, the citizens of Los Angeles revealed just how ambivalent they are about abortion. Sixty-one percent of those polled said abortion is morally wrong, whereas 57 percent of them said abortion should remain a woman's decision. The statistics became more inconsistent when pollsters raised questions about rape, incest, and parental authority.[101]

Unless their hot passions are brought under reason's cool control, people will be unable to sort through their conflicting feelings about abortion. And until states have some clear sense of where majority sentiment really rests, they will continue to play it safe, tending to experiment with restrictive rather than permissive abortion legislation.

Interestingly, and as a side point, not only will women's rights and well-being be thereby threatened; so too will researchers' rights and society's well-being. Since most of the fetal tissue used in organ transplantation and research is gained through abortions, fetal-tissue transplantation and research are fraught with many of the same questions that the abortion debate poses. Researchers are asked to weigh the life, dignity, and comfort of the fetus against the life, dignity, and comfort of others, and the same pro-life groups that oppose abortion also oppose the use of aborted fetuses for organ transplants and tissue research.[102] As they see it, researchers who use aborted fetuses for these purportedly noble ends are nonetheless complicit in an immoral act, and their complicity will have the effect of legitimating and even encouraging abortion.[103]

Women's, Minorities', and Men's Attitudes Toward Abortion

Many women, especially women who identify themselves as feminists, believe that the abortion debate should not center around the question of whether fetuses are the moral equivalent of born human beings but around the fact that fertilized eggs develop into infants inside the bodies of women. Writes Ellen Willis:

Pregnancy and birth are active processes in which a woman's body shelters, nourishes, and expels a new life; for nine months she is immersed in the most intimate possible relationship with another being. The growing fetus makes considerable demands on her physical and emotional resources, culminating in the cataclysmic experience of birth. And childbearing has unpredictable consequences; it always entails some risk of injury or death.[104]

A mother herself, Willis argues that as a result of her experiences during pregnancy and childbirth, the key question in the abortion debate should be, "Can it be moral, under any circumstances, to make a woman bear a child against her will?"[105] If women are ever to have the same degree of autonomy as men have, says Willis, they must have the power to say no to potential life.

In recent years, women have been especially worried that increased concern about fetal life will lead to decreased interest in women's rights. Particular interest has been paid to cases such as that of Marla Pitchford. While a student at Western Kentucky University, Pitchford became pregnant early in 1978. She discussed the situation with her boyfriend, also a student and, because he did not want the child, they decided to go to an abortion clinic (their funds were very limited). However, Pitchford had by now entered her twenty-fourth week of pregnancy, and Kentucky had a statute allowing only licensed physicians to perform an abortion after the eighteenth week. The clinics Pitchford and her boyfriend approached did not have a licensed physician on staff, and so they began to panic. In desperation, Pitchford attempted a self-induced abortion by inserting a knitting needle into her womb. She ended up in the hospital where she delivered a dead fetus together with the knitting needle. Charges were brought against Pitchford for violation of the Kentucky statute, which, by the way, had been created to protect women from dangerous abortions. Although Pitchford could have received a sentence of anywhere from 10 to 20 years, she was acquitted by reason of insanity. Pitchford claimed at the trial, "I just wasn't thinking rationally ... I felt like dying.'[106]

The Pitchford case is particularly significant in light of the fact that drugs such as RU 486 facilitate self-abortion. Unlike other morning-after pills, which must be taken immediately after having sexual intercourse, Ru 486 can be taken up to 10 days after a missed period to induce menstruation and terminate a possible pregnancy. Preliminary testing has also shown it to have fewer side effects than other similar drugs. On the one hand, many pro-choice groups see RU 486 as a great advance in the freedom of women to choose what to do with their bodies. Putting RU 486 on the market would allow women to decide freely, without societal pressures, whether they wish to be pregnant. On the other hand, many pro-life groups claim that RU 486, especially when it is described as a contra-gestion pill rather than an abortion pill, will encourage a careless and morally unreflective use of the pill to terminate pregnancy.[107]

RU 486, widely available in France, has been approved for use in other European countries but has not yet been marketed in them. It is also undergoing clinical trials in the United States as well as in several developing countries. No wonder that pro-life advocates feel driven to support legislation assigning the same moral and legal rights to concepti, embryos, and fetuses as is assigned to adult persons. If such legislation succeeds, however, women who seek abortions either will have illegal abortions—at best by securing RU 486 on the black market, at worst by submitting their bodies to back-alley abortionists—or they will carry to term their unwanted pregnancies (assuming that medical science is not able to create and provide artificial wombs for unwanted concepti, embryos, and fetuses). As pro-choice advocates see it, even if this leads to increased respect for fetal life, it will not lead to increased respect for adult women's lives. In fact, it may lead to women being viewed as fetal containers.

In the same way that we can appreciate why pro-life advocates react so vehemently to RU 486 (its use may transform the decision to abort a fetus into something of minimal importance), we can also appreciate why pro-choice advocates react so strongly to women's loss of control over their own bodies (such an attitude toward women threatens to reinforce old stereotypes of women as mere sex objects or reproductive machines). It is not surprising, then, that many women's groups are once again asserting that women's rights must be honored at all cost.

Interestingly, not everyone is convinced that either women in particular or society in general will be well served by emphasizing women's rights, or anyone's rights for that matter. For example, political theorist Wendy Brown regrets that so much pro-choice rhetoric is phrased in what she terms the "protective," "defensive," and "isolating" language of rights, a language that suggests that if I have a right to something, my right will eventually and inevitably come into conflict with your right to the same thing or to something else.[108] The rhetoric of rights pits the right to choose against the right to life. However, the real question is not whose right is most fundamental, the woman's or the fetus's. Rather, the real question is whether a woman and those to whom she is related should bring a new life into their midst if they do not know whether that life can survive, let alone thrive there.

We are reminded here of psychologist Carol Gilligan's work. In the process of listening to what each of 29 women had to say about her decision to abort or not to abort her fetus, what Gilligan discovered was that no matter their age, social class, marital status, or ethnic background, all these women had a conception of the self different from that of the typical man. Whereas men tend to see the self as an autonomous, separate being, women tend to view the self as an interdependent being whose identity depends on others. These different views of the self, says Gilligan, account for at least four emphatic differences between the way in which men and women make moral decisions.

First, women tend to stress the moral agent's continuing relationships to others, whereas men tend to stress the agent's formal, abstract rights. Thus, the typical woman is prepared to forsake some of her rights if she can thereby cement a faltering, but extremely meaningful, human relationship. Second, when making a moral decision, women espouse a somewhat more consequential point of view, calculating the effects of the moral agent's action on all who will be touched by it, whereas men espouse a somewhat more nonconsequentialist point of view, according to which principles must be upheld even if some people get hurt in the process. Third, women are usually more willing to accept excuses for a moral agent's behavior, whereas men generally label behavior as morally inexcusable just because it is morally unjustifiable. (To *excuse* an act is to point to extenuating circumstances that mitigate its wrongness; to *justify* an act is to articulate reasons for its rightness.) Finally, women usually interpret a moral choice within the context of the historical circumstances that produced it, whereas men usually abstract that choice from its particularities and analyze it as if it represented some universal type of moral choice.

Gilligan best illustrates this point when discussing male and female responses to Lawrence Kohlberg's famous example of a moral dilemma in which Heinz cannot afford the drug his dying wife desperately needs to survive. Should he steal the drug or not? When presented with this problem, says Gilligan, boys approach it analytically as if they were solving a math problem. For example, a boy named Jake solves Heinz's dilemma by weighing the rights of the pharmacist to receive payment for his property against the rights of the wife to live: "A human life is worth more than money, and if the druggist only makes $1,000, he is still going to live, but if Heinz doesn't steal the drug, his wife is going to die."[109] In contrast, claims Gilligan, girls presented with this same problem approach it synthetically, as if they were resolving a human relations problem. For example, a girl named Amy urges Heinz to arrange a "heart-to-heart" talked with the druggist. She reasons that if the druggist knew that Heinz's wife will otherwise die, he would willingly give the drug to Heinz.[110] Gilligan's point in comparing responses such as those of Jake and Amy is not to devalue Jake's way of handling Heinz's dilemma; rather it is to show that although Amy and Jake handle Heinz's dilemma differently, Amy's mode of moral reasoning is just as valid.

Because Gilligan believes that women's style of moral reasoning diverges in several important ways from that of men, she rejects Kohlberg's scale of moral development as a universal standard on which to evaluate both men's and women's moral progress. Kohlberg's scale consists of six stages through which a person must pass if he or she is to become a fully functioning moral agent. Stage one is "the punishment and obedience orientation," wherein the child does as he or she is told. Stage two is "the instrumental relativist orientation": Based on a limited principle of reciprocity ("you scratch my back and I'll scratch yours"), the child does what satisfies his or her own needs and, occasionally, the needs of others. Stage three is "the interpersonal concordance or 'good boy–nice girl' orientation": The adolescent begins to do his or her duty, show respect for authority, and maintain the given social order for its own sake. Stage four is the "law and order orientation." Stage five is "the social-contract legalistic orientation," wherein the adult adopts an essentially utilitarian moral point of view according to which individuals are permitted to do as they please, provided that they refrain from harming people in the process. Stage six is "the universal ethical principle orientation": The adult adopts an essentially Kantian moral point of view that provides a moral perspective universal enough to serve as a critique of any conventional morality, including that of the United States. The adult is no longer ruled by self-interest, the opinion of others, or the force of legal convention, but by self-legislated and self-imposed universal principles, such as those of justice, reciprocity, and respect for the dignity of human beings as individual persons.[111]

Gilligan takes exception to Kohlberg's sixfold scale not because it reflects an immoral or amoral position, but because girls and women tested on it rarely get past stage three. As Gilligan sees it, women's low scores on Kohlberg's test have little to do with any deficiency in their ability to reason morally and much to do with the construction of Kohlberg's scale, a scale for which Gilligan has an alternative that, in her opinion, more adequately represents women's approach to moral reasoning. For Kohlberg, the moral self is an individual legislating absolute laws for everyone without exception. In contrast, for Gilligan, the moral self is an individual working with other individuals to identify mutually agreeable solutions to thorny human relations problems. Whereas Gilligan describes Kohlberg's "male" moral point of view as an ethics of justice, she describes her "female" moral point of view as an ethics of care. Gilligan believes that woman's moral development takes her from an egocentric, or selfish, position to an overly altruistic, or self-sacrificial, position and, finally, to a self-with-others position in which her interests count as much as anyone else's.

At level one, the least-developed level of moral sensibility, a woman's care is directed completely inward. She feels scared and vulnerable, in need of affection and approval. For example, the women in Gilligan's abortion study who felt alone in the world, helpless, and uncared for saw a baby as someone who would care for them, who would give them some love. However, as these women struggled through their abortion decisions, many came to describe as "selfish" the decision to bring a child into the world without having the material and psychological resources to care for him or her. In Gilligan's estimation, for a woman to come to this kind of conclusion is to reach level two of moral development.

At level two, a woman shifts from self-centeredness to other-directedness. She becomes the stereotypical nurturant woman, who subjugates her wants and needs to those of other people's and who claims that all she wants to do is what the other person wants. This is the kind of woman who, in Gilligan's study, would have her lover, husband, parents, or church tell her whether to have an abortion. According to Gilligan, a woman can suppress her wants and needs in the interest of sustaining a relationship for only so long before she starts feeling resentful. Thus, to develop as a moral person, a woman must take steps to avoid this destructive boiling point. She must, insists Gilligan, push beyond level two or three of moral development, where she will learn how to care for herself as well as others.

At level three, the decision to abort, for example, becomes a complex choice the woman must make about how best to care for the fetus, herself, and anyone likely to be affected by her decision. One of the women in Gilligan's study explained her decision to have an abortion as just such a choice: "I would not be doing myself or the child or the world any kind of favor having this child. I don't need to pay off my imaginary debts to the world through this child, and I don't think that it is right to bring a child into the world and use it for that purpose."[112] Thus, in Gilligan's view, a woman attains full moral stature when she stops vacillating between egoism and altruism, recognizing instead the falseness of this polarity and the depth of her connection to others and of their connection to her.

If Gilligan's understanding of women's moral development is correct, the abortion decision is always a traumatic one for a woman. As she goes about deciding whether to have an abortion, a woman is less likely to be thinking about her right to choose and more likely to be thinking about the life that she cannot, and perhaps must not, bring into the world. Paradoxically, the *Roe* v. *Wade* decision made it possible for many women to admit that whether or not it is their right to choose, abortion is not a choice that most women want to make. There is simply too much that is special about women's "unique capacity for gestation and birth, for transforming potential life into actual life"[113] to give it up without anguish. Regrettably, the time for such honest confessions may be coming to an end. The *Webster* decision is one that has apparently forced some women once again to use the protective, defensive, and isolating language of rights; to speak as if women's interests were somehow separate from the interests of the other actual or potential people to whom they are intimately related. Despite all that has happened, however, it may still not be too late for both pro-life and pro-choice advocates to learn new ways to speak to one another about what matters most to them. They may discover that they have more in common than the polemics of the abortion debate have led them to believe. Minimally, they all probably want to create a world in which women do not need abortions because they have good jobs, supportive families, adequate child-care facilities, and access to safe, effective, inexpensive, and aesthetically pleasing contraceptives. Pro-choice advocates need to remember that the first pro-life groups were not political groups (and certainly not terrorist groups) but service groups. Currently, there are at least 3000 emergency pregnancy centers in the United States, 20 percent of which offer not merely counseling and emergency funds to pregnant women but also hospital coverage, housing, job training, and postnatal care. Such services give disadvantaged women the opportunity to choose to continue their pregnancies, a choice that is no less significant than its opposite. Likewise, pro-life advocates need to realize that pro-choice supporters are not selfish, heartless baby-killers. On the contrary, many people who are pro-choice describe themselves as "schizophrenic" when it comes to the abortion decision: Although they do not want the state to interfere with a woman's decision to have an abortion, they do not want women to make that decision without recognizing all the values that are at stake.

Finally, no discussion of abortion would be complete without attending to the role men should or should not play in a woman's decision to abort. Carol Gilligan's study on abortion has been faulted precisely because she did not interview the 29 men who had obviously played a role in the pregnancies of the 29 women she did interview. What were these men's attitudes toward their girlfriends' and wives' abortion decisions? Were the men more or less inclined than the women to choose abortion over pregnancy? Did they view the women's abortion decisions as decisions that should have been made jointly with them? Finally, did they support or abandon the women during the abortion procedure or continuing pregnancy? Why or why not?

For a variety of reasons, men's role in the abortion decision is controversial. Pro-choice advocates fear that if any concession is made in the direction of saying that men have a moral right to participate in women's abortion decisions, then spousal notification and consent laws will become the order of the day. These people may be right, and yet because procreation is an activity that involves men as well as women, we may be obliged to admit that, ideally, men and women should make abortion as well as contraception and sterilization decisions together.

In a recent *Time* magazine article, parents were asked what advice they would give their teenage daughter if she became pregnant. Fourteen percent responded, "Marry the father"; 22 percent said, "Raise the child alone"; 15 percent said, "Give the child up for adoption"; and 11 percent said, "Get an abortion." Asked what advice they would give their teenage son if he impregnated someone, these same parents replied as follows: 20 percent responded, "Marry the mother"; 7 percent said, "Help pay for an abortion"; 52 percent said, "Help pay for medical expenses and child support"; and 1 percent said, "Try to get out of the situation."[114] Clearly, parents want their sons to act responsibly; only 1 percent of them are encouraging their sons to view pregnancy as the girl's problem. But, if this is so, let us assume for a moment that the girl wants the baby but the boy does not. If she goes ahead with the pregnancy, she will be choosing fatherhood for him. To be sure, he helped choose motherhood for her when they engaged in unprotected sexual intercourse. If he had wanted to guard against fatherhood, he could have used a contraceptive, urged her to use one, or simply refrained from sexual intercourse. Likewise, if the girl had wanted to guard against motherhood, she could have used a contraceptive, urged him to use one, or simply refrained from sexual intercourse. At this point, however, the girl is pregnant and, if she chooses to be a mother, the boy will become a father, whether or not this is his desire. Similarly, if the girl chooses not to be a mother, the boy cannot become a father, even if he very much wants to be one. Although few of us would want the state to empower this boy to force the girl to carry the fetus to term, few of us have absolutely no sympathy for him.

Because the fetus is within the woman's womb, the decision regarding abortion is most properly hers. Whether she likes it or not, in choosing for herself, she will choose for others. We have been so busy debating the abortion decision that we have failed to pay adequate attention to the ways in which this decision, more than most others, reveals how the act of procreation makes men and women interdependent. If a man and a woman are not committed enough to each other to regard themselves as a "we," loving and responsible enough to make the abortion decision together, then the way for them to avoid mutual disappointment, anger, and even hate is to practice birth control.

7 Fertility and Infertility

After reading reports of burgeoning world population, overcrowding, and unwanted children, it may be hard to believe that anyone has trouble getting pregnant, but the fact is that many people do. Among a normal population of couples trying to achieve pregnancy, only 20 percent will conceive a child in the first month of concerted effort and deliver a child 9 months later. In each succeeding month, just 20 percent of those remaining will conceive and have a baby. Many factors can interfere with fertilization, a carefully orchestrated event that can take place only during a specific 10- to 15-hour interval once a month. One reason for the low rate is that, even if fertilization does occur, researchers estimate that only 30 percent or so of successful fertilizations end in successful pregnancies and births.[1]

For most couples, such statistics are of little concern and pregnancy, if desired, will be achieved within 1 year. However, for the approximately 15 to 20 percent of American married couples in whom infertility has been diagnosed, that year will be one of frustration as each month conception fails to occur.[2] Studies indicate that the actual incidence of infertility has increased by less than one percentage point over the past two decades; nonetheless, the demand for infertility services is mushrooming.[3] Among the causes of increased requests for infertility services in the 1980s were (1) delayed childbearing patterns, (2) a decreasing supply of infants available for adoption, (3) an increasing number of physicians providing infertility services, (4) a growing pronatalist movement, and (5) significant advances in reproductive technology.[4]

The term *infertility* is used when a couple fails to achieve a pregnancy within 1 year of unprotected intercourse. There are two broad categories of infertility: *Primary infertility* is diagnosed when a couple has never successfully conceived, whereas *secondary infertility* is diagnosed when a couple has successfully conceived at least once. When a person's infertile condition is irreversible by known therapeutic intervention (e.g., when a woman is born without ovaries, or a man without functional testes), she or he is sterile.[5] Finally, the term *surgical sterility* is applied only to an infertile condition that was created surgically and is largely irreversible by known therapeutic intervention (e.g., when a woman has undergone a tubal ligation, or when a man has undergone a vasectomy).

That the term *infertility* is applied to couples rather than to individuals is of considerable significance. Although the root of a couple's reproductive difficulties may rest with one of the partners, very often it rests with both of them or between them, as in cases of reproductive incompatibility (each member of the couple could beget children with a different partner but, for some reason, not with his or her own partner).

Infertile couples often seek professional help. The fertility specialist takes both the man's and the woman's complete medical history, gives each of them a complete physical examination and, if indicated, performs certain tests on one or both of them. If the specialist identifies the cause(s) of the couple's infertility, she or he often can prescribe treatment to overcome the couple's reproductive difficulties successfully. In some cases, medication, hormonal therapy, surgery, or psychological counseling can help a couple overcome their infertility; in other cases, however, only the newer technologies of artificial insemination, in vitro fertilization or embryo transfer can be of service. Because we will be discussing each of these newer technologies in subsequent chapters, we will concentrate here on more traditional techniques for the diagnosis and treatment of infertility.[6] The female and male factors of fertility will be considered successively, but it is important to remember their interconnectedness.

Female Fertility

Compared to the reproductive lifetime of a man (reports of paternity at ages beyond 90 years have been made), the reproductive lifetime of a woman is relatively short. After puberty, female fecundity lasts perhaps 35 or 40 years, declining rather steadily after the age of 30 and more certainly after the age of 35. Because an increasing number of contemporary women are delaying childbearing until their thirties, these women may have a harder time getting pregnant than younger women.

A woman's ability to conceive and bear children depends on a complex array of anatomical, hormonal, and timing factors. There are six important stages of the female reproductive process that must be properly carried out and coordinated for a successful pregnancy. They are: (1) ovulation, (2) the interaction of the sperm and cervical mucus, (3) the actual fertilization, (4) tubal transport of the egg (before and after fertilization), (5) embryo implantation, and (6) maintenance of the developing fetus within the uterus. These stages are somewhat arbitrary, for many interconnections and interdependencies exist among them.

Ovulation and Anovulation

Ovulation

Ovulation occurs when a mature egg is released from the ovary and transported by the fallopian tubes to the uterus. Normally, women ovulate once every menstrual cycle, generally 14 days before the onset of their next menstrual cycle. Only at the time of ovulation or, more accurately, during the 10 to 15 hours after the actual release of the egg can fertilization occur. Thus, couples who wish to conceive a child must take care to have sexual intercourse during the woman's fertile period.

Anovulation and Amenorrhea

As we noted in chapter 3, the female ovulatory cycle is regulated by the interplay of five principal hormones: gonadotropin-releasing hormone (GnRH) from the hypothalamus; follicle-stimulating (FSH) and luteinizing (LH) hormones from the pituitary; estrogen from the ovarian follicle cells; and progesterone from the corpus luteum (and, if fertilization occurs, from the placenta). When a woman's hormonal balance is disrupted, anovulation (absence of ovulation) and amenorrhea (defined as "cessation of menstruation for 6 months or more") may result.

Among the major causes of ovulatory problems are certain externally produced conditions. For example, serious female athletes, extreme dieters, and women suffering from nutritional imbalances may cease ovulating and menstruating as a natural protection against pregnancy, which cannot be supported by their low percentages of body fat. Not surprisingly, women who have systemic diseases or infections, especially of the liver or kidney, are also prone to anovulation and amenorrhea. Both prescription and over-the-counter medications and illicit drugs, such as the central nervous system depressants heroin and marijuana, may also interfere with ovulation. Finally, emotional stress is a factor that has been cited in connection with hormonal imbalances, but it is difficult to determine whether stress causes the imbalance or whether, instead, the imbalance causes the stress.[7] In any event, if the cause of the ovulatory disorder is externally produced, it can usually be eliminated.

Sometimes there are structural problems with the endocrine glands themselves, including not only the hypothalamus, pituitary, and ovaries, but also the thyroid and adrenal glands. The latter two glands produce thyroid hormone, necessary for proper hormone metabolism throughout the body, and androgens (including testosterone), necessary for the development of appropriate sex characteristics. Physicians can correct most hormonal deficiencies with hormone supplements once they are properly diagnosed, and excesses can be reduced with medication. One of the the most common hormonal excesses is hyperprolactinemia, an elevated level of the hormone prolactin in the body. Produced by the pituitary, prolactin is responsible for milk production and suppresses ovulation. Women with pituitary tumors or other pituitary disorders, hypothyroidism, high adrenal androgen levels, or kidney disease are particularly susceptible to hyperprolactinemia. If a physician treats this condition with a prolactin-reducing medication such as bromocriptine (Parlodel), she or he can frequently restore the woman's fertility.

The most definitive, and probably the most distressing, cause of anovulation in women of reproductive age is premature ovarian failure: Either the ovaries have been severely damaged or the supply of eggs has simply been exhausted before the normal time for menopause. To determine whether a woman's ovaries have failed, the physician needs to know whether her ovaries are producing estrogen (a healthy sign). Using the progesterone withdrawal test, the physician administers a progesterone injection to the woman or asks her to take progesterone orally for 5 to 10 days. If the woman menstruates 14 to 20 days after she has absorbed the progesterone into her system, this is a good sign. The endometrium would not have built up if estrogen were not present to act in concert with the progesterone. Thus, the physician is able to deduce that the woman's ovaries are producing estrogen and that her ovulation problem probably is attributable to a pituitary malfunction: The pituitary is not releasing enough LH at the right time to stimulate the follicle to release its egg.[8] This is a condition the physician usually can treat effectively.

If the woman does not menstruate, however, the physician will check the woman's FSH and LH blood levels. Since estrogen levels regulate FSH and LH secretions, the pituitary gland will respond to low estrogen levels by releasing as much FSH and LH as possible in order to stimulate the ovaries to produce more estrogen. When the ovaries are damaged or failing, the FSH and LH levels will become very high in a futile effort to elicit estrogen production. Blood levels of FSH and LH in excess of

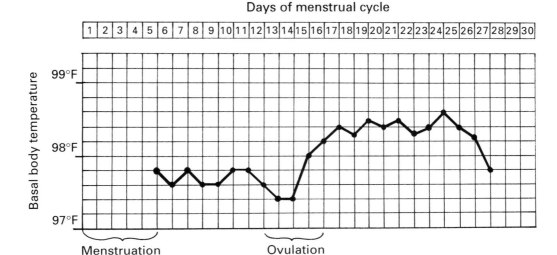

Figure 7.1 A representation of the basal body temperature chart for tracking the time of the month when ovulation will take place.

40 international units call for a diagnosis of ovarian failure. However, because this diagnosis is so serious and the condition essentially irreversible if due to a depletion of eggs, physicians ordinarily check a woman's FSH and LH blood levels several times to confirm their findings[9]

In addition to the progesterone withdrawal test, other tests for ovulation include the reading of basal body temperature charts, cervical mucus smears, and endometrial biopsies. Approximately midway through a normal menstrual cycle, a woman's body temperature rises 0.5 or so degrees in response to the progesterone produced by the corpus luteum. This dramatic temperature rise is illustrated in figure 7.1. Ovulation actually occurs 2 or 3 days prior to the temperature rise (these days are when the woman is most fertile) and remains so elevated until the corpus luteum deteriorates and her next period begins. The physician asks the woman to keep a chart of her body temperature over two or three cycles in the same way as would a woman practicing the rhythm method of birth control. If the woman does not observe a consistent temperature rise over several menstrual cycles, she is probably not ovulating.

An examination of cervical mucus can also be a useful indicator of ovulation. Throughout most of the menstrual cycle, a woman's mucus is thick, opaque, and relatively difficult for the sperm to penetrate. As ovarian estrogen secretion increases, however, the mucus becomes thinner and more transparent and, when smeared on a glass plate, dries in a fern-like pattern. After ovulation, progesterone counteracts estrogen's effect, and the mucus once again thickens. Hence, if ferning is still observed late in the cycle, the doctor can infer that progesterone levels have not increased and that ovulation probably has not taken place.

An endometrial biopsy involves the removal and examination of a small piece of endometrial tissue, enabling the physician to determine whether the uterus is prepared to receive an embryo. The procedure is performed 1 to 3 days before the onset of a woman's menstrual period. A normal biopsy almost always indicates that ovulation has occurred, that the corpus luteum is functioning properly, and that embryo implantation can take place successfully in the uterus. The only exception to this is the rare case of "trapped-egg syndrome," or luteinized unruptured follicle, a condition in which the follicle develops into the corpus luteum but fails to release the mature egg despite LH stimulation. This abnormal condition is difficult to diagnose not only because the endometrial biopsy appears normal but also because the other ovulation indicators—the progesterone withdrawal test, basal body temperature chart, and cervical mucus smear —appear normal as well. If pregnancy does not occur after several cycles of treatment with medication for increasing FSH production, ultrasound visualization of the ovary just prior to and following the expected ovulatory event may be advised. Ultrasonography will show the developing follicle and subsequent development of the corpus luteum. Attempts to treat trapped-egg syndrome usually involve hormonal supplements of LH or FSH or both to stimulate follicle growth and ovulation.

Interaction of Sperm and Cervical Mucus

Located between the vagina and the uterus, the cervix is usually filled with a thick mucus that prevents foreign materials and microorganisms from entering the uterus. As mentioned earlier, during ovulation the estrogen causes the mucus to become thin, easing the passage of the sperm into the uterus. This thinned, somewhat watery mucus promotes fertilization in the following ways: (1) it shields the sperm from the uterus's protective mechanisms of high acidity and the white blood cells of the woman's immune system; (2) it regulates a steady influx of sperm into the uterus over the period of optimum fertility; (3) it filters out abnormal sperm; (4) it provides some nutrients for the sperm; and, finally, (5) it prevents bacterial contamination of the uterus.[10]

In 5 to 10 percent of infertile women, the mucus fails to perform these vital functions, and the sperm either are unable to reach the uterus or are so badly damaged in the attempt that they are no longer capable of participating in fertilization.[11] Usually the mucus's functional failure is related to its poor quality, a condition that is often the result of previous cervical surgery, in utero exposure to diethylstilbestrol (DES, a drug commonly prescribed in the 1950s and 1960s to prevent miscarriage, though it is no longer used for this purpose), or clomiphene citrate ovulation induction therapy (a procedure that stimulates the hypothalamus to pump out more GnRH, which in turn stimulates the pituitary to increase production of FSH and LH). However, the interaction problems between mucus and sperm may also be due to an infectious condition in either partner or an immune response of sperm antibody produced by either partner. In 40 percent of such cases, a low dosage of estrogen supplement will improve mucus volume and quality.[12]

The primary method of detecting mucus-sperm problems is the postcoital test. The physician directs the couple to have intercourse at the time of ovulation (as predicted by basal body temperature charts and the woman's recognition of maximum vaginal wetness) and to come to the office within 8 hours to have a sample of cervical mucus removed and analyzed. The mucus is placed on a glass slide and examined under a microscope to determine the relative quantities of sperm present, how vigorously the sperm seem to be moving in the mucus, and whether white blood cells are present, signifying infection. If a semen analysis has previously shown that the husband's semen is normal, then dead, agglutinated, or immobile sperm in the postcoital test indicate an infection or immunological incompatibility between the wife's mucus and the husband's sperm.

If he or she observes white blood cells, indicating infection in either or both partners, the physician will treat both partners with an antibiotic to ensure that the infection is not passed back and forth between them. Successful treatment of the infection often restores fertility.

If what is observed is not white blood cells but sperm clumping together or shaking spasmodically, the physician will conclude that the couple is suffering from immunological incompatibility rather than infection since spermatic clumping or shaking indicates the presence of antibodies. Although the body's immune system normally produces antibodies as part of its protection against invasive foreign elements, for some unexplained reason 4 percent of all men and 50 to 60 percent of men who have had vasectomies produce antibodies against their own sperm. In addition, approximately 30 percent of the women with unexplained fertility problems produce sperm antibodies.[13]

To determine whether it is the man or the woman who is the source of an infertile couple's antibodies, physicians ordinarily compare the results of a semen analysis with those of a postcoital test. If the sperm clump together or shake spasmodically only in the postcoital test, the woman is probably the source of the antibodies. To determine whether the antibodies are specific to her husband's semen, tests of her mucus mixed with donor semen are performed. Normal results of these tests indicate antibodies specific to the husband's semen. If, however, the man is producing the antibodies, tests of his semen with donor mucus (bovine mucus is commonly used) will show the characteristic sperm clumping and shaking of an immunological reaction.

When the man is the source of the sperm antibodies, fertility is reduced to a 15.3 percent pregnancy rate.[14] One way of treating male-produced sperm antibodies is intrauterine insemination with sperm that have been washed to remove the seminal proteins and prostaglandins to which antibodies are sensitive. By injecting this sperm directly into the uterus, the physician bypasses the antibodies that may be present in the cervical mucus. However, this treatment does not guarantee the infertile couple a successful fertilization and pregnancy because it may be difficult to wash off proteins tightly associated with the sperm membranes and because antibodies may be present in the uterus as well as in the cervical mucus. In rare cases, seminal proteins and prostaglandins that are not completely removed by the washing process may cause cramping in the uterus, or unwanted bacteria may cause infection. If intrauterine insemination with sperm is unsuccessful, a physician may decide to treat an infertile couple with in vitro fertilization. By introducing an already fertilized egg into the female reproductive tract, the physician avoids setting up sperm antibody reactions in his or her patient; however, in vitro fertilization may have other drawbacks, which we will discuss later.

The most conventional form of therapy for female-produced sperm antibodies is condom therapy. Direct contact and exchange of body fluids is eliminated by the use of condoms for 3 to 6 months to suppress the production of antibodies. If all goes well, the level of antibodies in the woman will subside enough so that sperm can reach the egg when condom-free intercourse is resumed.

Another form of therapy for women who produce sperm antibodies is currently being studied and involves the administration of high doses of steroids to these women. The steroids suppress antibody production. Female producers of sperm antibodies are known to be at a higher risk for spontaneous abortion once fertilization has been achieved, but preliminary results indicate that this risk is reduced with steroid therapy.[15]

A final treatment method when female-produced sperm antibodies are the problem is artificial insemination with donor sperm (AID). If a woman's antibodies are specific to her husband's sperm, she should be able to become pregnant with a donor's sperm unless other abnormalities are present. Of course, AID is the treatment of choice only if both the husband and wife have no personal reservations about having a child to whom the husband is not genetically related.

Fertilization

From 50 to 100 million sperm are expelled in an average ejaculation. However, only several hundred of this huge number will reach the area of the egg in the fallopian tubes and, if all goes normally, only one of these sperm actually will penetrate and fertilize the egg. Sometimes the sperm will have difficulty penetrating the egg. This condition can be diagnosed by either the sperm penetration assay or the acrosin test.

The sperm penetration assay is the older of these two procedures and involves the incubation of human sperm with hamster eggs that have been specially treated to remove the zona pellucida. Under normal circumstances, protein differences in the zona pellucida of the human egg and the hamster egg prevent the human sperm from attaching to the hamster egg. The actual egg cell membranes are more similar, however, and sperm that can penetrate the hamster egg's membranes would be expected to penetrate a human egg's membranes as well.

The newer of these two procedures, the acrosin test, simply measures the biochemical activity of the enzyme acrosin, necessary for penetrating the zona pellucida and the egg cell membranes. Because the activity of acrosin is noticeably lower in men whose sperm are unable to penetrate the egg, a low acrosin reading indicates a sperm penetration problem.

Recently developed techniques help sperm penetrate the tough outer shell of the egg. These micromethods involve drilling, blasting, and cracking. In the microinjection technique, researchers draw sperm into a very fine needle and, after piercing the egg's zona pellucida, release the sperm into the underlying space.

Tubal Transport

Both before and after fertilization, transport of the egg from the ovaries to the uterus is dependent on the fallopian tubes functioning properly. Indeed, tubal problems are a leading cause of infertility in women. When ovulation occurs, the egg is pushed out onto the surface of the ovary, and the fimbriae on the end of the fallopian tube draw it to the tube entrance. As soon as it enters the tube, the rhythmic contractions of the muscular tube walls and the sweeping motion of the cilia on its inner lining propel the egg in the direction of the uterus. If it occurs, fertilization usually takes place in the first half of the egg's journey when it is closer to the ovary than to the uterus.

When tube walls are damaged, with resulting adhesions to the abdominal walls or scar tissue, the tube may be unable to contract regularly or the egg's path may be obstructed. If the fertilized egg encounters these difficulties, an ectopic pregnancy may result, inducing a great deal of pain and usually necessitating abortive surgery. Damaged cilia resulting from infections, abdominal surgery, or an earlier ectopic pregnancy can also prevent travel of both egg and sperm. Infection or irritation can affect the fimbriae too, causing the petal-like projections to close in on themselves, much like the closing of a tulip at night. When the tube end is so blocked, fluid buildup inside the tube will cause it to swell, injuring the delicate cilia.

Many conditions can lead to an impairment of the tubes, including a ruptured appendix, pelvic inflammatory disease, gynecological surgery, bowel surgery, endometriosis, in utero DES exposure, and prior ectopic pregnancy. When a tubal problem is suspected, the physician may recommend radiography of the reproductive tract, known as hysterosalpingography (HSG). Three to six days after the termination of a woman's menstrual period, an opaque dye is injected into the uterus. Subsequent x-ray films will reveal an outline of the interior of the uterus and tubes. Although this test is repeated two or three times to ensure accuracy, the physician generally is able to detect blockages, swellings, and other distortions on first inspection. Since the dye used in the HSG test occasionally dislodges material blocking the tube, the test itself sometimes has therapeutic as well as diagnostic value. Occasionally, HSGs may be complicated by excessive pain, bleeding, or infection. Physicians are careful not to use HSG on women who are allergic to iodine or other components of radiopaque dyes or on women who have had prior pelvic or tubal infections.

Laparoscopy is a more invasive procedure for examining a possible case of impaired tubes. The physician places a small telescope (the laparoscope) into a cut made in the belly button and, through another opening made just above the pubic bone, inserts a probe for handling the organs within the abdomen. To gain a less obstructed view of the reproductive tract, the physician pumps carbon dioxide into the woman's abdominal cavity, pushing the walls up and away from the organs of interest. In addition to using laparoscopy for visualization, physicians sometimes use it to perform minor surgical operations with a laser or specialized surgical knife. With this instrument, physicians often are able to remove both slight adhesions between the tubes and the abdominal walls and small patches of endometriosis. However, they are not able to correct more extensive damage with it, and so they must resort to full-scale abdominal surgery (laparotomy) in those instances. Thick adhesions, closed fimbriae, obstructed or deformed fallopian tubes, ovarian cysts, and large endometrial implants are some of the conditions that call for laparotomy. If a tube is irreparably damaged, it may sometimes be completely removed to give preference to the other tube; however, whatever affected one tube is not likely to have left the other completely unscathed.

Embryo Implantation

Once fertilized, the egg undergoes several successive cell divisions as it makes its way down the fallopian tube to the uterus. At the end of its approximately 3-day journey, the 16 to 32 cells that make up the developing embryo are known as the *blastocyst*. By the time the blastocyst reaches the uterus, estrogen and progesterone should have completed their preparation of the uterine lining for implantation. The endometrium should be thick and lush with many blood vessels, ready to provide a nutrient-rich environment for the embryo. If for some reason, the uterine wall is not adequately prepared, the blastocyst will not implant and subsequent development of a placenta will not occur. As a result, the uterine lining will deteriorate and be shed, along with the unviable embryo, in the next menstrual cycle. Thus, it is crucial that the corpus luteum secrete enough progesterone and build up the endometrial tissue at the right time. When the corpus luteum fails to secrete adequate progesterone or is late in initiating production of it, the resulting condition is known as *luteal phase defect* (LPD). LPD is observed in 3 to 5 percent of the women with fertility problems and is blamed for one-third of repeated early spontaneous abortions.[16]

Physicians can diagnose LPD by (1) monitoring a woman's blood progesterone levels over several days or (2) performing an endometrial biopsy, a procedure that permits direct observation of the development of the uterine lining. Since hormonal defects at one or more of the many steps of the interrelated endocrine pathways can cause LPD, therapeutic strategies are planned accordingly. Treatments include progesterone suppositories, the administration of human chorionic gonadotropin to promote corpus luteum activity, and FSH and LH supplements to promote proper follicular development, ovulation, and subsequent corpus luteum formation. Barring the presence of other abnormalities, the chances for pregnancy after therapy for LPD are approximately 50 percent.[17]

Pregnancy Maintenance

Looking back from the point of implantation, we can appreciate what a difficult course the sperm and egg, both alone and together, have had to travel, yet their odyssey is not over for there are still almost 9 full months before the process of human reproduction is complete. The blastocyst must develop into a mature fetus with the physiological and cerebral capacities to survive independently of the mother. When we reflect on our biological complexity, 9 months' time for all this development does not seem very long, nor is the small margin for error surprising. Researchers estimate that approximately 15 percent of the eggs exposed to sperm never divide, another 15 percent do not implant and, of the ones that do implant, 41 percent subsequently perish. All in all, only 30 percent of the fertilized eggs actually survive until birth.[18]

Miscarriages that take place before the first 20 weeks of gestation are known as *spontaneous abortions*. The great majority occur during the first trimester (3 months) of pregnancy, sometimes even before the woman realizes that she is pregnant. Spontaneous abortions after the twelfth week are rarer and usually elicit more concern. For most women, one or two early losses is not a major cause for concern. The spontaneous abortion rate for women has been found to be virtually the same after one abortion as before none—between 20 and 30 percent. (Women older than 30 years would be expected to be on the higher end of the scale.) However, after two losses, the odds for a third loss increase to 38 percent and remain high thereafter.[19]

Recurrent, or *habitual*, *abortion* refers to the situation in which a woman suffers three or more consecutive spontaneous abortions. Recurrent abortion is designated as *primary* when the woman has never carried a child to term and *secondary* when she has previously given birth successfully. If a woman appears to be experiencing recurrent abortions, especially if one occurred late in the pregnancy or if a previous birth was abnormal, she should be referred to a fertility specialist for consultation and testing. Women with a family history of spontaneous abortions should also probably see a specialist after only one or two early losses.

The possible causes of spontaneous abortion are many. Some problems are due to environmental factors that are relatively easy to adjust. Smoking, for example, is believed to incur a 25 percent greater risk of abortion and is connected with low birth weight as well. Nicotine tends to constrict placental blood vessels, and the presence of carbon monoxide tends to decrease the oxygen-carrying capacity of the blood. Either one of these two conditions can lead to oxygen deprivation of the fetus.[20]

Immoderate alcohol consumption, many drugs (licit as well as illicit), and excessive caffeine intake are all suspected of promoting pregnancy loss. Finally, workplace hazards (e.g., certain toxic chemicals) also may jeopardize a woman's pregnancy. It is advisable to note the chemicals to which one is regularly exposed and to consult with a physician.

The most common causes of spontaneous abortion are chromosomal defects. Between 40 and 60 percent of all first-trimester losses involve genetic abnormalities, arising either during the meiotic divisions of oogenesis or spermatogenesis or in the mitotic divisions following fertilization.[21] Abortion of genetically defective fetuses is a protective mechanism developed by the species to guard against the birth of individuals who would probably not survive outside the womb anyway. Although these chromosomal defects are numerous, three types are most common. The first is *autosomal trisomy*, the presence of three copies of a chromosome, though there should be only two. The second type of chromosomal defect is the *absence of one sex chromosome*. When a fetus with just one X chromosome does survive, it is born with a condition known as Turner's syndrome. The ovaries fail to develop, and such individuals are infertile. The third type is *polyploidy* (the presence of more than two complete sets of chromosomes), most commonly triploidy. Each of these three chromosomal abnormalities, as well as other rarer types, generally occurs as the result of random errors in meiosis or mitosis or after exposure to toxic substances.[22] Women younger than 17 or older than 35 and men older than 55 are believed to be more prone to errors in oogenesis and spermatogenesis.[23]

Aside from limiting one's exposure to toxins, the only treatment physicians can recommend for random chromosomal defects is to try again. Amniocentesis may be advised in subsequent pregnancies because there is an increased risk of chromosomal abnormalities occurring again. Sometimes, the parent carries a defect that is indistinguishable phenotypically but is passed on through the gamete to the progeny. For example, whereas a defect such as a balanced translocation does no harm to the parent, the offspring has just half of that parent's chromosomes and the defect is not balanced. Indeed, the resulting condition may be lethal. If one parent has a chromosomal anomaly that is always passed on to the offspring in a lethal form, a genetic counselor may suggest the use of donor eggs or donor sperm in conjunction with some version of one of the new reproductive technologies (e.g., AID, in vitro fertilization).

Yet another cause of spontaneous abortion is congenital defects of the uterine structure. Found in 1 of 600 women, such defects probably cause 10 to 15 percent of recurrent abortions.[24] There are several types of struc-

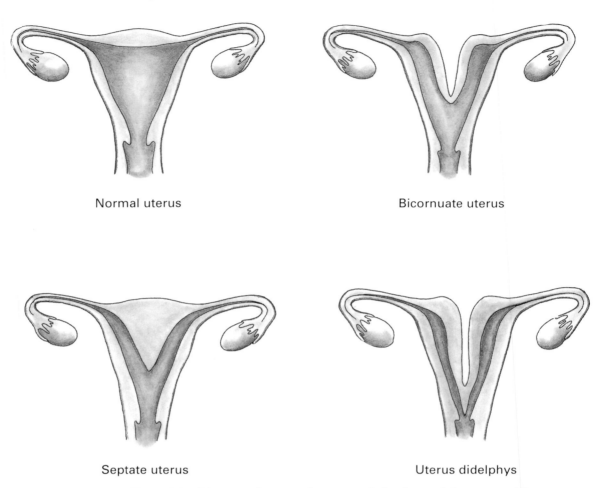

Normal uterus

Bicornuate uterus

Septate uterus

Uterus didelphys

Figure 7.2 Diagram of a normal uterus and the shape of the uterus with congenital abnormalities.

tural anomalies, of which the most common are the septate uterus, the bicornuate uterus, and the didelphic uterus (figure 7.2). In most cases, uterine structural abnormalities do not cause primary infertility and, depending on the particular defect, may not cause secondary infertility either. For example, the bicornuate uterus, the most common anomaly, is not usually a cause of recurrent abortion but instead is frequently associated with premature births and malpresentations. On the other hand, up to 90 percent of the women with septate uteruses are believed to be susceptible to recurrent abortion.[25] So too are the women whose uterine structural abnormalities were caused by in utero exposure to DES. Approximately 70 percent of women born to mothers taking DES have been found to possess, among other defects, T-shaped uteruses that often cannot support pregnancy.

Physicians usually suspect uterine deformities after a woman experiences a single second-trimester abortion or after a woman experiences more than one first-trimester abortion. Physicians can confirm their suspicions in one of several ways: by HSG (radiography of the reproductive tract), by hysteroscopy (insertion of a telescopic tube into the uterus through the cervix), or by laparoscopy (viewing the external shape of the uterus through an abdominal incision). If she or he determines that a septate uterus is causing recurrent abortion, the physician may pass scissors through the hysteroscope and cut away the excess tissue of the septum (simultaneous viewing through a laparoscope ensures the integrity of the external uterine wall). Rates of success, as measured by the incidence of full-term pregnancy after this surgery, are very high.

Another uterine abnormality is the presence of leiomyomas, or fibroids, in the uterine wall. These benign tumors are common, especially in black women, who have been found to be nine times more likely to have them than white women.[26] More often than not, women with leiomyomas have normal pregnancies, but sometimes, depending on the size, number, and location of these tumors, problems arise. Infertility, spontaneous abortion, and premature and otherwise abnormal birth have all been associated with uterine fibroids. The tumors are believed to interfere with pregnancy by marring implantation sites, thereby hindering nutritional intake by the fetus. Large myomas may also distort the shape of the uterus. Unless it is virtually certain that myomas are the primary cause of abortion or are so large as to endanger the integrity of the entire uterus, physicians do not usually advise surgery to remove them. Because this type of surgery (myomectomy) can cause abdominal adhesions worse than the conditions remedied, it is to be avoided if at all possible. Also, fibroids often grow back and, if severe, a hysterectomy may be advised. Nevertheless, in cases where myomectomies have been performed, pregnancy rates have improved to almost 50 percent depending on the woman's age at the time of surgery.[27] If the myomectomy causes significant weakening of the uterine wall, delivery by cesarean section is recommended.

Still another abortion-threatening uterine anomaly is the intrauterine adhesion. This type of adhesion is most frequently caused by prior dilation and curettage, especially that used in an early elective abortion. The most common symptom of intrauterine adhesion is an abnormal menstrual pattern, usually amenorrhea. Hysteroscopy is currently the best method of diagnosing intrauterine adhesion and also can be used to lyse adhesions when such action is deemed necessary. The lysis of adhesions is followed by temporary insertion of an intrauterine device to hold the uterine walls apart and prevent recurrent adhesion. Estrogen and progesterone supplements then are administered for 60 days to help build up the woman's endometrium again. Pregnancy results after such treatment are excellent.

Premature deliveries or second-trimester abortions are often symptoms of an incompetent cervix. The typical scenario is painless dilation of the cervix, spontaneous rupture of the membranes, and quick delivery of a living fetus who immediately dies.[28] The defect may have resulted from earlier surgery on the cervix, damage occurring at childbirth, or in utero DES exposure.[29] Treatment of this condition takes place during pregnancy. Approximately 14 weeks into the pregnancy, the physician does an ultrasound examination to verify normal pregnancy and then sutures the cervix closed. At approximately 38 to 39 weeks of gestation, the physician removes the stitch to permit vaginal delivery. The success rate is approximately 80 percent.[30]

For many years, physicians assumed that hormone deficiencies were the root of pregnancy mishaps, and treatment was planned accordingly. Among the most deleterious of these hormonal treatments was the administration of DES to thousands of women during the 1950s and 1960s, with the aim of preventing subsequent miscarriages. Studies later showed that the drug was ineffective and, in fact, caused several congenital defects in individuals exposed to it in utero. Ironically, one of the deleterious consequences was a higher incidence of spontaneous abortion in DES-affected women. A much safer hormonal treatment is progesterone therapy, used when a woman's natural progesterone levels are too low to sustain a full-term pregnancy. This is analogous to the treatment of LPD already discussed.

Recently, attention has turned to the possible role of the immune system in many previously unexplained pregnancy losses. Normally, the immune system will recognize foreign substances in the body and attack them. We might expect, then, that the fetus, with half of its genes from the father, would be a prime target for immunological assault. However, the body has somehow developed a mechanism whereby the special mother-fetus relationship is protected from attack.

Although the details of this mechanism are unknown, speculations abound. Some researchers believe that elevated levels of progesterone, secreted by the corpus luteum and placenta, depress the sensitivity of the female immune system[31] and enable it to tolerate foreign substances. Other researchers believe that the maternal immune system produces special antibodies that attach to and cover up the antigens on the fetus and placenta, preventing recognition and attack by lymphocytes and macrophages. They reason that were these special antibodies not produced, immunological attack on the fetus and subsequent abortion would result because antibodies attached to antigens normally invite attack. This may be the case when the father's and mother's genetic contributions are so similar that the maternal immune system cannot make antibodies specific for the paternal antigens. Nonetheless, this remains a matter of speculation as relatively little is known about the role of immunology with respect to recurrent abortion, and many more studies must be done before appropriate treatment regimens can be established. Until then, AID may be a viable option for couples afflicted with recurrent abortion apparently linked to immunological disorders.

Another likely cause of spontaneous abortion is uterine infection, but there is little solid evidence that demonstrates a causal connection between uterine infection and a spontaneous abortion. For example, mycoplasma is more often found in the uterine environments of recurrent aborters than in nonaborters, but researchers have been unable to establish concrete links between the two phenomena. Nevertheless, physicians often prescribe antibiotics for both the male and the female partner in cases of unexplained recurrent abortion, and frequently pregnancy ensues, but whether because of the antibiotic or mere luck is unknown.

Some systemic diseases are associated with increased incidence of pregnancy loss. Lupus erythematosus, a degenerative disease of the connective tissue, is one whose connection to recurrent abortion is fairly well documented. So too are hypothyroidism and kidney disease, especially when accompanied by hypertension.[32] Diabetes has long been cited as a cause of spontaneous abortion, but reliable studies have failed to validate that claim. Endometriosis also is suspected of playing a role in recurrent abortion, because endometrial tissue produces prostaglandins that may induce premature contractions in the smooth muscles of the uterus. When treated or brought under control, however, these and other related conditions do not preclude a normal pregnancy.

In investigating the causes of spontaneous abortion, we must not ignore the possible role of the genetic father. In cases of genetic defect, there is a 50 percent chance that the problem had its origins in the father's sperm. Some researchers have noted an increased incidence of abortion in cases where the male's sperm count exceeds 250 million per milliliter.[33] Other researchers have speculated that male semen may transport pregnancy-threatening drugs and hormones into the woman's vagina, where they are quickly absorbed by the woman's circulatory system. Although this phenomenon has not been definitively observed in humans yet, it has been observed in several animal studies.[34]

Another possible cause of recurrent abortion is psychological stress. Although significant proof of the connection between stress and recurrent abortion is lacking, many researchers are convinced that psychological stress is the cause of a multitude of physical harms. After a woman has experienced two or three spontaneous abortions, she and her partner may wish to examine the everyday rhythm of their lives. Work- or home-related stress, professional and personal disappointments, including the disappointment of failed pregnancies, may negatively affect the overall physical well-being of a pregnant woman and make her a likely candidate for a spontaneous abortion.

Whereas any pregnancy loss that occurs up to the twentieth week of gestation is called a *spontaneous abortion* or *miscarriage*, a pregnancy loss that occurs between the twentieth week and full term is called a *stillbirth*. Six of every thousand babies are stillborn.[35] In most cases, stillbirths are not associated with infertility but with isolated events such as toxemia, Rh factors, anemia, umbilical cord and placental mishaps, and implantation problems.[36] Newborn death, where the baby lives just up to birth, is another tragedy considered a onetime occurrence rather than an infertility problem. Usually, the baby dies because it is born prematurely, before it is able to function outside the womb. The causes for premature birth are many, including genetic factors, reproductive structural abnormalities, infection, and poor maternal health.

Clearly, spontaneous abortion is a cause for concern. Nevertheless, most spontaneous abortions are isolated events and are in no way a certain indicator of permanent infertility. Indeed, the chance for successful pregnancy after three consecutive spontaneous abortions, even in the absence of treatment, is 50 to 70 percent.[37]

Diagnostic Technology Used to Determine the Status of Pregnancy

Ultrasonography

Ultrasonography has become a very important diagnostic tool in medicine since its introduction as a method of soft-tissue imagery. Before we can appreciate how an ultrasonogram is obtained, we must understand some of the properties of sound. Sound is a mechanical vibration that is transmitted through matter. It is perceptible to the human ear if its frequency is between 16,000 and 20,000 cycles per second. Ultrasound is simply sound with a frequency in excess of 20,000 cycles per second.

Table 7.1 The velocity of ultrasound waves in various biological and non-biological materials

Material	Velocity (m/sec)
Biological	
Fat	1450
Vitreous humor of eye	1520
Human soft tissue, mean value	1540
Brain	1541
Liver	1549
Kidney	1561
Spleen	1566
Blood	1570
Muscle	1585
Lens of eye	1620
Skull bone	4080
Nonbiological	
Air	331
Pure water	1430
Sea water	1510
Plastic	2500
Metal	5000

From B. B. Goldberg, M. N. Kotler, M. C. Ziskin, and R. D. Waxham, *Diagnostic Uses of Ultrasound* (New York: Grune and Stratton, 1975) 6.

All sound is propagated through a medium in the form of a mechanical vibration of the particles of that medium. The velocity with which sound travels depends on the elasticity and the density of the medium. The density is the mass per unit volume, and the elasticity is a measure of how strong the connections are between the particles of the material. From the data in table 7.1, we can see that the velocity of sound varies enormously from air to water to metal but varies much less, although significantly, in various tissues and organs.

As sound propagates through matter, its intensity progressively decreases, largely due to the absorption of the sound energy as heat. The amount of sound energy absorbed depends on the viscosity of the tissue. In other words, the more "rigid" are the tissues, the greater is the viscosity and the greater the sound absorption. The high frequencies of ultrasound are useful in probing soft tissue at various distances.

Table 7.2 Magnitude of reflection of ultrasound waves at various biological interfaces

Interface	Percent Reflection
Blood–brain	0.3
Blood–kidney	0.7
Water–brain	3.2
Blood–fat	7.9
Muscle–fat	10.0
Muscle–bone	64.6
Brain–skull bone	66.1
Water–skull bone	68.4
Air–any soft tissue	100.0

From B. B. Goldberg, M. N. Kotler, M. C. Ziskin, and R. D. Waxham, *Diagnostic Uses of Ultrasound* (New York: Grune and Stratton, 1975) 22.

When a sound beam encounters a boundary between two tissues, a portion of the sound is reflected back and the rest is transmitted through the tissue. Since ultrasonic probes monitor the sound reflected back to a sensing device, the magnitude of the reflection at various biological interfaces allows the technique to be used in these cases. Table 7.2 shows the different degrees to which sound is reflected at various biological boundaries. Because sound is virtually 100 percent reflected from an air-tissue boundary, ultrasound cannot penetrate beyond the first air layer encountered. This means that the sound cannot penetrate the air-filled lungs, the gas-filled intestinal lumen or urinary bladder, or the gas layer between the ultrasonic probe and the surface of the body. For this reason, the patient is usually asked to maintain a full bladder for the abdominal ultrasound scan and a mineral oil or a water-soluble gel is used to provide an air-free contact between the probe and the body.

The operation of an ultrasonicator involves the generation of an ultrasonic pulse, the detection of ultrasound reflected off the biological interfaces, and the electronic processing of the detected signals into a meaningful three-dimensional picture of the organs or tissues. The high resolution that can be achieved allows the physician to observe the presence of very small anatomical structures and, with certain modifications, the movement of the organs and tissues. The sound is actually generated by the piezoelectric effect, which involves inducing a mechanical deformation of a crystal by applying an alternating voltage to it. The deformation of the crystal gives rise to the vibrations of the air molecules and establishes sound. The reflected sound is detected in just the opposite way: The sound causes the deformation of a crystal, which in turn induces a voltage. In practice, the generating and detecting crystals are mounted in an object called a *transducer probe*. This is the object that is moved over the surface of the body during an ultrasound scan.

Examination of a pregnant woman with ultrasound allows the physician to detect the gestational sac as early as the fifth week and, in almost all cases, by the eighth week. At this stage of pregnancy, ultrasound can detect certain abnormalities of the gestational sac which indicate that a spontaneous abortion may take place. Later in pregnancy, ultrasound can detect the fetal orientation; internal fetal head and body structures, including fetal heart beat; the presence of multiple fetuses; the age of the fetus (from the size of the gestational sac); the presence of an extrauterine pregnancy; and a variety of fetal abnormalities including hydrocephalus (an abnormally large head) and anencephalus (the absence of a head).[38]

Amniocentesis

Amniocentesis is a remarkable diagnostic tool. First, it can detect several sex-linked or sex-specific diseases such as hemophilia and Duchenne type muscular dystrophy. Second, it can reveal severe chromosomal abnormalities, consisting of chromosomes that are misshapen or the presence of too many or too few chromosomes. The most common example of this is Down's syndrome, in which one extra chromosome results in a child who is mentally retarded and who usually suffers from internal problems such as congenital heart disease or esophageal blockage. Third, it can reveal enzymatic abnormalities, in which enzymes are missing or are present in abnormal concentrations. The most common example of this is Tay-Sachs disease, a fatal disorder caused by genetic biochemical imbalances. Finally, it can detect 90 percent of neural tube defects such as anencephaly and spina bifida.

Physicians usually perform amniocentesis 16 to 17 weeks after the pregnant woman's last menstrual period to ensure that there is enough fluid to remove some safely for the tests. First, the physician views the uterus with ultrasound to determine its position. Next, she or he inserts a long needle through the pregnant woman's abdomen into the amniotic sac and removes approximately 25 mL of amniotic fluid together with some cells that have come loose from the fetus, as shown in figure 7.3. Then, the physician orders a series of biochemical assays on some of this fluid, reserving most of it for a 2- to 4-week incubation process that allows the living cells to multiply. After incubation, laboratory technicians stain and examine the

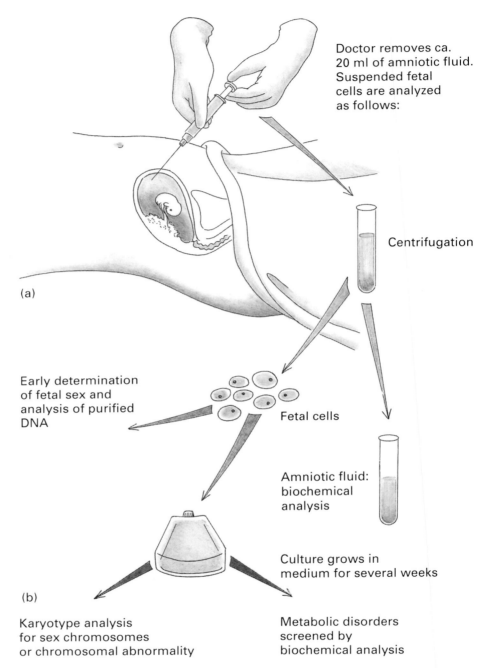

Doctor removes ca. 20 ml of amniotic fluid. Suspended fetal cells are analyzed as follows:

(a)

Centrifugation

Early determination of fetal sex and analysis of purified DNA

Fetal cells

Amniotic fluid: biochemical analysis

Culture grows in medium for several weeks

(b)

Karyotype analysis for sex chromosomes or chromosomal abnormality

Metabolic disorders screened by biochemical analysis

Figure 7.3 Amniocentesis. The method of (a) drawing amniotic fluid and (b) culturing the cells to determine the physiological and genetic state of the fetus.

cells' chromosomes to determine whether the fetus is normal and genetically healthy.

Amniocentesis is not as risky as once believed, but it still does present a slight risk of spontaneous abortion or rupturing of the amniotic sac. For this reason, physicians usually perform amniocentesis only on women who are more likely to deliver genetically abnormal children: women 35 years or older, women who have a history of genetic problems, or women who have already delivered a child with genetic abnormalities.[39] Given the risks that amniocentesis poses, most physicians are reluctant to perform it simply to reveal the sex of the fetus.

Chorionic Villi Sampling

Chorionic villi sampling (CVS) gives results similar to those obtained with amniocentesis. Because cells in the developing placenta have the same chromosomes as the fetus, if the physician can remove a small sample from the placenta surface (chorionic villi) without jeopardizing placental function or fetal development, she or he can learn much about the condition of the fetus.

To obtain a tiny sample of chorionic villi, the physician inserts a narrow flexible tube through the cervical canal and guides it to the placenta under ultrasonography. A placenta sample is obtained by vacuum aspiration, and chromosome analysis is then carried out in the laboratory.[40] The advantage of CVS is that it can be done 7 weeks earlier than amniocentesis and, because a larger sample of fetal cells is obtained, less time is necessary for the cells to multiply in culture. Overall, the results of CVS are usually available 2 months earlier than those of amniocentesis, a definite advantage if a woman is contemplating an abortion. However, because the risk to the fetus may be slightly higher with CVS than with amniocentesis, the test is used more cautiously than amniocentesis.[41]

Male Fertility

The role of the man in infertility has often been downplayed, and fertility testing on the woman often proceeds for extended periods of time before attention is turned to the man as the possible source of the problem. Indeed, it has been observed that in some 40 to 50 percent of infertile couples, problems of the male partner have contributed at least in part to the difficulties.[42] Given this statistic, fertility specialists now advise that the primary test for male fertility, the semen analysis, be performed as the first procedure in any fertility investigation. It is quick and inexpensive and, if a disorder is detected, the couple can be spared extensive and often expensive testing of the female partner.

Semen Analysis

Semen analysis should be performed even if the male partner has fathered children in the past, for changes may have occurred to impair his fertility. The man masturbates into a glass jar and brings the semen sample into the clinical laboratory within 1 hour of ejaculation. The ejaculate should be collected at a time that is commensurate with the average frequency of ejaculation because altering his normal ejaculatory pattern may undermine the infertility investigation.

In the laboratory, the technician examines the specimen for volume and quality of seminal fluid, concentration of sperm, motility, and morphology. The average volume per ejaculate is between 1 and 3.5 mL. A low volume may indicate that there is not enough seminal fluid to carry the sperm to the woman's cervix or that there is not enough seminal fluid to protect the sperm against the acidity of the vagina. A high ejaculate volume may indicate a sperm concentration that is too diluted. Because the first ejaculate fraction usually contains the most sperm, a physician may advise couples to practice coitus interruptus if the male has a high ejaculate volume. By withholding later fractions, further dilution can be avoided.

The concentration of sperm within an ejaculate can vary widely, even from the same individual. Hence a semen analysis should be repeated at least once, if not more often. Temporary illness or exposure to toxic substances may distort test results, and it may take time for normal sperm production to return after such distortions. Assuming that a man's sperm are healthy, only sperm counts consistently lower than 20 million sperm per milliliter suggest that fertility may be impaired. However, it is important to remember that many men who have sperm counts of less than 20 million have successfully fathered children, and so the figure must be considered somewhat arbitrary.

After ejaculation, semen coagulates within the vagina for 15 to 20 minutes, presumably to prevent the newly arrived sperm from leaking out. Within an hour, however, the semen should liquefy, allowing the sperm to start their journey up through the woman's reproductive tract. Sometimes though, the semen does not liquefy enough or at all, owing to some problem with the prostate gland, which secretes the chemical necessary for liquefaction. Another problem with the semen may be insufficient buffering action to protect the sperm from the acidity of the female reproductive tract. Furthermore, if many white blood cells are seen in the semen, it is likely that an infection is present.

Sperm Motility

To reach the egg, sperm must be able to propel themselves up the fallopian tubes, rapidly whipping their long tails back and forth. If more than half of the sperm in a sample are slow or have trouble moving in a straight line, fertility may be impaired. Clumping or frenetic trembling of sperm may indicate the presence of sperm antibodies. Mobility is of course connected with morphology, or shape. A normal sperm has an oval head and thin tail approximately ten times longer than the head. Abnormal sperm may have deformed heads or curled or kinked tails, as illustrated in figure 7.4. All men produce some abnormal sperm, and only when a man's per-

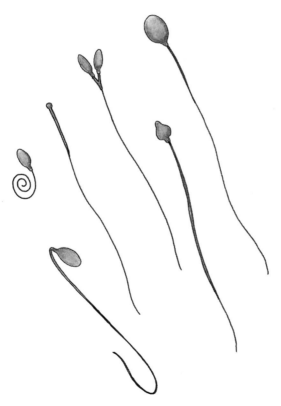

Figure 7.4   Sketch of various types of abnormal sperm.

centage of abnormal sperm is consistently greater than 40 percent is there any cause for concern.

Sperm Production

A diagnosis of poor sperm production (quantity and quality) is cause for the fertility specialist to examine both the endocrine system regulating production and the actual production site within the testes. Most of the hormones that regulate the female system are present in the male system, but they affect men differently from women.

Just as in the female system, regular pulses of GnRH from the hypothalamus stimulate the pituitary gland to produce FSH and LH in the male system. Instead of acting on ovaries, however, these hormones stimulate the male gonads, the testes. The LH induces the production of testosterone, which causes male secondary sex characteristics to develop and which, together with FSH, instructs the testes to produce sperm. In general, hormone deficiencies do not play as large a role in male infertility as they do in female infertility.[43] However, disorders associated with impaired thyroid, adrenal, hypothalamus, and pituitary activity do exist and, if properly diagnosed, can sometimes be alleviated with hormone supplements, surgical intervention, or radiation if tumors are present.

Testicular Abnormalities

If the man's hormonal signals seem to be operating properly, the physician will turn attention to the testes themselves for clues to the cause of poor sperm production. Elevated FSH levels are often a sign of at least partial testicular failure. Sensing abnormal sperm production, the pituitary increases its output of FSH in order to stimulate testicular function. Problems with the testes may be a result of genetic abnormalities, illness, drugs, heat, varicoceles (varicose veins in the scrotum), accidental surgical or physical injury, or toxins in the environment. Unfortunately, men with abnormal testes resulting from genetic defects cannot usually be helped; the physical apparatus needed for sperm production is simply not present, and nothing can replace it. In such cases, couples who desire children may resort to artificial insemination by donor sperm or, perhaps, to adoption.

Infections and diseases are other common causes of testicular impairment, temporary or permanent. The culprits include adult mumps, tuberculosis, gonorrhea, syphilis, smallpox, typhoid, influenza, and hepatic and kidney diseases. If arrested early, the damage that these illnesses cause may be alleviated, but sometimes the testes have atrophied so much that normal sperm production is irretrievably lost.

Occasionally, the medications used in the treatment of illness can hamper sperm production. Researchers have observed that some cancer-fighting drugs cause complete testicular failure. The use of illicit drugs and alcohol are suspected of interfering with fertility as well. So too can excessive heat interfere with sperm production. Even normal body temperature is too high for the delicate testicular tissues; it is for this reason that the testes are in the scrotum, hanging away from the body and thereby remaining cooler by 1 or 2 degrees. High temperatures seem to induce the production of malformed sperm with lowered motility. For some infertile men, elevated temperatures in the environment are to blame, and fertility may be restored simply by making adjustments in the environment—switching from a job as a foundry worker or wearing loose-fitting instead of tight-fitting underwear and pants.

Heat also seems to be one direct cause of the type of infertility that sometimes ensues from having undescended testicles as a child. Normally, the testes have descended in male infants by the age of 1 year, and surgery is needed to correct those few cases where descent is late (8 of 1000 male children[44]). If the surgery is delayed until after the age of 6, however, irreversible damage to the testes due to the exposure to the body's high temperature is likely. In addition to infertility, such men are at a much higher than average risk for testicular cancer.

Elevated temperatures may play a role in impairment of fertility by varicoceles as well. Varicoceles are pools of blood that arise when veins in the scrotum swell owing to malfunctioning valves. These valves normally prevent the backflow of blood. Because of the vascular structure around the testes, varicoceles usually occur on the left side. Often visible as swellings or blue venous networks, they are actually quite common, found in 10 to 15 percent of normal men as well as in 25 percent or more of infertile men.[45] The heat of the accumulated blood, as well as the increased concentration of toxic substances that are not being drained away, are believed to be the means by which varicoceles compromise sperm production.

Varicoceles can be treated fairly simply by surgery. The surgeon makes an incision in the groin and through it ties off the vein feeding into the varicocele. Approximately 50 percent of the time, affected couples will achieve pregnancy after varicocele surgery. However, many physicians believe that varicocele surgery is unnecessary and seek to improve semen quality by means of drug or hormone therapy, or by washing and preparing the sperm for artificial insemination.

Physical injury to the testes, from internal or external sources, is yet another cause of infertility. A particularly common problem, especially during puberty, is torsion of the testes due to a malformation in the tissue supporting the gonads. Great pain and swelling ensue because the blood supply to the gonads is cut off by twisted blood vessels. Surgery to relieve the torsion must be performed immediately to stem the irreversible cell degeneration resulting from the constricted blood supply. Even if only one side is affected, the surgeon will regularly secure both testes, since many individuals who experience torsion on one side are more vulnerable than average to experience it on the other side as well. Similarly, if one testicle is so damaged as to be nonfunctional, the surgeon generally recommends its complete removal to avert a degenerative influence on its partner.

Toxins in the work or home environment can interfere with normal sperm production. Lead, pesticides, mercury, solvents, and many other chemicals affect spermatogenesis and, if exposure is not reduced or eliminated, can cause permanent infertility. Excessive exposure of the gonads to radiation can have similar effects.

Sperm Transport

If biopsies indicate that normal sperm production is occurring in the testes but the semen analysis reveals a low or absent sperm count, then the physician deduces that the patient has a sperm transport problem. Seven percent of infertile men have some type of sperm transport disorder.[46] Perhaps the epididymis or the vas deferens are obstructed or deformed. Testing the semen for fructose, which is produced and introduced into the semen by the seminal vesicles, is a simple way to check for the possibility of an abnormal or absent (due to a congenital defect) vas deferens.

Scarring and blockage of the transport apparatus leading from the testes can result from infection. The seminal vesicles, prostate, and ejaculatory ducts as well as the vas deferens and epididymis can be affected by maladies such as prostatitis, gonorrhea, and tuberculosis. The end of the epididymis closest to the vas deferens is the most common site of impairment. Microsurgery to repair the tiny tubules of the epididymis can be difficult but is successful in 50 to 70 percent of attempts.[47]

Vasectomies, both deliberate and accidental (due to injury or surgical error), are the most common sources of infertility. Reversal by microsurgery is usually successful at reestablishing fertility in 70 to 90 percent of cases if performed within 10 years of the original vasectomy.[48] After 10 years, mounting pressure from blocked sperm may lead to ruptures in the epididymis's walls, which can be very difficult, if not impossible, to repair.

When the vas deferens is completely absent or impossible to repair, some surgeons may attempt a new technique that constructs an artificial pouch to collect sperm directly from the testes. The collected sperm can then be removed and prepared for artificial insemination. Results thus far have not been very encouraging; sperm that have not passed through the epididymis do not yet seem to have adequate motility to swim up to and fertilize the egg.

Impotence

Perhaps the most conspicuous cause of male infertility is impotence, the inability to maintain an erection and ejaculate during intercourse. Impotence may occur because of physiological or psychological impediments; often the second kind of problems will compound the first. Along with ejaculatory disturbances and other sexual problems, impotence accounts for approximately 10 percent of male infertility.[49] *Organic impotence* and *physical impotence* are terms used to describe impotence due to the body's physical inability to respond to sexual stimulation because of impaired hormonal systems, impaired neural paths, or abnormal reproductive organ development. Organic impotence can be congenital or can be brought on later by illness, exposure to toxins, drugs, surgery, or injury. Hormonal imbalances can often be alleviated by hormone supplements, and impotence due to infection or disease, depending on its nature and duration, can often be treated with medication. Likewise, cessation of exposure to toxins and some drugs can result in recovered sexual capabilities, again depending on the particular case. When physical impotence is irreversible, due to irreparable physical damage to the erectile tissue, penile implants have been found to be a safe and effective recourse for restoring sexual satisfaction. Women whose husbands use such implants claim that they cannot tell the difference from a normal erection. However, penile implants do not necessarily result in fertility; other problems may still exist to prevent the fathering of a child.

Psychological impotence occurs when the organic requirements for erection and ejaculation exist, but mental and emotional stress prevents their employment. Often, physical difficulties with erection and ejaculation will lead to psychological disturbances, causing impotence where there really is not sufficient physical cause for it. Counseling and adjustments in sexual techniques can often help to overcome this type of impotence.

Ejaculatory disturbances include premature ejaculation, in which ejaculation occurs before the penis is fully inserted in the vagina, and ejaculatory incompetence, where ejaculation does not occur at all during intercourse. Both of these disorders have some psychological roots and, like psychological impotence, can often be overcome with counseling and revisions in coital technique. Another type of ejaculatory disturbance is retrograde ejaculation, where ejaculation occurs into the bladder, instead of out of the penis. Normally, the bladder sphincter closes at the time of ejaculation, to prevent the mixing of urine and semen. The sphincter may become impaired as a result of diabetes, neurological disorders, and abdominal surgeries in the area of the sphincter. Retrograde ejaculation may be controlled by medication to contract the sphincter or, occasionally, surgery can correct the broken valve. The most common solution to achieve pregnancy, however, is the collection of the sperm from the urine for use in artificial insemination. Artificial insemination also may be employed using semen obtained by artificial or electrical stimulation of ejaculation from organically impotent men.

Conclusion

Clearly, many infertile men and women are willing to undergo considerable inconvenience, discomfort, and even pain to conceive a child to whom they are genetically related. Some critics argue that society should be focusing more on ways to prevent infertility than on ways to cure it. The critics are probably correct to emphasize preventive over curative medicine. Nevertheless, not all types of infertility are amenable to prevention; some require a cure, and for this reason alone funds should be earmarked for infertility research.

Other critics worry that "baby hunger" is not an altogether healthy desire. Why do so many people believe that they cannot be happy unless they beget, bear, and rear at least one child genetically related to them? Why won't adoption or foster parenting do? Infertile couples respond impatiently, even angrily, to these critics. As they see it, their infertility constitutes a deprivation of a very cruel sort, and if medical technology has the means to help them reproduce, then they wish to use those means. As wonderful as it may be to adopt or to foster parent a child, there remains in many people's minds something very special about a man and a woman conceiving a child who is not only a concrete sign of their love but also a biological connection to the future, a way to go on living after one's death.

Admittedly, society has sometimes overemphasized the importance of having genetic children. Women have been told that unless they experience pregnancy and motherhood, they can never be "real" women. Men have been told that there is no greater ego boost than creating a child in one's own image and likeness and seeing to it that the child inherits all of one's considerable possessions as well as one's family name. That both of these social messages are misguided is obvious. A woman does not need to produce a child to become a full person; she is a full person in and of herself. Likewise, a man should not view a child, male or female, as a reflection of himself or as proof of his potency. To do this is to treat his child as an object and to fail to realize that children are about love and not power. Nevertheless, there is nothing wrong with wanting a genetic child, provided that one is ready, willing, and able to assume the responsibilities as well as the rights of parenthood. Rather than faulting infertile people for wanting babies too much, society should make certain that no one takes advantage of infertile people by raising their hopes falsely, for example, or by charging them high fees for medical services that simply cannot deliver what is promised.

8 Artificial Insemination

Contraception, sterilization, and abortion are three reproduction-controlling techniques that enable people to determine when, where, with whom and, most importantly, *whether* they will bring children into the world. However, as we know, preventing unwanted pregnancies is not a problem for everyone. Even though human reproduction seems highly successful in practice—after all, millions of babies are born every year—in fact, it has a high failure rate. For every 100 human eggs that come in contact with sperm in the course of natural fertilization, only 84 are actually fertilized and only 69 are implanted. Of the original 100 eggs, 42 survive the first week of pregnancy, 37 survive through the sixth week, and only 31 survive to birth. In sum, the reproductive failure rate is approximately 69 percent! The fact that nearly 15 percent of all couples are infertile because of physiological problems such as ovaries that fail to release eggs, blocked or scarred fallopian tubes, and abnormal sperm production, compounded by the fact that only three of ten fertilized eggs come to term, explains why the demand for reproductive-aiding technologies is already strong and likely to grow.[1-4]

Diagnostic Kits to Aid Reproduction

In addition to the many sophisticated reproduction-aiding technologies that have been developed to help infertile couples, a number of valuable, relatively simple, self-contained diagnostic kits also have become available. Since a kit was developed to enable diabetics to monitor their own blood glucose level, people have been using kits to measure the levels of certain chemicals and drugs in their blood or urine.

Home diagnostic kits that predict the day of ovulation are available at pharmacies. These kits measure the level of luteinizing hormone (LH) that surges 12 to 36 hours before ovulation. Because the couple has advanced notice that ovulation is about to occur, they can plan sexual intercourse accordingly.

The first of these LH-measuring diagnostic kits—First Response by Tambrands and Ovutime by Ortho—employed a multistep immunological assay, the *enzyme-linked immunosorbent assay* (ELISA). The ELISA procedure is based on the specific interaction between a monoclonal antibody and LH. An antibody is a protein that normally acts to defend the body by binding to foreign molecules and cells. Monoclonal antibodies are antibodies secreted by laboratory-prepared cells that are hybrids of tumor cells and antibody-producing cells (lymphocytes). Monoclonal antibodies are produced to bind specifically to particular biological molecules such as hormones. For example, a monoclonal antibody is produced specifically for LH. It is then attached to an enzyme, which is a protein capable of changing the structure of other molecules called *substrates*. When this enzyme modifies the substrates used in the ELISA solution, new molecules are produced that cause its color to change.

A First Response or Ovutime kit contains (1) a solid plastic strip to which the monoclonal antibodies specific for LH have been attached; (2) a sample of monoclonal antibodies (the same kind attached to the plastic strip) with an attached enzyme; and (3) a solution of the substrate that the enzyme can modify. The woman tests her LH level by executing the following procedure:

1. She places the plastic strip with the attached monoclonal antibodies into a sample of her urine. At this time, any LH present binds to the monoclonal antibodies and is removed from the urine.

2. She removes the plastic strip from the urine and washes it thoroughly to remove anything in her urine sample that may interfere with the test.

3. She places the plastic strip in the solution containing the monoclonal antibodies with the enzyme attached. These monoclonal antibodies will bind to the plastic strip wherever LH molecules are located. This will form a sandwich-like complex.

4. Finally, she places the plastic strip with all the attached molecules into a solution of the substrate. The substrate is modified by the enzyme attached through the sandwich to the plastic strip. As a result, the solution changes color. For the substrate to be modified (and for the solution to change color), the enzyme has to be present, and for the enzyme to be present, it has to be linked through the monoclonal anti-

body to the LH. This sequence of events is the key to the assay. The intensity of the color is dependent on the amount of enzyme, which is directly dependent on the amount of LH present. If no LH is present in the urine, then none can bind to the first monoclonal antibody and none of the monoclonal antibody–enzyme complex can bind to the LH (because none is present); if no enzymes are present, then none of the substrate can be modified, so no change in color can occur.

These kits have been further refined, becoming even simpler to use and more rapid. Clearplan Easy, one of the new kits presently available in pharmacies, employs a sandwich immunoassay that uses blue latex microbeads in an ingenious way to allow the procedure to be completed with one step.[5] As in ELISA, the principle of Clearplan Easy's sandwich assay involves the formation of a complex (figure 8.1a). Each test strip consists of a plastic strip with an absorbent wick at one end and two windows in the middle. The wick is attached to a porous membrane with three separate zones of antibodies (figure 8.1b).

The woman holds the wick in a stream of her urine for 5 seconds. As the wick becomes saturated, the urine passes by capillary action into zone 1. This zone contains monoclonal antibodies to LH. The antibodies are attached to blue latex microbeads. As the urine interacts with these antibodies, it carries them along to zone 2. If LH is present in the urine, a complex between the LH and the antibodies to LH will be formed (figure 8.1b, positive). In zone 2, additional antibodies to LH are immobilized in the membrane. As the urine flows past zone 2, antibodies from zone 1, carrying the blue latex microbeads, which are complexed with LH, bind to this second antibody and become attached to the membrane. This is the sandwich from which the assay gets its name. Specifically, it is a sandwich of blue latex microbeads–LH antibody–LH molecule from urine–LH antibody immobilized on membrane. The result is a blue line in the test window.

Whether or not the urine contains LH, the urine flowing on the test strip contains antibodies bound to the blue latex microbeads which it picked up from zone 1. As the urine continues to flow, it carries these antibodies into zone 3. Zone 3 contains another type of antibody specific for the LH antibody. Since these two antibodies will interact whether or not LH is present, a blue band forms in zone 3 as a control that the test was performed correctly. The arrangement of zones 2 and 3 allows companies the flexibility to create different signals to indicate the test result. One common indicator is a plus for a positive test and a minus for a negative test.

Basis for the sandwich immunoassay

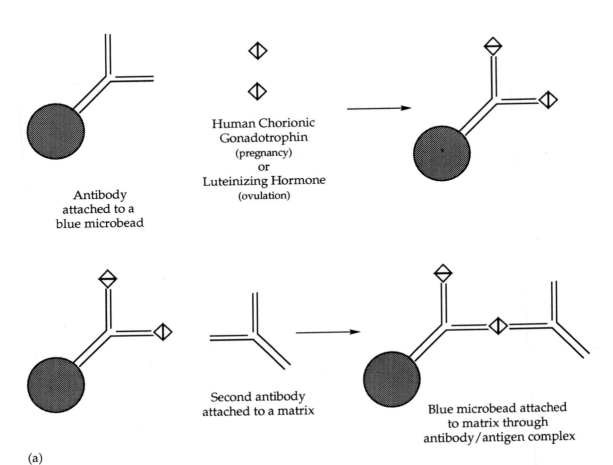

Antibody
attached to a
blue microbead

Human Chorionic
Gonadotrophin
(pregnancy)
or
Luteinizing Hormone
(ovulation)

Second antibody
attached to a matrix

Blue microbead attached
to matrix through
antibody/antigen complex

(a)

Figure 8.1 Schematic of the sandwich immunoassay for predicting ovulation and pregnancy. (a) The biochemical basis for the sandwich assay involving the binding of the hormone to an antibody attached to a microbead with subsequent formation of a sandwich complex. (b) Representation of the sandwich immunoassay for both the positive and negative cases. (See text for details.)

Sandwich immunoassay

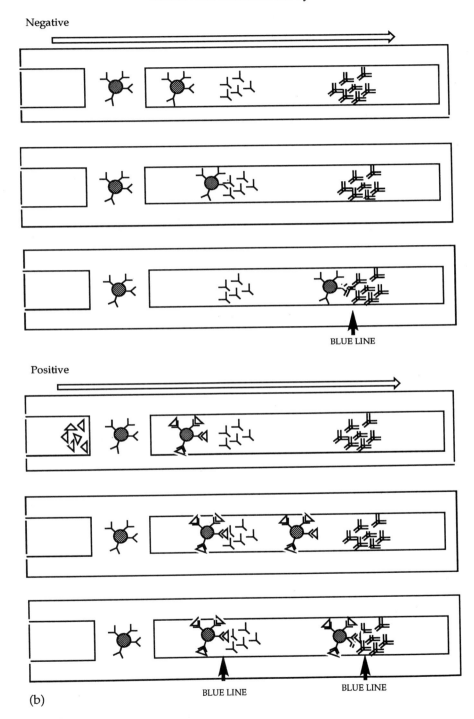

(b)

While these tests were designed to be performed by a nonscientifically trained person, they are the same tests that have been used by physicians, laboratories, and fertility clinics to predict ovulation. Variations on the test allow it to be used to determine if a woman is pregnant. Thus, even though these tests are simple and safe to perform they represent a sophisticated technological development that empowers people to control their reproductive lives without the direct intervention of experts.

Another type of diagnostic kit, Ovuplan, was developed by Personal Diagnostics but has yet to be marketed. This kit involves a completely different approach. It consists of a monitor with a memory function and disposable test packets. A woman uses the test packets to measure four enzymes in her saliva that vary with her ovulation cycle: peroxidase, alkaline phosphatase, glucosaminidase, and β-glucuronidase. For 1 month, the woman uses the sponge in the test packet to analyze samples of her saliva on a daily basis. The monitor reads and stores the results. After a month, the monitor analyzes the data and suggests a "fertility window" to be sampled during the next menstrual cycle. After 3 months of collecting and analyzing the data, the monitor predicts a 2-day period of peak fertility. Once again, this very sophisticated technological development could provide people with additional control over their reproductive lives.

Another diagnostic device, the Rabbit Ovulation Computer (manufactured by Rabbit Computers), is based on the basal body temperature method. On the first day of her cycle, the woman enters the date into the computer. Then on the next day, the woman places a sensor under her tongue and the computer detects her basal body temperature. After doing this for a number of cycles, the computer charts her ovulatory history and the microchip computes the days she is likely to be fertile. With the basal body temperature information, the computer also can tell whether the woman has signs of infertility, irregularity, or early menopause.

The Technology of Artificial Insemination and Sperm Banking

Because it is a fairly simple medical procedure, artificial insemination is the most widely used reproduction-aiding technology today. Although artificial insemination did not become a widely accepted treatment for human infertility until fairly recently, it had long been used to facilitate animal breeding. The first reported use of artificial insemination in humans was with a husband's sperm in 1790. Nearly a century was to pass, however, before a donor's sperm was used in the artificial insemination of a human. This occurred in 1884 when a wealthy Philadelphia merchant sought the aid of a physician to overcome the infertility that prevented him and his wife from having children.

The physician, Dr. William Pancoast, was a full professor of descriptive and surgical anatomy at Jefferson Medical College. Pancoast brought the couple's infertility to the attention of 6 student doctors in his anatomy class. Reasoning that either the woman or the man was the cause of the couple's infertility, Dr. Pancoast first conducted a complete physical examination of the woman. He concluded that she was in good reproductive health and capable of begetting and bearing a child. Pancoast's subsequent examination of the man revealed that he was the cause of the infertility, and extensive medical treatment failed to improve either the quality or quantity of his sperm. When everything else that could be tried had failed, Dr. Pancoast's students proposed that a "hired man" might be used. Dr. Pancoast took his students' proposal seriously. Without the consent of the couple, he injected semen from one of his students into the woman's womb during a routine examination. The woman became pregnant and a healthy son was born to the couple, albeit at the cost of their informed consent.[6]

Despite the fact that Dr. Pancoast's ethics were suspect, his experiment was a success. By the end of the nineteenth century, artificial insemination by husband or by donor was practiced by many physicians, if somewhat surreptitiously. In the United States alone, 10,000 children were conceived by artificial insemination before 1941, and 1000 to 2000 children were conceived by artificial insemination each year between 1941 and 1963. By 1982, 20,000 children annually were born as a result of artificial insemination.[7]

Types of Artificial Insemination

There are two variations of the artificial insemination (AI) procedure, one in which the sperm used comes from the husband or male partner (artificial insemination by husband [AIH]) and the other in which the sperm comes from a donor (artificial insemination by donor [AID], *not* to be confused with the sexually transmitted disease, acquired immunodeficiency syndrome [AIDS]). From a biological point of view, the source of the sperm is irrelevant. AI is the most reasonable treatment for a number of male infertility problems such as when there are no sperm in the ejaculate (azoospermia), when the sperm are reduced in number or quality (asthenospermia), or when the sperm are either dead or abnormal. Some of these problems may arise from a lack of production of sperm in the testis or an obstruction in the male genital tract.[8]

AIH is considered to be the most reasonable treatment when the husband's sperm are normal and able to fertilize the egg, but the sperm count is low. We mentioned earlier that a man with a normal sperm count ejaculates between 50 to 100 million sperm into the vagina. Apparently, this astronomical number of sperm is necessary for fertility. Even minor decreases in this number are likely to result in infertility. Thus, if a man has low sperm production, the physician must collect and pool a number of his patient's sperm samples before they can be used for AI. A new technique that may eventually alleviate the need for pooling multiple samples if the problem involves an obstruction in the genital tract is called *microsurgical sperm aspiration*. This procedure consists of microsurgical scrotal exploration and identification of the regions of the epididymis. A small incision is made in the epididymis, at the distal end if possible, and the milky contents are removed with a small pipet. If necessary, the sperm are then treated to improve their quality before they are used for AI.[9]

AID is indicated when the husband is so infertile that pooling his sperm is not of much use, when there is an Rh incompatibility, or when the husband suffers from a serious hereditary disorder. A minority of AID practitioners believe that, under certain circumstances, a small amount of the husband's sperm should be mixed with the donor's so the husband can feel that there is a possibility that he is the father. The majority of AID practitioners, however, oppose sperm-mixing as a deceptive, often harmful stratagem. If the husband needs to believe that his AID child may really be his genetic progeny, there is some reason to fear that his interest in perpetuating his genes is stronger than his interest in rearing a child.

AID also may be indicated when a single woman wants to have a child. Some AID practitioners object to artificially inseminating single women, but it is not clear on what they base their objection. Perhaps they reason that AID is a treatment for infertility, a condition from which the single women who seek their services do not suffer. More likely, they may be basing their opposition to artificially inseminating single women not on a medical reason but on a moral one; for example, they may believe children should not deliberately be conceived by a single parent.

In most cases of AI, the sperm is injected directly into the female genital tract, and no preliminary treatment of the semen is necessary. For example, pretreatment to ensure the capacitation of the sperm is not necessary as it is with other reproduction-aiding technologies, which take place outside of the body. Indeed, AI is so simple that home insemination kits may soon be commercially available.

A number of procedures have been developed to improve the quality of the sperm sample if quality is a problem. Generally, these involve washing and concentrating the semen on a gradient of a Percoll-containing solution to "increase the sperm fertilizability."[10]

Although the sperm are usually introduced into the vagina, new procedures have been developed for intrauterine insemination[11] and for hysteroscopic insemination into the fallopian tube.[12]

Sperm Banking

Simply because AI can be performed easily does not mean it is without its peculiar technological complexities. Because it is sometimes difficult to produce fresh sperm on demand and to screen them instantaneously for genetic abnormalities, the technology of AI significantly advanced when researchers developed ways to freeze sperm without harming their cellular structure. One relatively simple technique uses glycerol to prevent the formation of cell-damaging ice structures. In this procedure, a laboratory technician places a semen sample in a special vial designed to withstand extremes of temperature and suspends it over liquid nitrogen to achieve an initial freezing temperature of $-76°C$. In another procedure, called the *dry-ice pellet method*, the concentrated sperm sample is mixed with the cryomedium and then dropped into hollows of a dry-ice block without precooling.[13] After the sample is frozen, it is lowered into the liquid nitrogen where it is maintained indefinitely at $-196°C$. The average survival rate of nitrogen-frozen and thawed sperm is approximately 67 percent. Far from being a risky procedure, the freezing and thawing process of cryopreservation kills off abnormal sperm while safeguarding normal sperm. As a result, children conceived with frozen sperm have a lower incidence of birth defects and spontaneous abortions than children conceived with fresh sperm. With the increase in sexually transmitted diseases, and especially AIDS, essentially all AID is done with sperm that has been frozen and thoroughly tested.

There are approximately 400 hospital-based sperm banks in the United States. In addition, there are a growing number of commercial sperm banks that sell sperm to AID practitioners. Finally, there are a few sperm banks that have made a name for themselves because of their clientele or special purposes. One of these is The Sperm Bank of Northern California, a feminist-run facility that is committed to providing AID to any and all healthy women, including single and lesbian women. Another of these is The Repository for Germinal Choice, a facility that is dedicated to obtaining sperm from persons of prominence, achievement, and genius who are asked to donate their reproductive cells so that specially selected infertile couples can use them to produce "superior" children. Inaccurately known as the *"Nobel Prize–Winners" Spermbank* (a prize winner has yet to make a contribution), The Respository for Germinal Choice nonetheless prides itself on its eugenic mission. Perhaps it is the dubious nature of its mission that accounts for the fact that only 100 Germinal Choice babies were created during the bank's first 10 years of existence.[14]

Nonmedical Issues Regarding Artificial Insemination

AI is an increasingly acceptable way for an infertile couple to bring into the world a new life that could not have been conceived otherwise. George Annas reports that by 1980, in addition to the children conceived by AIH, there were 250,000 children conceived by AID.[15] Nevertheless, despite its popularity, AI still raises several ethical, legal, and social questions that affect such important human relationships as those between (1) the attending physician, the sperm donor, and the recipient; (2) the recipient and her partner or the sperm donor; (3) the sperm donor and his genetic child; and, finally, (4) the legal father and his legal child. The ultimate justification for AI will depend, then, on whether its consequences are more beneficial than harmful for society and also on whether it accords with individuals' rights.

The Ethics of Artificial Insemination

Ethical Arguments Against Artificial Insemination

Although most ethicists believe that AI is morally permissible, traditional natural-law theorists regard it as intrinsically wrong. So opposed is this comparatively small group of theorists to AI that they reject not only AID but also AIH. They reject AIH because it uses what they consider a "bad means" (namely, masturbation) to serve a "good end" (namely, procreation). The fact that most ethicists accept masturbation as a legitimate way to release sexual tension does not affect the traditional natural-law theorists' condemnation of it as a "solitary and essentially individualistic use" of a sexual organ meant to be exercised "in a joint and common act."[16]

Unwilling to challenge their colleagues' moral assessment of masturbation but wanting to assist infertile couples, less traditional natural-law theorists have suggested several alternatives to masturbation: (1) aspiration of sperm by puncturing a testicle and the epididymis; (2) coitus interruptus; (3) intercourse with condoms; (4) postcoital aspiration of sperm from the vagina; and (5) postcoital use of containers such as the "tassette."[17] The first of these alternatives, aspiration of sperm by puncturing a testicle and the epididymis, certainly provides no pleasure to the man. Nevertheless, this surgical alternative to masturbation has been rejected by the strictest natural-law theorists who argue that what is evil is not so much the pleasure that ordinarily results to the man from masturbation but rather the removal of sperm from his generative organs, a removal that supposedly breaks the natural line from sperm production to the procreative act. Whether sperm are removed from a man's body by masturbation or by surgery, they are removed from his body unnaturally.[18] The second and third alternatives, coitus interruptus and intercourse with condoms, are also rejected by the strictest natural-law theorists on the grounds that the "determining factor of true coitus"—namely, ejaculation into the vagina—is missing in them.[19] The last two alternatives to masturbation, postcoital aspiration of sperm from the vagina and postcoital use of containers such as the tassette, are accepted even by the strictest natural-law theorists, since the full act of coitus precedes the removal of the sperm from the woman's vagina.

If natural-law theorists are divided on the issue of masturbation, they tend to be united on their overall negative assessment of AIH and AID. They reject AIH on the grounds that "to reduce the shared life of a married couple and the act of married love to a mere organic activity for transmitting semen would be like turning the domestic home, the sanctuary of the family, into a biological laboratory."[20] They reject AID on the grounds that it necessitates the unjustified, indeed adulterous intrusion of a third party (the sperm donor) into the marital relationship.

Critics challenge the natural-law theorists' rejection of AIH, noting that although AIH has little to do with expressing a couple's psychological and spiritual intimacy, it has much to do with expressing their desire to beget, bear, and rear a child together, a process that will unify them more than any one act of so-called natural sexual intercourse. These same critics also challenge the natural-law theorists' third-party intrusion argument, observing that it depends on an odd definition of adultery as "the uniting of sperm and ovum of two people one of whom is married but not to the other."[21] Ordinarily, persons do not associate acts of adultery with the process of fertilization. As they see it, adultery occurs not when a physician dispassionately inserts a syringe full of an anonymous donor's sperm into a married woman's vagina but when a married person engages in more or less passionate sexual intercourse with someone to whom she or he is not married.

The fact that it is a mistake to define AID as a type of adultery does not mean, however, that AID in no way constitutes a third-party intrusion into the marital relationship. Some infertile couples choose AID over adoption because they believe that they will be able to love a child who is genetically related to at least one of them (the wife) more than a child who is genetically related to neither of them. But things do not always work out as planned. When a couple adopts a child, both the father and the mother stand in the same relation to it; if they choose, both parents can spend approximately the same amount of time caring for the child, feeling equally close to him or her. In contrast, when a couple has a child by AID, the mother is the child's begetter, bearer, and rearer; the father is only the child's rearer. For couples who are convinced that parenthood consists essentially in the rearing of a child, this asymmetry does not present a problem, but for couples who have mixed feelings about what makes a parent a "real" parent, this asymmetry can generate marital problems.[22]

Even if AID does not often cause marital problems, natural-law theorists insist that it almost always engenders a secrecy antithetical to the social values of openness, honesty, and truthfulness on which well-functioning family life rests.[23] For similar reasons, rights-oriented ethicists object to the secrecy that surrounds AID. They argue that such laudable goals as shielding the infertile couple from gossip, safeguarding the sperm donor's reputation, and protecting the psychological security of the child do not justify lying to the child about his or her genetic roots. When parents lie to their AID child, they see themselves as lying to secure happiness for both their child and themselves. What they do not see, says the rights-oriented ethicist, is that in lying to their AID child, they are undermining the child's autonomy. They are depriving their child of the opportunity to choose deliberately who he or she wishes to regard as the real father.[24]

Other types of manipulation occur when only one member of an infertile couple knows that the child is an AID child or when only one member of an infertile couple knows the identity of the AID donor. For example, rather than telling her husband that he is infertile and incapable of begetting a child, a wife may ask a physician to arrange AID for her. If she conceives, her husband will assume that the child is his genetic child and, supposedly, the family will live as it would if the child had been conceived normally. For another example, rather than discussing possible sperm donors with his wife, a husband may ask a physician to inseminate his wife with the sperm of his brother; indeed, in post World War II America such requests were made with some frequency by infertile Jewish men who were understandably concerned about maintaining their family blood lines.[25] Writing about such a case, an attending physician expressed "no regrets" about his silence, since "happy family relationships" resulted.[26] But, queries the rights-oriented ethicist, what happens in those cases where "happy family relationships" do not result? Is the attending physician's act of deception suddenly unjustified, or is it simply the case that acts of deception are always wrong even when the deceived parties are happier as a result of having had the wool pulled over their eyes?

As we have seen, rights-oriented ethicists emphasize the fact that deception is always wrong even if it has happy consequences. Although natural-law theorists agree with this viewpoint, they believe that, as it turns out, deception almost always has unhappy consequences. When a child discovers that her father is not her genetic father, or a husband discovers that his child is not his genetic child, or a wife discovers that the genetic father of her child is not an anonymous sperm donor but her brother-in-law, feelings of betrayal are likely to surface. Should these feelings grow strong, the family unit will fray around the edges and even weaken at its core, leading to alienation, separation, and perhaps divorce.

The conviction that AID weakens the family is manifest in the Feversham Committee's 1960 decision to condemn AID. Appointed by Great Britain's House of Lords, this committee concurred with the then Archbishop of Canterbury that AID fails to create bona fide families—that is, families consisting of two parents and the children begotten by them. Not only does AID lead to "irregular" families in which the rearing father is not the genetic father; it opens the way "for the bearing of children by unmarried women."[27]

To be sure, the Feversham Committee's 1960 recommendation was neither universally applauded nor ultimately accepted. Critics objected to its narrow definition of the family in general and to its implicit condemnation of single mothers in particular. Nevertheless, many of these same critics found themselves in agreement with the Feversham Committee when it went on to express concern about AID's eugenic implications. There are, the committee said, at least two reasons to fault infertile couples who prefer AID to adoption on the grounds that AID children are supposedly a better genetic bet than adopted children. First, such couples may be acting against their own announced best interests. Contrary to some reports, AID actually guarantees very little in the way of superior genes.[28] Screening of sperm donors remains rather basic. Provided that a man is not seropositive for the human immunodeficiency virus and is not a carrier of a major genetic disease, his sperm will probably pass muster. The fact that some AID practitioners often use the sperm of medical school students may be a source of comfort to some couples, but it really should not be. Frequently, these sperm are used without any attempts to screen them.[29] Second, such couples may be acting not only imprudently but also immorally or selfishly. Rather than adopting existing babies who are in great need of loving parents, they prefer to conceive special babies genetically related to the female member of the couple.

In response to these objections to AID, philosopher Peter Singer and physician Deane Wells agree that screening techniques for sperm donors need to be improved, but they refuse to concede that AID couples, who desire to have normal or even "better than normal" children, are any more selfish than most other couples. As Singer and Wells see it, it is one thing for a couple to want a healthy child and quite another for a couple to want a handicapped child that is likely to make intense demands on their financial, physical, psychological, or spiritual resources.[30] Certainly, fertile couples who give birth to demanding children are not free to abandon them, but neither are they required to beget or to adopt children that they believe will be exceptionally challenging to rear. Thus, say Singer and Wells, infertile couples who express a preference for healthy children should not be condemned for seeking to escape a burden that many fertile couples would not intentionally or knowingly shoulder.

Whatever the merits of Singer and Well's line of reasoning, however, many people find distinctions between normal and abnormal, healthy and handicapped, easy and difficult babies invidious. Babies, they insist, are intrinsically valuable persons, not instrumentally valuable things. They are not some sort of consumer good, investment option, or living testimony to their parents' supposed genetic superiority. No doubt, the insistence that babies are persons, worthy of society's respect and consideration, largely explains concerns about AID's eugenic implications, as does the fact that some of the original proponents of sperm banks were also key figures in the germinal choice movement and in Eugenic Insemination by Deliberately Preferred Donors [EID].[31] Nevertheless, despite the establishment of some special sperm banks, most ordinary sperm banks are, as was noted earlier, simply hygienic laboratories from which physicians can withdraw a supply of sperm at approximately $77 per vial.[32] Indeed, most physicians are so uninterested in the eugenic implications of AID that they err in the direction of not caring enough about the quality of sperm they use. Too little rather than too much screening of sperm is the problem that preoccupies most concerned commentators.

Arguments For and Against Artificial Insemination

Utilitarians morally assess AIH by weighing its projected harmful results against its projected beneficial results. Provided that a couple will not experience any psychological or spiritual trauma as a result of using AIH, and provided that the manipulation of the sperm outside the husband's body does not lead to genetic defects, utilitarians find no moral problems with AIH. By using this relatively simple technique, a couple is able to increase its personal happiness.

When it comes to AID as opposed to AIH, however, utilitarians are divided with respect to its utility-maximizing tendencies. There are, after all, reasons to believe that AID may cause a whole range of psychological, social, and legal problems, and the responsible person will contemplate the negative as well as the positive features of AID before pronouncing on its overall unity.

First, AID can jeopardize spousal love by creating feelings of inadequacy, resentment, or asymmetry between a husband and wife, a possibility to which we previously alluded. According to some psychologists, AID fathers do not always love their AID children as much as they should. One AID father, to whom an AID son was born, confessed to his psychologist that he had hoped his wife would deliver a girl because in his mind "a son would highlight my loss because he wouldn't be a small version of me."[33] Frequently, when the AID mother senses that her husband is keeping their AID child at arm's length, she overcompensates by becoming totally devoted to their AID child, effectively blocking her husband from her emotional life.[34] So treated, the AID father is likely to fault his wife for caring nothing about his feelings and everything about *her* child's.

Second, AID can have long-range negative consequences for AID children. Judging it best to hide the AID "secret," some AID practitioners still advise AID couples not to tell their children about their genetic heritage. No matter what precautions are taken, however, such secrets do not usually remain secrets. Many AID children eventually find out that their rearing fathers are not their genetic fathers, and some of these children are traumatized by this discovery. Suzanne Rubin, an AID child herself, writes that:

No one considers how the child feels when she finds that her natural father was a $25 cup of sperm. The fantasies revolve around what the donor was thinking while he was filling the cup. There is no passion, no human contact in such a union; just cold calculation and manipulation of another person's life.[35]

Clearly distressed by the circumstances of her conception, Rubin concludes that healthy family relationships cannot be built on a "foundation of deliberate lies" and that the people who suffer the most in AID families are the children, some of whom never learn to cope with the sperm donor in their background.

Third, AID can have any number of deleterious effects on a sperm donor. For example, an anonymous sperm donor may feel guilty about having fathered a genetic child with whom he has no possibility of contact. Alternatively, an anonymous sperm donor may, as a result of a breach in confidentiality, suddenly find himself pursued by a child with whom he wants no relationship. Of equal concern is the AID donor's fear about possible disruption to his own family should one of his AID offspring have direct access to him or should his nonconsenting wife discover his involvement in sperm vending.[36] AID may also have a deleterious effect on the nonanonymous sperm donor who begins to see reflections of himself in the child he fathered. Wanting to be more than a name to his boy or girl, he may find himself rebuffed by the rearing parents who prefer that he have no contact with the child.

Finally, AID can result in still other unfortunate consequences. A sperm bank may negligently or recklessly sell defective sperm to a couple, or it may negligently or recklessly deliver the sperm of a white donor to a black couple who specifically asked for a black donor's sperm.[37] When a man and woman find themselves the parents of a child who fails to meet their fundamental expectations, they may be tempted to disavow the child as somehow not really theirs.

As strong as their case against AID seems, the utilitarians' case for AID seems equally strong. Utilitarian advocates of AID believe that its pitfalls have been greatly exaggerated. They argue that even if a few couples have marital or child-rearing problems subsequent to the birth of their AID child, most do not. They also observe that even if some husband-wife tensions and jealousies do accompany the begetting, bearing, and rearing of AID children, these tensions and jealousies are probably not much worse than those that ordinarily accompany the assumption of parental responsibilities. Provided that prospective AID parents are fully informed about this technology's negative as well as positive repercussions, and provided that both of them nonetheless give consent to it, there is no compelling moral reason to deny them AID, especially if they intend to be as honest with their AID child as they have been with each other.

Insofar as the problem of the deceived child is concerned, AID's utilitarian advocates concede that a policy of lying to AID children is wrong.

Not only are many AID children seriously distressed when they discover the truth about themselves; a policy of lying to these children undermines trust between *all* parents and children. After all, if children cannot trust their parents to tell them the truth, whom can they trust?

However, if a policy of lying to AID children causes such problems, the remedy for this unhappiness is not, say AID's utilitarian advocates, to create another kind of unhappiness by forbidding AID to infertile couples. Rather, it is to establish a policy of telling the truth to AID children even if such a policy triggers a degree of short-term suffering for some AID families. Although AID parents may have been able to excuse or justify the lies they told to their AID children in the past when a largely intolerant society made life difficult for children who were procreated in unorthodox ways, this particular excuse or justification is less available today. Increasingly, society accepts children who have been brought into the world through the use of reproduction-aiding technologies and, increasingly, society affirms the right not only of adopted children but also of AID children and children conceived by in vitro fertilization to know about their genetic origins. In fact, as things now stand, being an AID child can be more of an asset than a liability. Comments one AID daughter:

Knowing about my AID origin did nothing to alter my feelings for my family. Instead I felt grateful for the trouble they had taken to give me life. And they had given me such a strong set of roots, a rich and colorful heritage, a sense of being loved. With their adventure in biology, my parents had opened up the fairly rigid culture they had brought with them to this country. The secret knowledge of my "differentness" and my sister's may have helped our parents accept ... the few deviations from their norms that we argued for.[38]

To the degree that differentness is celebrated by a society, say AID's utilitarian advocates, lying to AID children is unnecessary.

With respect to the problem of the harmed anonymous sperm donor, AID's utilitarian advocates argue that very few sperm donors torment themselves about being deprived of contact with their genetic children. They sell their sperm and go home happy to have made a few dollars or to have contributed to the well-being of an infertile couple. If anonymous sperm donors are harmed in any way, it is as the result of breaches of confidentiality, but a proper balance can be struck between the AID child's interest in knowing about his or her genetic heritage and the sperm donor's interest in keeping his personal identity a secret from his genetic child. Whereas laws can permit AID children access to nonidentifying information about their genetic fathers (e.g., their medical histories), laws also can forbid these children access to identifying information about their genetic fathers (e.g., their names or photographs). Only in those cases where both the sperm donors and the sperm recipients (that is, the AID parents) mutually consent should exceptions to the no identifying information rule be made.

Finally, insofar as problems at the sperm bank are concerned, they can be resolved in a variety of ways. Legislators may hold the owners, managers, or employees of sperm banks liable for the mishandling of sperm or the mismatching of sperm donors and recipients.

The Legal Aspects of Artificial Insemination

AIH and the Law

Although AID presents more legal complications than does AIH, AIH is not without its own legal complexities. In a 1949 case, *L.* v. *L.*, a woman who had conceived a child through AIH sought an annulment on the grounds that AIH did not constitute consummation of the marriage. Reasoning that sexual intercourse is necessary for consummation, the English court granted her request.[39]

An even more instructive AIH case is a recent French one. Told that he had testicular cancer, Alain Parpalaix deposited his sperm in a sperm bank in 1981. After his death in 1983, his wife Corinne sought to secure his sperm so that she could be artificially inseminated with them. The sperm bank refused on the ground that her husband had left no instructions concerning what he wanted done with his sperm after his death. A Paris court ruled that Mrs. Parpalaix should be given the sperm, claiming that sperm "is a human secretion that contains the seed of life and is destined to create a human being" and that Mr. Parpalaix's decision to deposit his sperm constituted a "specific contract" with an implicit obligation for the sperm's conservation and for its eventual use.[40] Nevertheless, said this same court, it is unclear whether a child born well after his or her supposed father's death is his or her father's *legitimate* child. According to French common law, a woman's husband is the legal father of her child if that child is born within 300 days of a marriage. But if a child is born to a woman well after she has been widowed, then her child cannot claim her deceased husband as his or her legal father. Thus, any child conceived and borne by Mr. Parpalaix's widow is not, as a matter of common law, Mr. Parpalaix's child.

AID and the Law

Although AIH has generated several legal problems, AID has generated many more. Among these legal problems, the following four appear most often: (1) the claim that AID is a form of adultery; (2) the claim that AID children are illegitimate; (3) the claim that there are no clear rules governing the rights or duties of AID donors, recipients, and children; and (4) the claim that AID opens up new grounds for medical malpractice and medical products liability. Although the first two of these problems have been legally resolved, the third and the fourth have not.

AID as Adultery

For the first half of the twentieth century, many U.S. courts operated on an assumption they apparently borrowed from English Commonwealth courts that AID, without or even with the husband's consent, is a form of adultery. In 1921, for example, the Supreme Court of Ontario, Canada, ruled in a rather unusual case that AID *without* a husband's consent is adultery. Unable to consummate their marriage due to the wife's pain during sexual intercourse, a couple separated by mutual consent so that the wife could seek a cure for her disability in England. While in England, the wife concluded that she could overcome her disability in one of two ways: (1) through surgery or (2) by bearing a child through artificial insemination. She chose the second course of action and bore a child. Returning to Canada 6 years later, the wife discovered that her husband no longer wanted her. Consequently, the wife sued her husband for divorce and alimony, a suit that provoked him to countersue, arguing that alimony was inappropriate since his wife was adulterous.

Investigating this case (*Oxford* v. *Oxford*), the court reasoned that unless the woman could establish either that her husband had consented to AID, which he had not, or that AID does not constitute adultery, she would be found guilty of adultery. The wife's lawyer argued that since moral turpitude (fornicating with someone) is the "essential element of adultery," the wife was not guilty of adultery. In the course of making its ruling, however, the court rejected this understanding of adultery. Instead it offered a rather curious definition of adultery according to which adultery is not the voluntary surrender of one's *sexual* powers or facilities to another person but the voluntary surrender of one's *reproductive* powers or facilities to another.[41]

In 1954, this Canadian ruling was expanded in an Illinois action for visitation rights. According to the Illinois court, AID is adultery even when the husband consents to it: "Artificial insemination [by donor], with or without the consent of the husband, is contrary to public policy and good morals and constitutes adultery on the part of the mother. A child so conceived is not a child born in wedlock and is therefore illegitimate."[42]

More in accord with society's actual sentiments about AID was a 1958 Scottish case. In *MacLennon* v. *MacLennon*, a husband sued for divorce on the grounds of adultery because he had not consented to his wife's use of AID. The Scottish court held that for adultery to be committed, there must be two persons physically present and engaging in the sexual act with some degree of penetration of the vagina by the penis but not necessarily any deposit of sperm. Since artificial insemination never requires physical intimacy but always requires a deposit of sperm, the court reasoned that, whatever else AID may be, it is not an act of adultery.[43] This court's ruling apparently resolved, once and for all, that AID is not an act of adultery.

Legitimacy of AID Children

Not only did some past courts classify AID as adulterous; they also classified AID children as illegitimate. Traditionally, the begetter rather than the rearer of a child was regarded as his or her father. Thus, in common law, a child begotten through a genetic father not the mother's husband was considered illegitimate.

In the United States, a legal trend toward ruling that the rearing father is no less a father than the genetic father began in 1948. In a New York divorce case, *Strnad* v. *Strnad*, the wife sued to limit the husband's visitation rights to their AID child, a child who had been conceived with his consent. Although the court did not explicitly rule that the AID child was legitimate, it did hold that the exhusband, though not the genetic father of the child, was "entitled to the same rights as those acquired by a foster parent who has adopted a child, if not the same rights as those to which a natural parent under the circumstances would be entitled."[44]

Later, in a 1968 California case, a woman sued her exhusband for child support. He refused to support the child on the grounds that it was not his even though he had permitted his exwife to have the child by AID. The Supreme Court of California held that a child conceived through AID does not have a natural father in the person of the anonymous sperm donor. The child does, however, have a legal father in the person of the husband who consents to his wife's artificial insemination.[45]

Although more than 20 years have passed since *People* v. *Sorenson*, no comprehensive statute governing AID has been written. However, several states have enacted a variety of laws to regulate certain aspects of AID. Despite the variations in these laws, most states agree that (1) the husband must consent to AID; (2) the AID child is legitimate; (3) the wife must consent to AID; and (4) an authorized or licensed person must perform the artificial insemination. In addition, several states require the person performing the artificial insemination to certify the consent form and place it in a file. Finally, several states explicitly state that the sperm donor is not the natural father of the child.[46]

Although courts have been denying the parental role of sperm donors in recent years, and although great care is being taken lest sperm donors be named as plaintiffs in paternity suits, there are notable exceptions to this trend. Feminist Gena Corea argues that the parental rights of the sperm donor disappear or appear depending on the marital status of a woman. If a man donates his sperm to a married woman, his status shrivels to that of an anonymous "semen source" who "supplies a bodily fluid and, still nameless, disappears." In contrast, if a man donates his sperm to an unmarried woman his status quickly swells "to that of a father with rights over his issue."[47]

Two admittedly exceptional cases support Corea's argument. In 1977, a man gave some of his sperm to his woman friend who, after she was nearly 3 months pregnant, broke off all relations with him. Protesting that he did not want to break off relations with her, the mother of his genetic child, the genetic father sued for visitation rights. Significantly, a New Jersey court gave him not only the right to visit his genetic child but also the right to be designated his genetic child's legal father.[48] Three years later, in 1980, a homosexual who donated sperm to a lesbian friend filed a suit seeking both visitation and custody rights to his genetic child. In 1983, the California Supreme Court declared him to be the legal father of his genetic child and awarded him visitation rights on the grounds that every child should have a father—that is, a *man*—in his everyday life. What is highly problematic about these two decisions is that they failed to pay as much attention to the rights of the women involved as to those of the men. Single women who use AID may use it because they want neither husbands for themselves nor fathers for their children. They also may use it because they have not been able to find a suitable marital partner and they fear losing the opportunity to bear children. The marital status of a woman should not affect the parental status of a sperm donor. Clearly, the courts will need to resolve this issue in the near future as more unmarried as well as married women choose AID to serve their procreative purposes.

The Rights and Responsibilities of AID Participants and Recipients

Although the courts and legislatures have managed to establish the non-adulterous nature of AID and the legitimacy of AID children, they are still struggling to determine the rights and responsibilities of AID donors, recipients, and children. Nonetheless, even if the last word on these rights and responsibilities has not been uttered, it is still possible to identify the network of relationships AID creates.

AID donors

Until very recently, the law has focused almost exclusively on the rights and responsibilities of anonymous sperm donors, men who do not wish contact with AID recipients and AID children. Noted professor of British law, Dr. Glanville Williams, claims that the reasons for donor anonymity are twofold: the desire "to protect the donor's reputation" and the desire "to eliminate the risk of the wife transferring her affections to the donor."[49] But it is unlikely that today's sperm donors are really worried either about their reputations or about their being sexually harassed by the women who receive their gametes. Instead, today's sperm donors fear that their genetic children may eventually seek their financial or psychological support.

Currently, sperm donors sell their sperm on the condition that they remain anonymous. Although records usually are kept of AID transactions, donors are not told who their recipients are or vice versa. Nevertheless, it is not impossible for the identity of a sperm donor to be disclosed to his child because many standard consent forms govern only the donor-physician and recipient-physician relationships and not also the donor-child relationship. Thus, in the absence of clear legislation, if an otherwise fatherless AID child is able to establish the sperm donor's identity, that donor may be assigned the same rights and responsibilities as has a father of an illegitimate child.[50]

Another practice that directly affects anonymous sperm donors is the matter of payment for their sperm. Some critics argue that it is morally wrong for persons to sell their body parts, including their tissue. Some people object to such sales on the grounds that no one owns his or her body, that it is a gift from God to be disposed of according to divine plan. Other people object that although individuals have a right to sell whatever parts of themselves they wish to sell, such sales should nonetheless be prohibited because they easily lead to abuses. Great Britain, for example, which does not pay its blood donors, collects more and better blood than does the United States, where blood donors are usually paid.

Supposedly, payment to donors vastly increases the risks involved in transfusion, such as the transmission of hepatitis and, more recently, the dreaded AIDS virus. Indeed, infected blood tends to come from men who are desperate enough to sell their blood for money under the false pretense that it is healthy.[51] Since it is possible to sell sperm more frequently than blood, these same men also may be tempted to sell their genetic material even if they suspect or know that they carry a genetic defect. Thus, even if donors have a right to sell their sperm, that right is limited by the state's interest in preventing the birth of genetically defective babies. The issue, then, is not so much compensation or noncompensation of donors as it is appropriate criteria for donor selection.

Currently, donor selection is not a well-developed, carefully regulated practice. Approximately 80 percent of all AID practitioners use medical students as sperm donors, a tradition that critics claim is eugenically motivated. Comment Snowden and Mitchell: "If male medical students are known to possess particular social and psychological characteristics which are in some way distinctive, and if donors are being deliberately selected from this group, then eugenic selection is taking place in a planned way."[52] Defenders of the tradition argue that because these young men are knowledgeable about genetics, sexually responsible, and honest, they are ideal sperm donors. But evidence suggests that some medical students are just as human—that is, as ignorant, dishonest, and sexually irresponsible—as are other people, and thus AID practitioners should not exclusively, or nearly exclusively, rely on them for sperm.

Thus far we have discussed the possible rights and responsibilities of AID donors who wish to remain anonymous. Also of interest are the rights and responsibilities of AID donors who do not wish to remain anonymous or whose identity was never a secret. On an episode of the television program "St. Elsewhere," one of the medical residents donates sperm to the hospital's infertility program. Through a complicated chain of events, he discovers who his sperm recipient is and begins to follow her pregnancy obsessively. Eventually, he has himself assigned to her case, at which point he begins to act like an expectant father. The pregnant woman's husband is bewildered by the resident's inappropriate behavior and asks the chief of residents to remove him from his wife's case. As a result, the resident nearly has a nervous breakdown, protesting that the pregnant woman is carrying his child and that he has a right to be involved in his child's life. Of course, it is not at all clear that the resident has any such right. Many commentators believe that when a man sells or donates his sperm, he relinquishes his rights to establish a parental relationship with any subsequent child. It is as if he has given his sperm up for adoption. What this line of reasoning suggests is that *provided* the resident signed the appropriate informed consent forms voluntarily, he gave up any right he may have had to know and rear his genetic child.

AID recipients

Relatively little has been written about the responsibilities and rights of AID recipients. We do know, however, that more than 95 percent of the people who use donated sperm are infertile married couples and that they are frequently permitted to "special-order" sperm from a particular kind of donor. Sometimes a donor's sperm are given to more than one recipient, but Lilli Katz, an employee of the Fairfax Cryobank, claims that "there are some limits to the number of half brothers and half sisters" an AID child is likely to have. The rule of thumb for the use of any one man's sperm is ten pregnancies per geographical unit.[53]

As we noted previously, many infertile couples choose AID over adoption for a variety of reasons. They desire to have a child to whom at least one of them is genetically related, or they desire to appear "normal," or the woman desires not only to rear a child but also to beget and bear a child. The issue, of course, is whether these desires give AID recipients the *right* to have a child by artificial insemination. There is considerable debate about whether the right to procreate includes the right to procreate by "artificial" as well as "natural" means. Some theorists maintain that the more artificial and less natural a means of procreation is, the more the state may justifiably interfere in it. Such theorists argue that it is not unjustifiable to restrict the use of AID to married infertile couples only. Indeed, some AID practitioners already go further, claiming that it is their responsibility to decide which married infertile couples are to use AID. As they see it, no married infertile couple should be permitted to use AID unless the couple is strongly motivated and "childworthy," and unless the wife is a good risk as a child begetter, bearer, and rearer.[54]

The main problem with permitting AID practitioners to make such decisions is that what one AID practitioner may describe as a childworthy family, another AID practitioner may describe as a "child-unworthy" family. Admittedly, persons who wish to adopt children, for example, are screened just as rigorously as persons who wish to use AID. Nevertheless, it is probably discriminatory to require either prospective AID couples or prospective adoptive parents to meet standards for parenthood that persons who have children naturally are not required to meet. Just because a person is infertile, she or he should not be required to be a better parent than his or her fertile counterpart.

Other problems emerge when an unmarried woman or man wishes to use AID. For a variety of reasons, some courts and legislatures have serious reservations about permitting unmarried women to use AID. Twelve states currently require that AID be performed by a licensed physician or under his or her supervision,[55] and at least one state, Georgia, has ruled that any child born as the result of self-insemination is an illegitimate child.[56] Since many AID practitioners are not in favor of artificially inseminating single women, Georgia's statute and statutes like it have a deterrent effect on self-insemination. If she cares about her prospective child's legitimacy, an unmarried woman will think twice before she inseminates herself to conceive him or her.

Not all states require that physicians perform AID, however. In such states, the self-insemination movement has made enormous strides. Lesbian feminists have been at the forefront of this movement, but an increasing number of unmarried, heterosexual women are joining it. Career women who hear their biological clocks ticking but who are unready, unwilling, or unable to marry are especially attracted to AID. However, because it is difficult for unmarried women to identify and approach sperm donors, and because unmarried women often have difficulty securing sperm from sperm banks that require a physician's prescription, some feminists have established their own sperm banks. The Sperm Bank of Northern California is one such establishment. Its policies deviate from typical sperm banks in several ways. First, it provides sperm to any woman, regardless of her marital status, sexual preference, or physical disability. Second, it permits women to examine a catalogue of donor information and to select their own donor on the basis of this information. Third, it offers sperm donors release-of-information contracts, which give them the option to "legitimate" their genetic children when they reach majority.[57]

If more unmarried women wish to use AID in the future, there may be increased pressure to legally limit their access to it. But it is not clear whether it is constitutional to forbid unmarried women to use AID. To deprive unmarried women of AID may be to violate their right to privacy —that is, their right to decide whether to beget and bear children. It may also violate their right to the law's equal protection by forbidding them, but not married women, to use AID.[58] If the state may not forbid a woman, married or unmarried, to terminate a pregnancy absent a compelling state interest to do so, on what grounds may it forbid a woman, married or unmarried, to initiate a pregnancy absent a compelling state interest to do so?

Eager to prevent unmarried women from using AID, the state may claim that it has compelling interests to limit AID to married women only. Among the interests the state may point to are the following four: (1) its interest in population control; (2) its interest in encouraging two-parent families, (3) its interest in discouraging illegitimacy; and (4) its interest in preventing incestuous marriages.

Critics believe that none of these state interests are truly compelling. First, they reason that even if the state needs to limit population size, it may not do so by "irrationally focusing on one class"—in this instance, the very small class of unmarried women who wish to use AID. Second, they claim that the state is fighting a lost battle insofar as encouraging two-parent families is concerned. Divorce, separation, and desertion have killed the two-parent family, and forbidding AID to unmarried women is unlikely to resurrect it.[59] Third, they point out that the state's main reason for discouraging illegitimacy is that illegitimate children constitute an economic drain on society; fatherless children are supposedly penniless children. However, the unmarried women who use AID are typically career women capable of supporting a child. Finally, they argue that for the state to claim that its interest in preventing incestuous marriages is served by the prohibition of AID to unmarried women is "fanciful." Even admitting the rare chance of 2 AID children of the same anonymous donor meeting and marrying each other, the state has other, less restrictive means of preventing such incestuous relationships (e.g., a clearinghouse system for AID records).

The state may also argue that it has enough compelling interests to prohibit the use of AID by unmarried men. Artificially inseminated by a man's sperm, a so-called surrogate or contracted mother can carry the resultant child to term for the man with the understanding that she will relinquish her parental rights to the child on its birth. Were the state to block this sort of arrangement on the grounds that it is against the best interests of children because men are less suited than women to rear children, critics would reject this justification as sexist and, therefore, unable to withstand constitutional scrutiny.

AID children

Although adoptive parents are currently urged to inform their children of their adoptive status, AID parents are not always urged to inform their children of their AID status. What is more, although grown adopted children have, in many jurisdictions, the right to know certain facts about their genetic parents, sometimes even their identities, grown AID children do not have a similar right. The best explanation for this asymmetry is that whereas adoption is ruled by what is in the best interests of the child, AID is apparently ruled by what is in the best interests of the sperm donor. Were AID ruled by the child's best interests instead of the sperm donor's, say some critics, the AID child would be able to know the personal identity as well as the genetic history of the sperm donor.

One group that advocates full information disclosure to AID children is a London-based group of lesbian feminists called The Feminist Self-Insemination Group. These women, who use the sperm of a variety of men, tell their children as soon as possible that they were conceived through AID. Because their mode of conception is presented very matter-of-factly and positively to them, these AID children apparently accept it readily. When researchers asked one of them, a 4-year-old girl, if she planned to be a mother some day, she replied: "When I grow up I'll get a sperm and grow a baby in my tummy."[60] And because AID is presented as one way to challenge genetic purity by matching donors and recipients from very different backgrounds, these AID children seem able to transcend the barriers of race and class quickly. Overhearing that one of the middle-class white women in the self-insemination group had not found a sperm donor yet, a kindergarten boy solved her problem when he pointed outside and said, "The black workman fixing the windows outside could give you a seed."[61]

As wonderful as this policy of total openness about AID sounds, critics doubt that it always serves the best interests of AID children. First, the fact that sperm donors know their AID children could, as we have noted, lead them to demand visitation or custody rights. Unless the women to whom they gave their sperm are willing to relate to them on a day-to-day basis, however, stress and struggle rather than familial peace and harmony are likely to result. Second, the fact that AID children know their sperm donors could, as we have also noted, lead them to attempt what may be impossible—namely, to forge close bonds with men who want nothing to do with them.

But even if a policy of total openness does not always serve the best interests of AID children, a policy of limited openness probably does. An AID child may not have a right to know personal information about the sperm donor, but she or he probably has a right to know genetic information about the sperm donor so that the child can avoid or learn to live with inherited diseases or defects, for example. Thus, legislation is needed to strike a proper balance between sperm donors' and AID children's rights. If AID children have a right only to genetic information about sperm donors, AID recipients could be given this information at the time of their insemination. But, if AID children also have a right to personal information about sperm donors, they could receive this information either when they reach the age of majority or, more restrictively, when the sperm donors die or decide to disclose their identities voluntarily. In either event, AID children would not be permitted to make any financial claims on their genetic fathers. To be sure, there are no easy ways, short of using only the frozen sperm of deceased donors, to balance the sperm donor's interest in remaining anonymous against the AID child's interest in knowing about his or her past.[62]

AID practitioners

Of growing concern to policymakers and the public alike is the fact that not all AID practitioners are equally competent to practice AID. A 1979 study by Martin Curie-Cohen and two colleagues showed that most AID practitioners were "woefully deficient" in their knowledge of genetics.[63] Anywhere between 50 and 95 percent of all AID practitioners were unable to identify correctly those genetic diseases for which carriers can be genetically screened and, even when they knew how to make such identifications correctly, they sometimes failed to screen for possible carriers. Thus, while 95 percent of AID practitioners said they would reject a carrier of Tay-Sachs, fewer than 1 percent actually screened sperm donors for this carrier state.[64]

Underscreening of sperm donors remains a problem, but it is becoming less of a problem as AID practitioners shift from using fresh sperm to frozen sperm. In May 1979, the American Association of Tissue Banks (AATB) approved a set of provisional standards for the freezing and storing, or *cryobanking*, of human sperm. These standards maintain that the "ideal basis for proper donor selection requires personal, physical, and genetic examination and history of individuals, as well as in-depth semen analysis which includes microbial screening."[65] In addition, the standards enumerate medical and genetic criteria for donor rejection, outline the appropriate questions to ask in composing a genetic history, and recommend that all cryobanks be prepared to conduct whatever biochemical tests and chromosome tests a physician requests.

As good as the standards of the AATB are, there are a regrettable number of ways to avoid them. If AID practitioners fail to request necessary tests, there is not much that the AATB can do. Likewise, if some cryobanks fail to join AATB precisely because they do not want to be held to its standards—standards that cost commercial cryobanks profits because the more screening and testing they do, the more they must charge for their products[66]—the AATB has little recourse.

In the near future, however, AID practitioners and cryobanks may find it difficult to escape standards such as those of the AATB. Given that

AID is generally viewed as a medical treatment for infertility, the state will probably regard as negligent AID practitioners who fail to exercise due care in screening and testing sperm donors. A pertinent case in this respect is *Ravenis* v. *Detroit General Hospital*.[67] Subsequent to a corneal transplant, a patient developed ophthalmitis, which led to total loss of vision in the transplanted eye. The hospital was held liable for failure to supervise adequately the selection of the eye donor. The court determined from testimony that there were established medical criteria for determining the suitability of cadavers as eye donors and that the hospital was negligent for not having provided its staff with these guidelines. Although there are still no established medical criteria for determining the suitability of sperm donors, the proposed AATB standards are a move in this direction, a move affirmed by those who insist that AID services should be delivered in a manner "best calculated to maximize the interests of the child and not just those of the sperm donor."[68]

No matter what medical criteria are ultimately established for determining the suitability of sperm donors, however, sperm banks must also establish high standards of care for the sperm they choose to store. An increasing number of men are storing their sperm in banks to preserve them before undergoing a vasectomy or to protect them from the environmental hazards of industry, commerce, war, space flight, and "the as yet unassessed hazards of the chemical mutagens of modern life."[69] Such men demand that their sperm be handled with extreme care. If a man deposits his sperm for his own future use, he is likely to suffer trauma if his sperm are given away without his consent or if his sperm are negligently mislabeled, damaged, or destroyed. Of course, sperm banks are not charitable establishments. In the early 1970s, the Idant Corporation in New York City was charging $80 for testing, freezing, and storing three ejaculations for 6 months; $18 per year for continued storage; and $30 for a withdrawal. What happens, then, if a depositor fails to pay his annual fee? May the bank sell his sperm to an AID practitioner? May it destroy them? Or must the bank return the sperm to their depositor?[70] Given that issues such as these are likely to arise, we may soon see much more detailed legislation regulating the collection and storage of sperm.

Social Dimensions of Artificial Insemination

Currently, society's attitudes toward artificial insemination are relatively positive, especially among the couples who use it. Approximately 172,000 American women went to physicians for artificial insemination in 1987.[71]

Although artificial insemination is not always successful (success rates vary from 38 to 57 percent),[72] in 1987 some 35,000 children were born as a result of AIH performed by some 11,000 physicians (these live births represent 37.7 percent of the cases in which AIH was tried).[73] If these statistics are accurate, most of the women who go to physicians for artificial insemination go for AIH rather than AID. This speculation fits Corea's observation that the practice of AID has developed at a "snail's pace."[74] For example, in Holland there were fewer than 10 AID births annually from when the practice began in 1948 until 1960; and although 5000 to 7000 AID children per year were being born in the United States by 1960, that number had increased to only 6000 to 10,000 AID children per year by 1980.[75] The number of AID children is probably something on the order of 20,000 yearly now but, given the high rate of male infertility, we would expect the number of AID children to be higher than this.

Men's and Women's Varying Attitudes Toward AID

Men's Attitudes

Although statistical evidence is in short supply, there is anecdotal evidence to support the speculation that genetic fatherhood means more to men than genetic motherhood means to women. *If* men do, in fact, place a very high premium on being genetically related to their children, this could help explain why there are not more AID births than there are. As Corea sees it, however, there are no "ifs" about the value men place on genetic fatherhood. The slow development of AID is, she says, attributable to the fact that AID "poses a threat to the patriarchal family and to male dominance."[76] What men supposedly want is children, especially sons, to whom they are genetically related, children through whom they can achieve a corporeal immortality of sorts. Men who are obsessed with this notion of paternity can no more tolerate AID than rape or adultery. AID threatens them because it provides wives "with a means of rebellion."[77] In fact, in 1981, a male attorney expressed concern that if AID became the norm, the human male would cease to be "socially necessary." The human species, he reasoned, could easily be reproduced from frozen sperm or from live sperm taken from a small number of selected donors. No longer would women have any real need for men.[78]

As it stands, men may easily dismiss this lawyer's exaggerated fears about AID. Most women value men for more than the role they play in procreation. What is more, contrary to Corea's assertions, there is some evidence that relatively few *infertile* men have problems accepting AID. In one study that involved infertile couples, both the male and female members of the fertile couples *unanimously* endorsed people's right to have children by means of AID despite alarming overpopulation statistics. In addition, 86 percent of them denied that adoption or foster care is preferable to AID because it provides a home for an already existing child; 88 percent of them denied that husbands of wives who receive AID find it difficult to accept as their own any offspring produced; and 93 percent of them agreed that AID should be used as a reproductive option to avoid inheritable retardation or genetic diseases. Moreover, not one of these infertile couples believed that there is any analogy between adultery and AID; still, only 50 percent of them believed that lesbians should be permitted to conceive by means of AID.[79]

To be sure, some men may have serious reservations about AID. In the same study referred to above, *fertile* male and female medical students were surveyed with respect to their attitudes about AID. As is evidenced in table 8.1, the fertile male medical students were not nearly as receptive to AID as fertile female medical students were.[80] Although the significance of this gender gap is by no means clear, perhaps fertile men are less able

Table 8.1 Attitudes of fertile men and women toward the use of artifical insemination with donor sperm

Attitude	Men (N = 56)	Women (N = 57)
Lesbians should be permitted to conceive via AID	40%	60%
Given the state of overpopulation in the world, I do not approve of "artifically" encouraging new births.	70%	30%
I think that the husbands of wives who receive AID must have difficulty accepting as their own any offspring produced.	64%	36%
I believe that adoption or foster care is preferable to AID since it provides a home for a child already born.	65%	35%
I believe conceiving via artifical insemination with donor semen is like committing adultery.	87%	13%
I believe AID should be utilized as a reproductive option in cases where there is a danger of inheritable retardation or genetic disease.	15%	85%

than fertile women to appreciate that there is more to being a father (or mother) than transmitting one's genes to a future generation.

Women's Attitudes

Since women not only contribute half of the genes in AID but also are able to experience pregnancy, it is no wonder that they are often more receptive to AID than are men. Of course, this is not to say that women are especially pleased either with the way AID was practiced in the past or with the way it is practiced now. Earlier we noted that Dr. William Pancoast in 1884 artificially inseminated his unconscious patient without her consent. Although legal authorities spent decades debating whether AID is a form of adultery, they never described Dr. Pancoast as an adulterer or, more aptly, a rapist. Indeed, the eminent legal authority Glanville Williams once asserted that "the question whether artificial insemination performed without the woman's consent would be rape is too academic to be worth discussion."[81]

What disturbs many women about the practice of AID today, however, is that 61 percent of surveyed physicians said they would be likely to reject an unmarried recipient without a male partner. Despite the fact that the majority of American children live with only one parent, society continues to idealize the nuclear family—that is, a heterosexual couple with one or more children. Repeatedly, people simply assert that children need both a mother and a father if they are to be reared properly, though there is very little conclusive evidence to support this assertion. Given all the articles we read about women not being able to find men who are willing to commit to a long-term monogamous relationship, including articles that tell single women older than 40 that they have virtually no chance of finding a spouse, it is not surprising that some knowledgeable, well-situated young women wish to use AID. As these women view it, human relationships, especially familial relationships, are what make life meaningful, and the fact that a woman has not found a man with whom she wants to share her life is no reason why she must resign herself to a childless fate. If a financially and emotionally secure woman is permitted to adopt a child, she should be permitted to have a child by AID.

But even if some critics are willing to concede that a "good" single heterosexual woman can parent a child better than can a "bad" heterosexual couple, they are not as ready to concede that lesbians, single or coupled, can parent children effectively. Certainly, they are not ready to bestow their benediction on lesbians who wish to use AID. So biased is traditional society against lesbian mothers that it may be a mistake for them to use AID. Not only may they find unwanted men in their lives; they may also have to fight these men in court for the custody of their children. Lesbians are particularly concerned that the state will deprive them of custody on two grounds: (1) that their supposed "psychopathological" style of mothering deviates negatively from the "normal" style of mothering—that is, the kind of mothering heterosexual women do— and (2) that their children may "fall victims to negative psychosexual influences"—that is, that they may find lesbian sexuality preferable to heterosexuality for themselves.[82] To describe a lesbian life-style as "psychopathological" and a "negative psychosexual influence" is, of course, to describe it from a biased heterosexual point of view. Just because a woman is a heterosexual does not mean that she is qualified to rear a child, and just because a woman is a lesbian does not mean that she is not qualified to rear a child. Clearly, the fact that AID makes it possible for women to be single parents by free choice is a fact with which society must reckon. As feminists see it, however, the questions to ask are not ones about the future of the two-parent family but ones about whether it is better or worse for some women to be single parents and ones about whether it is better or worse for some children to have one parent rather than two.

Class, Racial, and Ethnic Concerns

Class Issues

Each of the 172,000 women who underwent artificial insemination in 1987 paid approximately $953; more than half of these women had insurance coverage that paid approximately 48 percent of the total cost.[83] For some couples, this is simply too much money to spend on getting pregnant. Absent a willing donor and a self-insemination kit, these couples are likely to give up trying. Interestingly, 5.6 percent of these 172,000 women were single. Although solid evidence is unavailable, anecdotal evidence suggests that most of these women were well-to-do. For example, there is a case of a lesbian woman, of middle-class background and high professional standing, who decided she wanted to become a mother.[84] Her wish was fulfilled when she was impregnated using AID. Unlike a rich single woman, however, a poor single woman may not be able to satisfy her longing for a child by using AID unless she is willing to inseminate herself artificially with an acquaintance's sperm. Moreover, unlike a rich single woman, a poor single woman may not have enough money to support her AID child once he or she is born. In fact, she may have to go on welfare and stay on welfare to feed, clothe, and shelter him or her. As some critics see it, it is morally irresponsible for a poor single woman to use AID knowing full well that the only way she can support a child is by going on welfare. After all, say these critics, "many people who might prefer 4 children to the 1.8 national average limit their families because they are not able to support more children."[85]

Racial and Ethnic Concerns

Not only does artificial insemination remind us of the fact that reproductive freedom is limited by social and economic conditions; it also reminds us of certain racial and ethnic concerns. As we noted earlier, AID does have eugenic implications. As early as 1935, Dr. Herman J. Muller, a Marxist geneticist, began to talk about "germinal choice." As he saw it, better-quality children could be produced if women would allow themselves to be artificially inseminated with the sperm of "transcendentally estimable" men[86]—that is, men who were deemed great sometime after their death. When Dr. Jerome K. Sherman, a friend of Muller, developed a method of freezing human sperm, Muller was ecstatic because the success of his germinal choice program depended on the widespread availability of frozen, processed semen. Driven by visions of Mozarts, da Vincis, and Einsteins everywhere, Robert K. Graham, a wealthy businessman, established a sperm bank that he viewed as the means to make Muller's dreams come true. Only the sperm of Nobel Prize–winning men would be banked in his Herman J. Muller Repository for Germinal Choice. Planning to inseminate only highly intelligent women with these special sperm, Graham suffered considerable embarrassment when the mother of the first germinal-choice baby turned out to be a former convict and accused child abuser.[87] He suffered even more embarrassment when Muller's widow insisted that he stop using her husband's name for the repository. Apparently, Muller's widow was deeply disturbed that Graham had allied himself with Dr. William Shockley, a "scientist" she and many others regarded as racially biased. According to Shockley, there is a "basic, across-the-board genetic disadvantage in terms of capacity to develop intelligence and build societies on the part of the Negro races throughout the world."[88] Clearly, Negroes (sic) have no business depositing their sperm in select sperm banks, insisted Shockley. Only men with superior IQ scores should preserve their sperm.

Shockley's ideas about what counts as an ideal human being could not be further from feminist writer Marge Piercy's. In her novel, *Woman on the Edge of Time*, she envisions a society in which eggs as well as sperm are banked to preserve a full range of racial and ethnic characteristics so that society can celebrate difference in all its variety and beauty.[89] Clearly, society need not be alarmed by either the technique of artificial insemination or the fact that sperm can be banked for long periods of time. It does need to be concerned, however, about the ways in which artificial insemination and or cryopreservation can be used to limit individual freedom and to impede social justice.

9 In Vitro Fertilization and Embryo Transfer

With the exception of artificial insemination by donor (AID), in vitro fertilization (IVF) and embryo transfer are probably the most widely used and loudly publicized assisted reproductive techniques (ARTs).[1] After several years of clinical research, Drs. Patrick Steptoe and Robert Edwards managed not only to fertilize an egg externally and transfer an early embryo into a woman's womb but also to see that pregnancy through to term. Overlooked in the 1978 publicity surrounding the birth of the first test-tube baby, Louise Joy Brown, however, was the fact that Steptoe and Edwards were not the only researchers working in this area. A number of other similar projects were well under way before Louise's birth. For example, Landrum Shuttles and his associate externally fertilized an egg in 1972, but the experiment failed because one of Shuttles's associates who had moral and legal qualms about test-tube baby research decided to destroy the embryo.[2]

Whom to credit as the foremost pioneer(s) in IVF research is not the issue on which we wish to focus attention here, however. Rather, we are more interested in the political reactions to IVF research. Among other things, the sensationalized news coverage of the achievement of Steptoe and Edwards prompted the secretary of the then Department of Health, Education and Welfare (DHEW) to constitute an Ethics Advisory Board (EAB) to study the ethical, legal, and social aspects of IVF as well as its scientific aspects. Although the EAB concluded in 1979 that IVF did present some problems, it nonetheless recommended that IVF researchers not be denied federal monies for their clinical and basic research projects.[3]

Despite the EAB's recommendation, however, Congress did not then, and has not since, appropriated federal funds for IVF research. Apparently, Congressmen and Congresswomen have turned cold shoulders to U.S. reproductive researchers in order to appease powerful political lobbies such as the so-called right-to-life movement. Lacking adequate funds, American reproductive researchers have found it difficult to keep pace with foreign reproductive researchers whose work is government-supported. Nevertheless, they have managed to progress beyond simple IVF—in which a woman's eggs are removed, fertilized with her husband's sperm, and then placed in her uterus—to more complex forms of IVF that mix and match donors and recipients. So, for example, Mrs. Jones's egg may be fertilized in vitro with a donor's sperm and then inserted into her womb, or a donor's egg may be fertilized in vivo with Mr. Jones's sperm, after which the resulting embryo is flushed from the donor's womb and inserted in Mrs. Jones's womb.[4] In yet another scenario, the husband and wife contribute their sperm and egg, but the resulting embryo is carried by a third party who is, in a sense, donating the use of her womb. Still, insists Gary Hodgen, former Chief of Pregnancy Research at the National Institutes of Health (NIH), "If federal funding were there, every step of the process—from the quality of the egg and sperm to why some embryos are rejected by the womb while others are not—would be better understood."[5] Moreover, claims Hodgen, if federal funding were available, and if a newly constituted EAB (President Ronald Reagan disbanded the original EAB in 1980) were to lift the veil of secrecy that currently hides IVF, then the public would have the opportunity both to understand this technology from a scientific point of view and to hear vigorous debate on the more controversial ethical, legal, and social aspects of the new reproductive technologies.[6]

The Technology of In Vitro Fertilization

The terms *test-tube babies* and *in vitro fertilization* conjure up all sorts of Faustian, Frankensteinian, and *Brave New World* images, but these do not generally mirror the mundane realities of IVF. The phrase *in vitro fertilization*, which literally means "fertilization in glass," is simply used to denote all fertilization procedures that occur outside the human body.[7]

IVF Procedures

Four elements are necessary for IVF to take place: (1) ripe eggs ready to be fertilized, (2) sperm ready to initiate fertilization, (3) a medium in which to mix the egg and the sperm to achieve fertilization, and (4) a medium to support the development of the embryo.[8] If we recall the intricate hormonal control required for in vivo (internal) fertilization, we can easily appreciate why in vitro (external) fertilization is so difficult.[9] The developmental state of the egg and the uterus must be closely matched for an externally fertilized egg to be successfully implanted. When fertilization takes place within the body, the outer cells of the blastocyst secrete human chorionic gonadotropin (HCG), which causes the corpus luteum to be maintained. The corpus luteum continues to secrete progesterone, which acts on the uterine wall to induce its development and to sensitize the uterus for receptivity to the implantation of the blastocyst. During this time, no new egg follicles begin to mature and menstruation does not begin. To replicate these processes ex utero (outside the womb), physicians must treat their patients with hormones to prime the uterus to accept the embryo for implantation.

Collection of Eggs

The first step in preparing a human egg for fertilization in vitro is the collection of the preovulatory oocytes. Physicians must obtain these oocytes during their final stages of maturation just before ovulation,[10] when the beginning stages of meiosis have taken place and the cortical granules have developed to provide protection against fertilization by more than one sperm.[11]

There are two ways for physicians to predict whether an egg is ready for retrieval: (1) by becoming familiar with the rhythm of the woman's menstrual cycle or (2) by treating the woman with hormones that will better ensure follicle maturation and ovulation at a specific time.[12,13] Of these two methods, most physicians prefer the second because it is more predictable, although there is now a trend back to the natural cycle. The physician gives follicle-stimulating hormone (FSH) in a preparation called clomiphene (marketed as Clomid) to a woman soon after she has menstruated in order to promote the maturation of several follicles instead of just one.[14] Through the use of daily blood or urine tests for estrogens as well as pelvic examinations, the physician monitors the maturation of the follicles. To confirm the maturation, she or he uses ultrasonography to visualize the follicles on the surface of the ovaries. When these various tests and examinations indicate that the developing eggs have reached the correct stage of maturity, the physician stops FSH administration. Between days 11 and 14 of the cycle, the physician administers the hormone HCG to trigger release of the eggs from the follicles[15] but, before the eggs are released naturally into the fallopian tubes, the physician removes the eggs surgically.

Collection by laparoscopy

The actual retrieval of the eggs begins when the surgeon administers to the woman a general anesthetic in preparation for the recovery of the preovulatory oocytes. Extensive experience has shown that the highest rates of oocyte collection are achieved 32 hours after the HCG injection if the woman is receiving hormonal treatment or 18 to 27 hours after the luteinizing hormone (LH) surge if hormonal treatment is not employed.[16] The surgeon makes a small incision in the woman's abdomen near the navel, inserts a laparoscope, and then guides it through the abdominal cavity to the ovary. The laparoscope is a long, thin fiberoptic tube approximately 0.33 inches in diameter (containing a light and an optical system) that enables the physician to see the ovaries (see figures 3.10 and 3.11). Under these conditions, the ovaries appear as oval objects studded with small, bluish bulges, which are the follicles containing the eggs; the eggs themselves, which can be seen with the unaided eye, appear as cellular objects surrounded by starburst patterns of tiny follicular cells and mucus called the *cumulus mass*.[17] The viscosity of the cumulus mass is an indication of the stage of maturation of the oocyte. The surgeon inserts a long hollow needle through the metal tube holding the laparoscope to the targeted follicle.

Collection by transvaginal ultrasound-directed oocyte retrieval

A variation on the IVF procedure is called *transvaginal ultrasound-directed oocyte retrieval* (TUDOR). In this procedure, the eggs are obtained from the ovaries by inserting a needle through the vaginal wall rather than through the abdominal wall. Instead of a laparoscope, the movement of the needle is monitored with ultrasonography. Whereas the original procedure involved placement of the ultrasound probe on the abdomen, current technological developments allow the probe to be placed in the vagina. This brings it much closer to the ovary and provides a clearer picture for guiding the needle to the follicle. On the one hand, the procedure is more difficult for the physician to perform since she or he must guide the needle without puncturing anything vital. On the other hand, it is easier for the patient because it is generally performed under local anesthesia with no surgery. TUDOR is rapidly replacing laparoscopy. In 1985, approximately 94 percent of the egg retrievals were done with laparoscopy. Just 3 years later, in 1988, only 13 percent were done by laparoscopy and 86 percent were done with ultrasonography.[18]

In either situation, the physician generally uses a double aspirating needle or two separate needles to provide two channels,[19] one for aspiration and the other for flushing the follicle if the oocyte is not collected initially. As the surgeon punctures the bulging follicle with the needle, she or he gently suctions out the yellow-orange fluid in it.

As soon as the surgeon has suctioned this fluid, an embryologist examines it under a microscope to determine whether an egg is present.

Though an egg is not always present, in many cases one or more eggs are seen. When present, a technician immediately washes the eggs and then places them in petri dishes that contain a nutrient solution. From there the technician places the eggs in an incubator for between 4 and 8 hours. If the cells are not completely mature and ready for fertilization, they may be incubated for a few hours with some follicular fluid until maturation is completed. The entire egg collection procedure usually lasts approximately 30 minutes.

Collection of Sperm

Although most of the physician's attention is focused on the recruitment and incubation of the eggs, she or he must also obtain and treat sperm in preparation for in vitro fertilization. After the semen sample is collected by the husband or the donor by masturbation, it is washed in a liquid culture medium and spun in a centrifuge to separate the sperm from the seminal fluid. As valuable as the seminal fluid is to the sperm in certain ways, it contains some fertilization-inhibiting substances. This washing procedure simulates the conditions the sperm encounters in its journey through the vagina, cervix, uterus, and fallopian tubes. During this journey the sperm are bathed in secretions that remove these deleterious substances[20] and capacitate the sperm to penetrate the egg.[21] Finally, the concentrated sperm sample is covered with fresh culture media and put in an incubator for approximately 1 hour. During this time, the most active sperm swim out of the denser lower layer and into the upper layer of the medium, mimicking the condition in the female genital tract where the sperm must swim through the uterus and fallopian tubes.[22] The sperm in the upper layer of media are used to prepare the sample for IVF.

Clearly, the maintenance of the egg and the sperm ex utero is no simple matter. IVF researchers have yet to create and maintain an artificial environment that perfectly replicates in vivo conditions. For these researchers, the best indication that approximately natural conditions exist is the survival and continued viability of the egg and the sperm prior to and including the moment of fertilization.

Fertilization

The next step brings together the two reproductive cells for the process of fertilization. The technician removes the eggs from the incubator and places each one in a petri dish in a small droplet of media. He or she then pipettes a few drops of the highly concentrated sperm onto each egg.

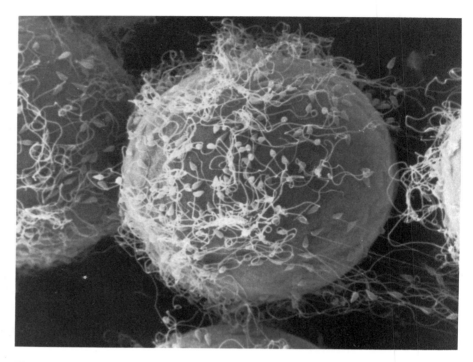

Figure 9.1 A scanning electron micrograph reveals thousands of sperm cells bound to the surface of an egg. (Courtesy of Dr. Mia Tegner, Scripps Institute of Oceanography)

Under these conditions, the concentration of the sperm is between 50,000 and 100,000 sperm per milliliter, which is only one-thousandth of the concentration in a fertile man's ejaculate. However, this concentration of sperm is more than enough because the physician applies it directly to the egg (figure 9.1), sometimes using a layer of inert paraffin oil to keep the sperm and egg in a small volume.[23] Finally, the physician places the mixture in a body-temperature incubator and, if all goes well, fertilization occurs within 24 hours after the sperm and egg are mixed (figures 9.2 and 9.3).[24]

Defects in sperm-oocyte interaction, which would normally lead to fertilization, are now recognized as one of the major causes of reproductive failure in the ARTs.[25] Fertilization is a very complex process involving many physiological steps, including binding of the sperm to the zona pellucida, passage of the sperm through the zona to the cell membrane, binding of the sperm to the membrane, penetration of the sperm into the oocyte, the decondensation of the sperm nucleus, the formation of pronuclei, and the formation of the embryo.[26]

The malfunction of any of these steps can prevent fertilization from taking place. Tests have been developed to assay for the success of each

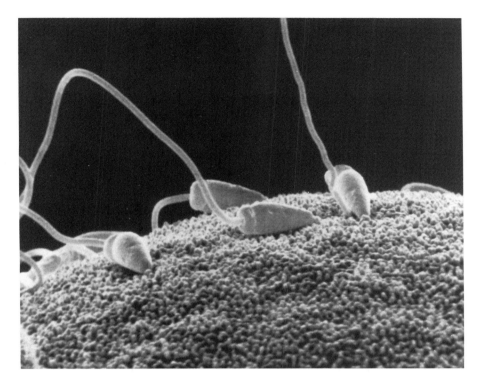

Figure 9.2 Sperm on the surface of the egg just before fertilization. (Courtesy of Professor E. William Byrd, Southwestern Medical Center at Dallas, The University of Texas)

step, and a number of procedures have been devised to treat the problems (see chapter 7). For example, the binding of the sperm to the zona is tested by the hemizona assay, and the ability of the sperm to penetrate the zona is monitored by the penetration assay. The ability of the sperm to penetrate the oocyte membrane can be tested using the hamster penetration assay. If the sperm is unable to perform adequately, new procedures are available to aid the process. The sperm can be placed directly into the egg with a very fine needle by microinjection. Alternatively, the egg can be subjected to zona drilling to provide holes in the zona and membrane to facilitate entry of the sperm into the interior of the cell.[27]

Incubation of the Embryo

Shortly after fertilization, the conceptus (a term that designates the embryo before the fourteenth day of its development when the primitive streak, the forerunner of the neural tube, appears) is placed in another medium that is specifically prepared to support embryonic development.

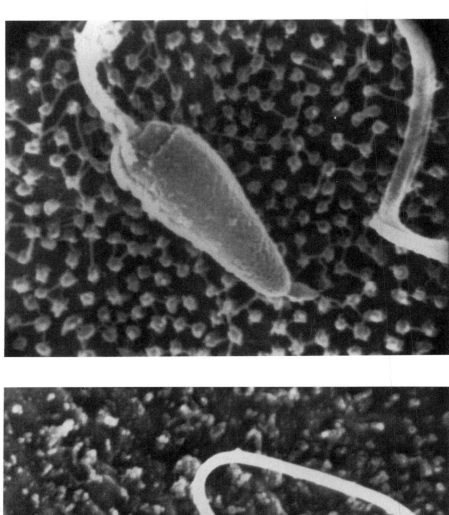

Figure 9.3 The moment of fertilization as the sperm penetrates the egg. (Courtesy of Dr. Mia Tegner, Scripps Institute of Oceanography)

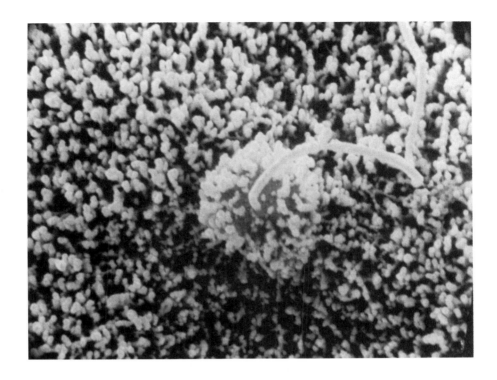

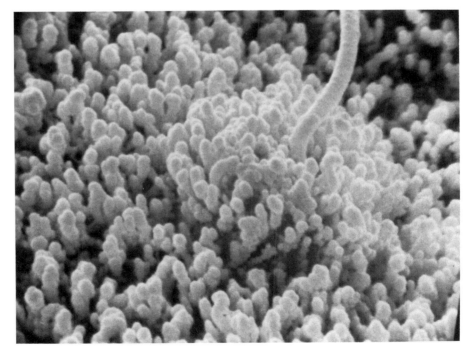

At this time, the pronucleus of the sperm and the egg merge to make the nucleus of the new cell and, for the most part, the subsequent embryo cleaves normally.[28] In general, those embryos that grow the fastest in vitro are apparently the best candidates for establishing pregnancy,[29] provided that the physician implants them in the uterus at precisely the right time. But physicians are not always able to judge how fast an embryo is growing or when a woman's uterus is most ready for implantation. If the embryo develops more slowly outside the fallopian tube, the physician might introduce the embryo into the uterus prematurely and the implantation reaction might not be triggered, or the physician might introduce the embryo too late and the uterus will have have passed the optimal time for implantation. This variable time scale may be synchronized through the administration of suitable hormones to the woman and careful regulation of the development of the embryo.

Recently, a novel procedure has been suggested to help promote development of the embryo and prepare it for introduction into the woman. The concept involves coculturing the embryos with human tubal epithelial cells to provide a more natural nutritional environment.[30]

Placing the Embryo in the Uterus

Two days after fertilization, the fertilized egg has developed into an embryo of at least two to eight cells called the *blastocyst*.[31] At this stage, reproductive researchers assume that the embryo is ready for introduction into the uterus of the mother.[32] The physician instructs the woman to assume a position believed to promote implantation: She kneels, sits back, then leans forward until her chest rests on her knees, extending her arms over her head and supporting some of her weight with her elbows. With the aid of a microscope, the physician draws the embryos into a long catheter[33] in a very small volume of media (between 0.03 and 0.10 mL). She or he introduces the catheter into the woman through a larger tube previously inserted into the uterus through the vagina and cervix and then flushes the embryos into the uterus. The woman slowly lowers herself into a lying position, taking care not to shift suddenly, which might lower the chance for implantation. She lies flat on her stomach for 4 hours before she is allowed to resume normal activity. Some reproductive researchers prefer to perform the embryo transfer during the evening because spontaneous contractility of the uterus, which might impede implantation, is lower at night.

The IVF technique has become so popular that there are more than 100 clinics operating in the United States and, according to one estimate, a new IVF baby is born every day somewhere in the world. These statistics may lead us to believe that IVF is a highly successful technique. In fact, it is not. Whereas 31 percent of natural fertilizations result in birth of a child, only 20 percent of IVF fertilizations do. This relatively low success rate can be increased, though, depending on how many IVF attempts a couple undergoes. At some clinics successful pregnancy rates (not to be confused with actual births) can soar as high as 50 percent. What cannot be ignored, however, are the emotional and financial costs associated with multiple IVF attempts that fail. A couple may spend thousands of dollars and much time traveling to and from distant IVF clinics only to lose the dream of ever having a child. Nevertheless, many couples are willing to risk this disappointment. In their view, they have nothing to lose and a great deal to gain. The demand for IVF is growing so rapidly in some areas that a corporation called *IVF Australia* has opened a chain of franchised clinics in the United States. According to the company, these clinics will offer personalized care that is not currently available in large, urban medical centers. Also, since the clinics will be local, there will be less disruption to the couple's home life and jobs.

Gamete Intrafallopian Transfer

Gamete intrafallopian transfer (GIFT) was developed to improve the relatively low success rate of the conventional IVF procedure and to decrease trauma to the potential mother. GIFT, the placement of the egg and sperm in the woman's fallopian tubes, attempts to mimic the normal physiological process. As in conventional IVF, the woman is treated with hormones to promote the development of a number of oocytes, and the eggs are obtained by laparoscopy. What distinguishes GIFT from IVF, however, is the fact that the laparoscope is not removed from the woman's body after the eggs are obtained. Instead the potential father's sperm is collected, concentrated, and mixed with the woman's eggs, and the mixture is then inserted through the laparoscope into the woman's fallopian tubes.

GIFT has clear advantages over both artificial insemination and IVF. Because the sperm is placed directly in the fallopian tubes, it does not have to travel through the cervix and the uterus. Thus, many opportunities for mishaps are eliminated. Another advantage of GIFT over IVF is that the fertilized eggs are allowed to develop in their natural environment before reaching the uterus and undergoing transplantation. Yet another advantage is that the entire procedure occurs in the space of 1 day. In IVF, the eggs are removed from the woman on one day and reimplanted on the next; in GIFT, the eggs are recovered, mixed with the sperm, and reimplanted on the same day. This feature of GIFT lowers the inconvenience to the woman and the cost to the couple. The pregnancy rate with GIFT is approximately 30 percent, with 40 to 50 percent or so of the births being twins. The problem of multiple births, which also characterizes IVF, is being studied. Because the problem has been linked to the implantation of multiple embryos, one possible solution is to put fewer eggs (in GIFT) or embryos (in IVF) back into the woman.

Tubal Embryo Transfer

Depending on circumstances, there are a number of variations on the basic procedures just discussed. Tubal embryo transfer (TET) involves the transfer of embryos formed in vitro into the fallopian tubes either with the laparoscopic method or with the transvaginal intrafallopian tubal transfer method.[34] As the name implies, the laparoscopic method is essentially the one described for GIFT except that embryos instead of the gametes are being placed in the fallopian tubes. The transvaginal intrafallopian tubal transfer method is essentially the same as the oocyte retrieval method except that the embryo is placed in the fallopian tube through the vagina. Regardless of the path of insertion, the basic differences among these techniques are that IVF involves the placement of 44- to 48-hour embryos, TET involves 20- to 24-hour embryos, and GIFT involves the introduction of gametes.[35] Other procedures that are slight variations of the TET methodology include zygote intrafallopian transfer (ZIFT) and pronuclear stage tubal transfer (PROST). The basis for all of these tubal embryo transfer procedures is the assumption that the fallopian tube plays a protective role for embryo development and eventual implantation, whereas the environment in the uterus may be deleterious to these developmental stages of the embryo.

The Technology of Embryo Transfer

Another type of technology that holds promise involves the transfer of an embryo from the womb of one woman into that of another.[36] In its simplest form, embryo transfer involves the transfer of a fertilized egg from a volunteer fertile donor to an infertile recipient after the donor has been artificially inseminated with the sperm of the recipient's husband. This form of reproductive-aiding technology is usually indicated when mature oocytes do not develop in the woman's ovaries. This technique is the converse to AID. Whereas the sperm are supplied by a male donor in

AID, the fertilized egg is supplied by a female donor in embryo transfer. There are many other variations of this basic procedure including IVF of the donor's egg, followed by implantation; the fertilization of the donor's egg, either in vitro or in vivo, with sperm from a donor, followed by transfer of the embryo to the infertile woman (called *embryo adoption*); and transfer of the fertilized egg from the uterus of a fertile woman, after insemination by her fertile husband, to the uterus of a contracted mother, a procedure indicated when the biological mother is physiologically unable to carry or give birth to the child.

No matter what form it takes, embryo transfer involves a number of basic steps. There must be careful synchronization of the ovulation times between the embryo donor and the recipient woman. Then, approximately 5 days after fertilization by the appropriate method, the donor's uterus is subjected to lavage (or a washing out) through a plastic tube called a *catheter*, and the embryo is recovered from the lavage fluid. Finally, the embryo is transferred to the recipient's uterus for implantation. Since the egg did not originate in the recipient, the embryo might be expected to elicit an immune response, but it seems to be unaffected by the maternal immune response.[37] Significantly, since pregnancy does not begin in a biological sense until implantation at the end of the second week, the embryo donor does not know whether she is pregnant (and, in fact, she is not even certain that fertilization took place) prior to the lavage, a psychological advantage that contracted mothers do not have.

Compared to IVF, embryo transfer is much easier. It can be done as an office procedure without anesthesia or surgery. However, the child will not be genetically related or, in some cases, gestationally related to the social mother. Thus, embryo transfer poses the same psychological problems to the social mother as its converse, AID, poses to the social father.

Increased demand for and use of embryo transfer has led to the development of embryo-freezing techniques. For the purposes of transfer, embryos may be obtained by either a lavage procedure or an IVF procedure. When a number of eggs are obtained and fertilized through IVF but only one is transferred to the woman, the remaining ones may be frozen. The availability of frozen embryos is particularly valuable in cases where an initial IVF attempt fails to result in pregnancy. One or more frozen embryos can be thawed and used in subsequent IVF attempts without subjecting the woman to another invasive laparoscopy.

Many new procedures, and improvements of the existing ones, are being developed to increase the success rate of IVF and related techniques. These procedures, which represent a major challenge to the whole field of assisted reproduction, include: embryo cryopreservation, oocyte donation, cryopreservation of oocytes, in vitro maturation of oocytes, monitoring sperm function, and microinjection of sperm.[38]

The Ethics of In Vitro Fertilization

The Moral Status of the Preimplantation Embryo

One of the most controversial ethical issues in the debate over IVF is the embryo's moral status, and here the embryo is generally a 2- to 3-day-old blastocyst consisting of approximately eight cells. Not surprisingly, the basic positions on the status of the early embryo are similar to those articulated in the abortion controversy: (1) from the moment of fertilization, the preimplantation embryo is truly human life; (2) at some point after fertilization, the preimplantation embryo is either truly human life or increasingly so; and (3) the preimplantation embryo is not truly human life. Whereas pro-life advocates agree with the first of these positions, pro-choice advocates tend to agree with the second or third of them. As a result, the pro-life camp insists that an in vitro embryo deserves the same protections that an in vivo embryo deserves. As we shall see, the pro-choice camp is less solicitous than pro-life advocates about protecting in vitro embryos, but this should not be surprising in light of the fact that they tend also to be less solicitous about protecting in vivo embryos.

Full-Protectionist Position

According to most natural-law theorists, preimplantation embryos have the same moral rights as adult persons. To make a distinction between a mere human being on the one hand and a full human person on the other, says the natural-law theorist, is to make a distinction that does not count. By virtue of the simple fact that an individual is a *Homo sapiens*, she or he is far more than a *mere* human being; rather, she or he is a potential human person—that is a human being with a capacity for sentience, self-consciousness, the ability to communicate, and rationality. It is this capacity, says the natural-law theorist, that makes all human beings, from the moment of conception, worthy of the respect and consideration accorded full human persons. If it is wrong to freeze, experiment on, and destroy adults, it is also wrong to freeze, experiment on, and destroy embryos. Indeed, the Rev. Donald McCarthy has even claimed that embryos have the right not to be created except as a consequence of "personal self-giving and conjugal love"[39] because no adult would choose to be born under anything less than these circumstances.

Although the "continuous-development argument" makes considerable sense, critics of it insist that it proves too much. If it is wrong to destroy any potential person, even a 2-, 4-, 8-, or 16-cell blastocyst, says philosopher Peter Singer, then it is probably wrong to prevent the union of an egg and sperm:

If the potential of the embryo is so crucial, why do all sides agree that they would not object to disposing of the egg and the sperm before *they have been combined? An egg and a drop of seminal fluid, viewed collectively, also have the potential to develop into a mature human being.*[40]

Singer's point may be extended even further. If techniques such as parthenogenesis (the production of offspring from egg cell only) and cloning (the production of offspring genetically identical to their parents from somatic cells) are ever developed, all our cells will have the potential for parenthood. Under such a set of circumstances, says the critic, even the staunchest supporter of the principle of potentiality will forsake it so that people can continue to move around freely without "murdering" thousands of potential persons as they slough off their cells.

Modified-Protectionist Position

Because the principle of potentiality can be extended to the point of absurdity, some rights-oriented ethicists as well as natural-law theorists espouse only a modified version of the full-protectionist position. Clifford Grobstein, for example, makes a distinction between nonsentient "human materials" such as cells, tissues, and organs that currently have no "reasonable prospect of possessing or developing sentient awareness" and "human beings or persons" that are sentient.[41] Grobstein admits that he is not certain when nonsentient embryos become sentient. Perhaps they become sentient 14 days or so after fertilization when the so-called primitive streak (the first indication of the development of a nervous system) begins to form, or perhaps they become sentient at approximately 6 weeks when the parts of the brain associated with consciousness begin to develop. In either event, says Grobstein, we do not owe the same kind of respect and consideration to a nonsentient embryo that we owe to a sentient embryo, infant, or adult.

From a less scientific perspective, Dr. Leon Kass, a rights-oriented ethicist, argues that although the process by which a preimplantation human embryo becomes an adult human person is a continuous one, embryos do not have precisely the same moral rights as adults. To decide —intentionally, recklessly, or negligently—to flush an eight-cell blastocyst down the drain rather than to place it in a woman's womb is not the equivalent of homicide. But, insists Kass, neither is it an inconsequential matter solely between a doctor and his plumber.[42] Early embryos deserve our respect because of their potentiality, even if, as the EAB said in 1979, "this respect does not necessarily encompass the full legal and moral rights attributed to persons."[43]

The Nonprotectionist Position

The nonprotectionist position, that preimplantation embryos have no rights, is most loudly voiced by philosopher Joseph Fletcher, who rejects the view that "the mere fact of fertilization results directly in a truly *human* being or at least a *nascent* human being" with a 'right to life'."[44] Fletcher comes close to supporting philosopher Michael Tooley's belief that given certain conditions, infanticide during at least the first week of life is as justified as abortion in vivo or in vitro, because only self-aware human beings are human persons with rights to life.[45] Nevertheless, both Fletcher and Tooley believe that once human material achieves sentience, it has an interest in not suffering pain and that this interest should be respected unless the rights of full human persons conflict with it.

The Problem of Surplus Embryos in a Clinical Context

Depending on whether an ethicist adopts a full-protectionist position, a modified-protectionist position (which, by the way, is probably the majority view), or a nonprotectionist position with respect to the status of the embryo, he or she will have a characteristic way to solve the so-called surplus embryo problem. When several eggs are harvested from a woman and fertilized, usually only three or four of the resulting embryos are returned to the woman's womb during each menstrual cycle. With luck, one of these embryos implants itself into the wall of the uterus and develops normally while the others are flushed out of the woman's system. Few ethicists condemn the loss of in vitro embryos that fail to implant, because their loss is analogous to that of in vivo embryos that fail to implant because of "natural" miscarriages. Many ethicists do condemn, however, the practice of returning some but not all of the embryos to the woman's womb either because they are not needed or because they have been deliberately treated for clinical or basic research purposes.

There have been several responses to ethicists' concerns about surplus embryos. The first is the avoid-the-issue response. To spare women the pain associated with repeated laparoscopies, physicians at the Norfolk, Virginia, Fertility Clinic, for example, used to "prime" their patients with drugs so that they would produce as many eggs as possible at one time.[46] After the external fertilization of these eggs, the physician placed all of them into the waiting women's wombs to increase their chances of becoming pregnant. Although the physicians realized that, as a result of their policy, some women might find themselves the mothers of triplets, quadruplets, quintuplets, or even sextuplets,[47] they insisted that what they most feared was not too many multiple births but too few successful pregnancies. However, when some researchers discovered that the drugs used to achieve superovulation actually impeded embryo implantation, Norfolk physicians stopped superovulating their patients and began placing only one or two in vitro embryos into a woman's womb per menstrual cycle. Provided that a woman's hormones are in balance and that her menstrual cycle is regular, a small number of fertilized eggs are as likely to implant as a large number of fertilized eggs. Thus, physicians need not create a large number of embryos for introduction into a woman's womb, and what is not created need never be destroyed.[48]

The second response to the problem of spare embryos is the technological-fix response. Because implantation may not occur even under ideal conditions, some women will have to submit to repeated laparoscopies. The solution, therefore, is to harvest and fertilize multiple eggs and to freeze spare embryos for future attempts at implantation. Although critics of IVF speculate that the frozen-embryo population may be largely defective, Australian and Dutch researchers have reported so much success with the technique of embryo freezing and transfer[49] that U.S. and British clinicians are confident of its safety.[50] Even so, a clinically proved, safe method for embryo freezing and transfer does not solve the problem of surplus embryos; it simply postpones it. Once the egg donor is impregnated, for example, she has no need for the surplus frozen embryos, and there is little reason to believe that scores of women, even infertile women, will request the transfer of surplus frozen embryos, genetically unrelated to them, into their wombs. This is not to say, however, that a so-called technological fix cannot ever resolve the problem of surplus embryos. If safe techniques for freezing eggs are perfected, then there will be no clinical reasons—other than a desire to detect genetic abnormalities as soon as possible—for producing surplus embryos. When a woman reaches the appropriate stage in her menstrual cycle, her physician will simply thaw one of her eggs, combine it with sperm, and place the resultant embryo in her womb.

The third response to the problem of surplus embryos is the acceptance approach ("Let's be honest; we're always going to have some surplus embryos"). Some IVF patients refuse to have more than one or two of their embryos placed in their wombs, and other IVF patients—the ones who become pregnant—usually have no use for their surplus embryos. When either of these events occurs, physicians will have to decide what to do with the unwanted embryos. They cannot stay frozen forever. At some point, physicians will either have to donate them to someone who wants to bear them or to discard them as no longer viable. But because some infertile couples wish to avoid the psychosocial complications of having unwanted genetic offspring in the world, they may insist that their physicians discard rather than donate their surplus embryos.[51] And because it is not clear what moral and legal rights infertile couples have with respect to their unwanted IVF embryos (are they akin to property rights or to parental rights?), says philosopher David T. Ozar, physicians may err in one of two ways: (1) in the direction of defect by discarding an embryo that is viable (capable of implanting in some woman's womb) or (2) in the direction of excess by securing an injunction that keeps the embryo frozen until it is no longer viable.[52]

Not only do IVF physicians sometime find themselves in charge of unwanted embryos; they sometimes find themselves in charge of embryos that are best described as abandoned or orphaned. During the 2- to 3-day span between egg retrieval from the woman's womb and embryo transfer into it, an infertile couple may decide to separate or divorce, or one or the other of them may get cold feet about parenting, have a debilitating accident, become fatally ill, or even die.[53]

For example, in 1981 Mario and Elva Rios entered an IVF program in Melbourne, Australia. Physicians there retrieved and fertilized with donor sperm several of Mrs. Rios's eggs. Although one of the resulting three embryos was placed in her womb, the other two were frozen for possible future use. When Mrs. Rios miscarried, she told her physicians that she was not emotionally ready for another cycle of IVF. After some discussion, she and her husband decided to fly to South America to adopt a child. Before she left on this trip, Mrs. Rios told the physicians at the Melbourne clinic to keep her frozen embryos for her should she ever decide to use them. Unfortunately, Mrs. Rios died before she had the opportunity to make this decision. In 1983, she, her husband, and their adopted child were killed in a plane crash. Because Mr. and Mrs. Rios were very wealthy, questions were immediately raised about the status of the orphaned embryos. Did they have the right to inherit the Rios estate? And who, after all, had the right to determine the embryos' future? Ozar, a modified protectionist with respect to the status of preimplantation embryos, comments:

If the Rioses were still alive, it would be natural to conclude, both in law and from an ethical perspective, that they, together with the doctors and researchers involved, are the responsible parties. With the Rioses now dead, should the executors appointed for the Rioses' estate or the Rioses' heirs [both of the Rioses had children from previous marriages] or possibly the state take over the Rioses' role in these decisions.[54]

As it so happened, a committee convened to answer these questions recommended that the embryos be discarded, but the state of Victoria rejected this recommendation, ruling that the embryos be implanted in a surrogate mother. Whether such an implantation actually took place is unknown. If it did not, physicians and researchers at the Melbourne clinic will eventually have to decide the fate of the orphaned embryos and, given that embryos deteriorate over time, the involved physicians and researchers may decide to discard them at some point.[55]

Discarding unwanted IVF embryos may be unjustified from both a rights-oriented and a utilitarian point of view. Kass argues that there are special ethical problems associated with discarding unwanted IVF embryos. Unlike embryos whose existence conflicts with the interests or rights of pregnant women, these ex utero embryos do not jeopardize anyone's health or welfare.[56] Thus, those who justify abortion on the grounds that a pregnant woman's right to life is stronger than that of an in vivo embryo may find it difficult to justify the willful killing of an ex utero embryo that is not impeding a pregnant woman's life. Also, unlike successfully aborted in vivo embryos, these ex utero embryos are viable in the sense that, given current technology, they have a chance of surviving if they are transferred into a woman's womb.[57] If one couple wishes to adopt another couple's unwanted IVF embryo, then they should be permitted to do so, says the rights-oriented ethicist, for it is one matter to kill an in vivo embryo to save its mother's life and quite another to let an ex utero embryo die when there is someone who is ready, willing, and able to bear and rear it.

Whereas the rights-oriented ethicist argues that it is unjustified to disregard an embryo's right to life when it is unnecessary to do so, the utilitarian simply argues that it is a disutilitarian waste to throw embryos away when people are eager to adopt them. A policy of embryo donation should be preferred unless the benefits that accrue to the adopted embryos and their adoptive parents fail to outweigh the harms that accrue to those IVF couples who want their embryos to be discarded rather than adopted.[58]

The Problem of Surplus Embryos in a Research Setting

If there are serious ethical problems about discarding embryos in the clinical context, there are equally serious problems about not discarding embryos in the research setting. Over the past decade, there has been much controversy about fetal research because of its alleged connections to abortion. In the context of fetal research, the DHEW defines a fetus as "the human from the time of implantation until determination is made following delivery that it is viable or possibly viable."[59] Once the fetus is viable, researchers may perform on it only those therapeutic or non-therapeutic experiments that they may also perform on a premature infant.

The DHEW also monitors researchers' experiments on nonviable fetuses. In general, it follows the 1976 guidelines of the National Commission for the Protection of Human Subjects, which approved certain kinds of therapeutic and nontherapeutic fetal research but only on the recommendation of an Institutional Review Board (IRB) and with the informed consent of both the fetus's father and mother. Among the kinds of nontherapeutic research the commission approved were in utero fetal research when (1) abortion is not planned, the risks are minimal, and there is no other way to obtain the knowledge, and (2) abortion is planned and the risks are minimal.[60] Critics of the commission's recommendations have objected that the fact that an abortion is planned does not justify dispensing with the "no other way to obtain the knowledge" requirement. They claim that just because a fetus is destined for abortion does not make it any less valuable than a fetus that is not destined for abortion.[61] Given this objection, it is not surprising that these same critics have expressed reservations about researchers using either unwanted surplus IVF embryos or deliberately created human embryos as desirable candidates for experimentation.

That full protectionists are opposed to experiments on spare embryos, but especially on deliberately created embryos, also is not surprising. As they see it, it is almost always wrong to experiment on children, infants, or embryos because these "persons" cannot consent to being used as research subjects. They maintain that there are only two exceptions to this no-experimentation rule. If parents or guardians (1) believe that experimentation may in some reasonable way serve the best interests of their young charges or (2) believe that their young charges would, if they could express themselves, choose to be experimented on for the sake of others, then they may give their consent to it. Provided that there is no way to ameliorate the degenerative condition that is killing their child, infant, or embryo, for example, parents or guardians may authorize a limited range of experiments—certainly not painful ones—to be performed on their young charges in order to bring some good out of a very bad state of affairs. The knowledge gained from such experiments may restore life or health to someone else's child, infant, or embryo. Nevertheless, even if full protectionists may permit certain experiments on doomed children, infants, or embryos, they do not permit the deliberate creation of embryos for purposes of experimentation. As these ethicists see it, it is one thing to make the best of a tragic situation and quite another to create a tragedy in order to make the best of it.

Non-protectionists have no objections either to experimenting on existent surplus embryos or to creating embryos deliberately for experimental uses. As they see it, only self-aware human beings can have interests, including the interest not to be used as an experimental subject. Because embryos are not self-aware, they are without interests. Therefore, researchers may experiment on them provided that these "human materials" (the nonprotectionist term for embryos) are not sentient—that is, capable of feeling pleasure or pain. As long as the researcher is confident that a 1-week-old embryo cannot feel pain, says the nonprotectionist, that researcher should proceed with his or her experiment. Some nonprotectionists go even further than this. They argue that it is less morally problematic to do research on an early embryo that feels no pain than on a full-grown animal that does feel pain.[62]

Most ethicists are neither full protectionists nor nonprotectionists; rather, they are modified protectionists who believe that the embryo is less than a fully human person though more than mere human materials. These moderates neither wholeheartedly endorse nor adamantly oppose experimental research on existing surplus embryos or deliberately created embryos. In lawyer John Robertson's view, for example, experimentation is permissible provided that (1) "the expected benefits of research outweigh the symbolic gain in respect for human life that a ban on all embryo research seeks;" (2) the embryos are under a specific age; and (3) the embryos have been obtained in an appropriate way.[63]

Currently, the U.S. government specifies a 14-day limit on embryo research, after which time the embryo must be discarded. This cutoff point is intended to avoid the possibility of doing research on an embryo that possesses a rudimentary nervous system and thus might feel pain; it also demonstrates respect for the embryo. However, many researchers believe this cutoff point is excessively restrictive because the embryo is unlikely to feel pain until it is much older. As a result of this federal restriction and others like it, many researchers have left the public sector for the private sector in order to continue more freely their experimentation on embryos.[64] For example, Gary Hodgen, formerly a public employee at the NIH, is now doing independent in vitro work supported by a $1.5 million research grant from a private Massachusetts-based firm. Among his projects are the following: (1) an attempt to engineer genetically the hormones used to stimulate follicles; (2) an exploration of the ovarian process that causes an egg to mature; and (3) a series of experiments to learn how to identify those IVF embryos most likely to survive in the womb. Significantly, Hodgen uses only what he regards as politically safe strategies in his experimentation on embryos. Instead of using invasive strategies, Hodgen uses a needle-in-a-haystack approach, looking "for a molecular marker released into the spent [IVF] culture medium—either a unique substance or a different amount of some common chemical released by the embryos that survive."[65] In others words, rather than experimenting on the embryo itself, Hodgen focuses only on its environment to minimize negative reactions from local pro-life groups, for example.

The Effects of IVF on Fundamental Familial Relationships

Thus far we have focused on ethical issues surrounding the IVF embryo in either the clinical or research setting, but critics of IVF have raised other, more general concerns about it. As in the case of AID, critics of IVF argue that IVF is especially problematic from a moral point of view when it requires a couple to use a third party in order to procreate. Although some critics are willing to accept IVF in which the husband's sperm and the wife's eggs are used, they are not willing to accept IVF in which donors' eggs, sperm, or embryos are used. As many traditionalists see it, whenever a donor enters the picture, there is the possibility of family discord: The parent who lacks a genetic connection to the child may not feel as close to him or her as the parent who has such a connection. Over time the "deficient" parent may become alienated from the child or jealous of the other parent. The strength of this objection is, of course, dependent on its dubious empirical truth. After all, women who marry widowers with children often come to love these children as much as does their genetic father, and men who marry divorced women with children are capable of loving these children despite their lack of genetic connection to them.

Another objection to IVF is a natural-law objection. If it is wrong to separate sex from procreation, it is equally wrong to separate procreation from sex. Physician Leon Kass, for example, claims that there is "wisdom in that mystery of nature which joins the pleasure of sex, the communication of love, and the desire for children in the very activity by which we continue the chain of human existence."[66] As he sees it, "making babies in laboratories—even 'perfect' babies—"[67] spoils or "degrades" one of the most beautiful experiences a man and a woman can have—namely, weaving a continuous line from their mutual act of sexual intercourse, to the union of their genetic material, to the embryonic development and birthing of their child and, finally, to the rearing of that child.

Since Kass realizes that not all married couples are physically capable of weaving a continuous line between begetting, bearing, and rearing children, he accepts adoption (a process that breaks the line between rearing children on the one hand and begetting and bearing them on the other). He also accepts IVF as a "court of last resort" provided that the egg and sperm belong to the wife and husband, respectively, and that the embryo is implanted in the wife. Although such a couple is not able to join their two separate bodies in an act of sexual intercourse that produces "a child who is flesh of their separate flesh made one," says Kass, they nonetheless beget, bear, and rear a child genetically related to both of them, "someone who descends and comes after, someone who will replace oneself in the family line to preserve the family tree by new sproutings and branchings."[68] What Kass is unwilling to accept, however, are those forms of IVF that involve egg donation, sperm donation, or embryo donation. To break the line between begetting a child on the one hand and bearing it on the other is a rupture that Kass is not prepared to justify morally.

Although Kass's concerns about preserving the continuum between begetting, bearing, and rearing children are legitimate ones, it is doubtful that, simply because IVF exists, men and women are going to choose an artificial mode of reproduction over a natural one. After all, how many healthy people choose intravenous feeding over chewing and swallowing simply because it is possible for them to eat through their veins instead of by mouth? Admittedly, the new reproductive technologies may one day be able to promise couples something Nature was never able to promise them: namely, healthy babies. In fact, scientists at Britain's Clinical Research Center have already found a way to perform genetic tests for cystic fibrosis on preimplantation embryos.[69] As techniques for genetic screening are perfected, prospective parents may increasingly choose artificial over natural means of procreation; that is, they may choose IVF over in vivo fertilization so that researchers can screen their embryos for defects, discarding any imperfect ones. But not all prospective parents will necessarily embrace artificial procreation. Some of them will want to procreate the old-fashioned way. Indeed, some of them may even want to beget and bear so-called imperfect babies, babies who resemble them precisely because of their imperfections. Then the ethical question will become whether these holdouts have the right to have an imperfect child naturally when they have the means to have a perfect child artificially.[70]

More than likely, a rights-oriented thinker will argue that couples do not have a duty to produce the best child they can possibly produce. After all, even if a child has some physical or mental limitations, she or he is no less a person than a so-called perfect child. Nevertheless, the rights-oriented thinker will probably concede that there is a difference between procreating a less than perfect child, on the one hand, and a child so imperfect that it cannot achieve any discernible measure of personal happiness and developmental satisfaction, on the other. If treating persons with respect and consideration means anything, it must mean to create and maintain conditions that permit persons to exercise their rights, conditions such as a sound mind and a sound body. If so, prospective parents may have a moral obligation to beget and bear children artificially if that is the best way to bring into existence persons who are capable of exercising their rights.

Related to the objections that IVF breaks the continuum between begetting, bearing, and rearing a child and that it provides people with the opportunity to custom-design their children is the objection that at least some forms of IVF jeopardize the parent-child relationship. As we noted earlier, all sorts of variations on standard IVF, where the sperm and egg of a married couple are conjoined in vitro and then implanted in the womb of the female partner, are now being practiced. Up to 5 different parents can be involved in the begetting, bearing, and rearing of a child: the man who donates his sperm and the woman who donates her eggs; the woman who carries the fertilized egg to term; and the man and woman who will rear the child after its birth. Faced with 5 parents, a child may wonder to whom she or he is primarily related: To the begetters? The bearers? The rearers? Some critics maintain that children will lack a sense of identity if their rearers are not also their begetters and bearers, but this objection arises only in societies that put a premium on having children that are (1) gestationally related to their female rearers and (2) genetically related to their male and female rearers. It does not arise in societies that put less of a premium on genetic or gestational bonds. In fact, such societies are more likely to reason, as did the ancient

Greek philosopher Plato, that if any factor creates social disorder, it is the fact the genetic parents are so attached to their genetic children that they automatically put their interest ahead of other competing social interests. Thus, Plato recommended that the rulers of his ideal republic relinquish their children at birth to be reared collectively in state-run nurseries. Never were these parents to be told who their genetic children were.[71] Such a policy strikes critics as cruel but, as Plato saw it, provided that children are reared attentively by their caretakers, it matters not whether their caretakers are genetically related to them.

Even if there were not strong arguments against the selective use of IVF, there may be strong arguments against its indiscriminate use. For example, were there, as philosopher D. Gareth-Jones worries, a "wholesale transfer of procreation to the laboratory," then "the justification and support which biological parenthood gives to the monogamous marriage" could be undermined.[72] Supposedly, what holds many marriages together is the fact that both parents are biologically related to their children and therefore interested in staying with their children "through thick and through thin." But, ask the critics, is it so much that natural parents find it difficult to live apart from their natural children, or is it simply that parents find it difficult to live apart from their children, whether or not their children are genetically related to them? In sum, are biological facts (consanguinity) always (or usually) more capable of holding a family together than are social intentions (a professed desire to rear a child)?

IVF, Reasonable Risk Assumption, and Informed Consent

As some ethicists see it, the major moral issues to address in any discussion of GIFT, IVF, and embryo transfer are the risk-benefit ratios and whether their users know how risky these technologies are. Scant attention has been paid to the risks of clinical GIFT, IVF, and embryo transfer, but such risks do exist. GIFT carries the risks of multiple pregnancy and of general anesthesia. These risks as well as the risk of having to undergo the cycle of harvesting eggs, fertilization, and implantation four or more times (unless, of course, cryopreserved embryos are used) or of experiencing a life-threatening ectopic pregnancy (the Office of Technology Assessment estimates that tubal pregnancies occur in 2 to 17 percent of IVF procedures) attend IVF.[73] Finally, the possibility of both a spontaneous abortion and the birth of a defective child may be slightly higher than average for an IVF-initiated pregnancy and perhaps also for a GIFT-initiated pregnancy.[74] Whether an infertile couple, especially its female member, should take any of these risks is a matter for ethical discussion.

In general, if it is to be morally justified, a risk assumption must be reasonable. According to philosopher Joel Feinberg, several factors affect the reasonability of a risk assumption:

1. The degree of probability that harm to oneself will result from a given course of action

2. The seriousness of the harm being risked

3. The degree of probability that the goal inclining one to shoulder the risk will, in fact, result from the course of action

4. The value or importance of achieving that goal—that is, just how worthwhile it is to one

5. The necessity of the risk—that is, the availability or absence of alternative, less risky, means to the desired goal.[75]

Thus, an infertile couple should be informed about all the risks that GIFT or IVF poses before the partners decide to go ahead with the procedure. In particular, the woman should be aware of these risks since it is primarily her body that will suffer any negative consequences. Given that a woman will probably experience considerable pain and discomfort throughout an IVF program and that there is only a 25 percent chance that she will, after repeated hospital stays, a time expenditure of $4\frac{1}{2}$ years, and a cash expenditure of approximately $25,000, achieve pregnancy, a decision to use IVF may be unreasonable.[74] In contrast, given that all other alternative means to having a child have been exhausted and that the infertile couple wants a baby more than anything else in the world, a decision to use IVF may be very reasonable.

A similar line of reasoning would apply to a couple's decision to use GIFT, except that GIFT is not only less risky than IVF but also less expensive (an average cost of $3,500) and more successful (an average 29 percent pregnancy rate, ranging from 10 percent to 56 percent effectiveness based on the type of infertility). The only benefit that GIFT lacks is that, unlike IVF, GIFT does not permit either diagnosis of genetic or chromosomal abnormalities in preimplantation embryos or identification of defects in the fertilizing ability of gametes.[77]

What looks like a reasonable risk on the surface, however, may not really be reasonable if it has not been voluntarily accepted. The assumption of a risk is fully voluntary, according to Feinberg, only if one assumes the risk with informed consent, aware of all relevant facts and known contingencies and unaffected by any external coercive pressure or internal compulsion. "Neurotic compulsion, misinformation, excitement or impetuousness, clouded judgment (as, from alcohol or drugs), or immature or defective faculties or reasoning"[78] are among the factors that tend to defeat ascriptions of full responsibility. Because we are always lacking something in the way of knowledge and power, our choices are never perfectly voluntary. Nevertheless, we can make a distinction between choices that are almost certainly voluntary and choices that are almost certainly involuntary. An infertile couple will be able to give its informed consent to IVF or GIFT, for example, provided that (1) the couple's physician tells his or her patients about the risks as well as the benefits of these procedures and (2) no one pressures, badgers, or otherwise coerces the partners into using these procedures.

Unfortunately, informed consent has not always been the rule in clinical IVF research. According to some reports, Lesley Brown, mother of the world's first test-tube baby, had assumed that IVF was a well-developed technique and that hundreds of test-tube babies had been born prior to her setting foot in the clinic of Drs. Steptoe and Edwards. No one told her just how physically and psychologically draining IVF can be when all does not go well,[79] and so she consented to IVF without an adequate appreciation of the hardships she would be asked to bear.

Furthermore, even if a woman adequately appreciates the hardships IVF can entail, the mere fact that she decides to go ahead anyway does not conclusively establish the voluntariness of her decision. If a woman is made to feel that she is "next to nothing" without a child, that her husband will leave her if she cannot produce an heir, and that her old age will be lonely,[80] her decision to use IVF or GIFT may be far less than a fully voluntary one. Although no gunman points a pistol at her head as she signs the consent papers, a host of psychological mechanisms stand ready to punish her should she waver. In assessing how informed a woman's consent to IVF really is, we must weigh these psychological pressures against two facts. First, as IVF and GIFT techniques are developed, women are subjected to less pain and discomfort, to fewer major medical risks, and to fewer disappointments as the rate of successful embryo transfers, implantations, and births increases. Second, as women become more self-confident, they are choosing to use reproduction-aiding technology not because other people have told them that they must have a child in order to establish their womanhood but because they themselves very much want to have a child. As a result of these two developments, an increasing number of women are able to choose IVF and GIFT voluntarily.

Issues of informed consent also arise in connection with both egg and embryo donation. Because she must undergo laparoscopy, an egg donor assumes considerable risks, risks that seem all the greater because she assumes them not to increase her own chances of gaining a much-wanted child but to increase another woman's chances of doing so. In contrast to an egg donor, an embryo donor risks both less and more: She risks less than the egg donor in that she undergoes no surgical procedures, agreeing only to in vivo artificial insemination followed by embryo transfer. She risks more than the egg donor, however, in that an unwanted pregnancy is sometimes the result of an unsuccessful embryo transfer or flushing. Although the specially designed catheter used to wash out the embryo donor's uterus generally works effectively, occasionally an embryo does implant in the donor's uterus. Clearly, embryo donation and egg donation pose major health risks to embryo and egg donors, risks that sperm donors do not have to shoulder. Nevertheless, provided that egg and embryo donors understand and are willing to take the risks that attend IVF in particular, their decision to sell or share their genetic material or progeny is no less voluntary than sperm donors' decision to sell or share their sperm.

Another set of sensitive problems centers around the potential child. The potential offspring of IVF confront several physical and psychological risks, and they do not have the ability either to understand the nature of these risks or to shoulder them voluntarily. For this reason, theologian Paul Ramsey objects that IVF amounts to unethical nontherapeutic experimentation on unborn children without their consent.[81] Ramsey's accusation of "unethical nontherapeutic experimentation" may make sense in the basic research context. These researchers use either existent surplus embryos or even deliberately created embryos for experimental purposes with the intention of destroying or discarding them after a short period of time.[82] On the one hand, if we view these early embryos merely as human materials, then researchers are not required to secure their informed consent (assuming this were possible) because mere matter is without interests (that is, desires, wants, needs); at most, the researchers are required to secure the informed consent of the egg and sperm donors, who may have an interest in the ultimate disposition of their reproductive gametes. On the other hand, if we view these early embryos as human persons, then whatever informed consent standards apply to infants most likely apply to these embryos, with the added complication that, if they have been created solely for experimental purposes, their genetic parents may not want to act in their best interests.

Even if Ramsey's objection makes sense in the research context, however, it may not make sense in the clinical context. As IVF supporters see it, clinical IVF is not nontherapeutic experimentation. IVF parents want to act in the best interests of their IVF embryos because the results of a successful IVF cycle is a child who receives the benefit of life, a benefit that she or he would not otherwise have. Other IVF supporters add the condition, however, that in order to be justified, IVF must offer to a child not simply life but a life that is worth living. Although lawyer John A. Robertson agrees that it is wrong to use techniques that can cause a child to be born damaged, he nonetheless argues that if the only way to give a child life is by risking some damage to it, then it is permissible to use IVF provided that the damage risked to the child is not so great that she or he would be unwilling to live with it.[83] In any case, as presently practiced, IVF has shown no higher rate of congenital deformity than occurs with coital reproduction.[84] Thus, there are no strong utilitarian arguments against IVF on the grounds that it poses too many physical risks.

Even if it does not pose serious physical risks, IVF may pose serious psychological risks. As Robertson sees it, the possibility of psychological harms due to conceiving and implanting embryos posthumously, donating sperm, eggs, or embryos anonymously, or serving as surrogates contractually have been exaggerated. When it comes to posthumous conception, for example, Robertson does not believe that being born 50 to 100 years after one's genetic parents have died or being raised by a mother and a father in their eighties is worse than not having been born at all. However, he does admit the following:

The conclusion that offspring are better off from long storage does not fully dispel the discomfort felt at the idea of posthumous conception and implantation, or embryo transfer after long periods of cryopreservation. The idea of postponing conception or implantation until long after the gene source's death is new and strange. Even if no harm to offspring is shown, our concept of birth and parentage is severely tested. The technology thus presents a novel situation that tests our understanding of reproductive responsibility and the welfare of offspring.[85]

Provided that people meet well IVF's challenges of reproductive responsibility, Robertson and other IVF advocates believe that, at least in the clinical context, IVF serves to further rather than to frustrate IVF embryos' best interests.

Legal Aspects of In Vitro Fertilization and Embryo Transfer

Constitutional Issues Related to Clinical Applications of IVF and Embryo Transfer

Although few states have enacted legislation or promulgated regulations directly governing human IVF or embryo transfer, existing laws on (1) artificial insemination and (2) research involving human fetuses suggest ways in which IVF legislation may be constructed in the future. Were laws banning IVF passed, however, they would probably be challenged on constitutional grounds. Indeed, in Illinois where legislation sought simply to regulate and not to ban IVF, it has been so challenged. In 1979, Illinois legislators made any physician who undertakes an IVF procedure the legal custodian of the embryo and liable for possible prosecution under an 1877 child-abuse statute. As a result, many Illinois physicians decided not to practice IVF, although the state attorney general assured them that most simple IVF procedures would not violate the statute. Concerned about the chilling effect of the statute on these physicians, an infertile couple challenged the Illinois attempt at regulation as unconstitutional. On behalf of the class of infertile people, they argued that such restrictions on IVF violate infertile people's fundamental right of privacy.[86] Should the couple's class action succeed, then Illinois would have to show that anti-IVF legislation is not only necessary to protect a "compelling state interest" but that it is the least restrictive way to do so.[87] However, should the couple's class action fail, then Illinois would need to demonstrate only that its anti-IVF legislation is rationally related to a constitutionally permissible purpose it chooses to pursue.[88]

No matter what the outcome of the Illinois couple's specific challenge, there is already some legal precedent on which to base a right to reproduce by means of reproduction-aiding technology. In a series of cases stretching over a 40-year period, the Supreme Court has ruled that, absent compelling state interests, the state may not (1) through sterilization, for example, deprive individuals of their right to procreate [*Skinner* v. *Oklahoma* (1942)];[89] (2) interfere with married couples' right to make procreative decisions [*Griswold* v. *Connecticut* (1965)];[90] and (3) interfere with unmarried individuals' as well as married couples' right to make procreative decisions [*Eisenstadt* v. *Baird* (1972)[91] and *Carey* v. *Population Service International* (1977)].[92]

Using these court cases as precedent, IVF proponents would seek to interpret them as broadly as possible. Specifically, they would argue that: (1) because *Skinner* regards the ability to procreate as a fundamental human good, then infertile individuals have a right to use whatever reproductive technologies will make them fertile; (2) because *Griswold* encompasses a married couple's decision to use contraceptive means not to conceive a child, it also encompasses their decision to use reproductive technologies to conceive a child; and (3) because *Eisenstadt* and *Carey* regard as personal and private any individual's decision to bear or not to bear or beget a child, they must also regard as personal and private any individual's decision about how to bear or beget a child. In contrast, using these same court cases as precedent, IVF opponents would seek to interpret them as narrowly as possible. Specifically, they would argue that (1) *Skinner* establishes only the right of certain fertile persons to remain fertile and not also the right of infertile persons to make themselves fertile; (2) *Griswold* establishes only a married couple's right to use contraceptives to prevent conception and not also a married couple's right to use reproduction-aiding technologies to cause conception; and (3) *Eisenstadt* and *Carey* regard as personal and private only procreative decisions that involve the act of sexual intercourse and not also procreative decisions that involve acts of AID, IVF, and so on.

Chances are that even a broad Constitutional reading of cases such as *Skinner, Griswold, Eisenstadt,* and *Carey* would initially limit the right to use IVF, for example, to a husband and wife when the egg and sperm are donated by the husband and wife, the embryo is implanted in the wife, and procreation by the couple is impossible without IVF. Where there is absence of marriage, of a genetic link, of a gestational link, or of necessity, the case for IVF will be weakened. Therefore, a homosexual who wished to transfer an embryo fertilized in vitro from his sperm and a donor's egg to the womb of a contracted mother would have difficulty establishing that his right to privacy encompasses his decision to beget a child by such means.

No doubt, critics might object that laws preventing homosexuals from using IVF violate these men's right to beget a genetic child. After all, how are men who eschew sexual relations with women supposed to procreate except through technological means? A right to beget a genetic child is probably the dimension of the right to privacy most amenable to a narrow constitutional reading. In the same way that any purported fundamental right to life-sustaining food does not necessarily support a right to life-enhancing foods such as caviar, morels, and truffles, the right to beget genetic children probably encompasses access only to those means of procreation without which an individual cannot procreate. Because, in principle, a homosexual man could procreate through sexual intercourse, the argument could be made that he does not need to use IVF to beget a child.

Constitutional Issues Related to Basic Research Involving IVF or Embryo Culture

Because the state has sought to regulate reproduction-aiding research in many ways, researchers have argued that the state is violating their right to seek new knowledge. As most constitutional lawyers see it, however, even if researchers have a free-speech right to choose a research goal, they do not also have a right to pursue that goal with any research method they choose to use.[93] In the same way that the free-speech right to believe a religious teaching does not entail the right to engage in harmful religious practices, the right to seek knowledge does not entail the right to use harmful research methods:

The state may not interfere with the researcher's choice of the end or topic of research, but it may regulate only the methods used in the research, in order to protect interests in health, order and safety with which unrestricted research might conflict. Such restrictions are valid if they are reasonably related to protection of nonspeech interests and are not so vague and over broad that they chill the exercise of protected speech.[94]

Thus, a state may legislate against the deliberate creation of research embryos if such legislation is "reasonably related" to the protection of some of its health, order, and safety interests. For example, the state may claim that the manipulation of reproductive tissues in vitro poses a safety threat or is inconsistent with the dignity that should be accorded potential human life.[95] Should researchers object that such restrictions violate their right to seek knowledge, the state will reply that researchers are free to seek knowledge using methods other than the restricted ones. Of course, what the state may not always understand is that research goals and research methods are often symbiotically related; that is, the research goal cannot be attained with any research method other than the proposed one. When this is the case, the state may need not simply a rational interest but a compelling interest, such as a "clear and present danger" to society, to restrict researchers' methods.

Like some researchers, some egg and sperm donors have claimed that the state may not regulate reproductive research. Of course, egg and sperm donors have different interests from researchers. Whereas the latter invoke constitutionally protected speech rights, the former invoke constitutionally protected privacy rights to control the use and implantation of their own genetic materials.[96] Nonetheless, it is not clear how far this right extends and what kind of right it is.

Some commentators are of the opinion that this right extends only to genetic materials within the body. Other commentators believe that this right extends to genetic materials outside the body but that it ends when a person donates or sells his or her genetic materials. Still others maintain that persons have no right to sell or even donate their genetic materials.[97]

Despite a severe shortage of donor organs, the state permits people to donate kidneys, livers, and hearts only under certain conditions, and it forbids people to sell them under any conditions. The only exception to this rule is the sale of blood and sperm. As the state sees it, to protect its citizens' interests in health and safety, it may forbid them to sell any of their vital organs. For example, an impoverished man with huge debts may feel compelled to sell his liver when such sale is in no way in his best interest. Although egg selling as well as sperm and blood selling are less hazardous to one's well-being than are kidney, liver, and heart selling, the state may have reasons to forbid or regulate even the sale of the former materials. For example, if screening techniques were unable to distinguish between defective and nondefective gametes, the state could justifiably ban the sale of eggs and sperm to protect buyers' health and safety interests. However, adequate screening techniques are available and the state already permits sperm and egg selling. The growing consensus is that once a person sells her or his gametes, she or he loses control over them unless her or his informed consent was not secured prior to the sale.

Rights of IVF Children

Insofar as IVF offspring are concerned, several legal remedies exist to succor their parents or them when, due to lack of informed consent, they have shouldered unreasonable risks or when, due to the intentional, reckless, or negligent conduct of IVF practitioners, they have been either harmed or put at excessive risk of harm. Physicians are required to secure their patients' informed consent to IVF, but it is not clear just how many of IVF's risks physicians must disclose to their prospective IVF patients. The majority view still holds that physicians need not disclose a known risk if a reasonable physician, exercising medical judgment for the benefit of the patient, would not disclose the risk. However, as we noted in chapter 4, this traditional standard for disclosure is being challenged. To safeguard themselves from liability, physicians should probably disclose those known IVF risks of which a reasonable patient would wish to be apprised.

Fearful that not even this level of disclosure may be enough, cautious lawyers advise physicians to disclose those known IVF risks of which unreasonable as well as reasonable patients would wish to be apprised.[98] For example, even though there is little empirical evidence that IVF treatment poses risks to IVF embryos, physicians should nonetheless discuss such remote possibilities on the slim chance that the embryo is born dead or defective. Only then, say cautious lawyers, will physicians have a defense if they are sued for either wrongful death or wrongful birth.

In a wrongful death suit, IVF parents might seek to recover damages for the personal suffering and economic losses sustained by them as a result of the death of their IVF child or even their unimplanted IVF embryo.[99] In *Del Zio* v. *Columbia Presbyterian Hospital*, for example, the jury returned a verdict for $50,000 in favor of prospective parents whose unimplanted embryo was deliberately destroyed by a member of the hospital staff.[100] In a wrongful birth suit, IVF parents might seek to recover similar damages where a deformed or abnormal child is born as a result of negligent medical advice or a decision to proceed with IVF.

Although there is less clear precedent for it, IVF infants themselves may also have a cause of action for either a wrongful birth or even a wrongful life suit. In a wrongful birth suit, the IVF infant sues on the basis of prenatal or even preconception injuries sustained by it.[101] In the early half of this century, courts routinely dismissed such suits on the grounds that until they reach the point of viability, fetuses are not separate organisms; rather, they are merely parts of their mothers. During the 1970s, however, civil courts began to accept conception as the point at which a fetus is a separate organism,[102] and this despite *Roe* v. *Wade's* 1973 emphasis on viability as the crucial moment in the fetus's development. Thus, in *Renslaw* v. *Mennonite Hospital*,[103] the Illinois Supreme Court upheld an infant's suit for injuries sustained as a result of a blood transfusion administered to its mother 8 years before its birth. Said the court: "We believe that there is a right to be born free from prenatal injuries foreseeably caused by a breach of duty to the child's mother."[104] But if such a ruling makes sense, it makes even more sense to uphold an infant's suit for injuries sustained as a result of a bungled IVF implantation, for example. The foreseeable harm to the child as a result of such negligent handling seems "more direct and substantial" than the foreseeable harm to the infant in the *Renslaw* case.[105]

Even if infants are increasingly able to bring successful wrongful birth suits, they have not been able to bring successful wrongful life suits in which they argue that, given their damaged condition, it would have been better for them not to be born at all. With one exception, which was later overruled, courts have rejected wrongful life suits either on the grounds that there exists no "fundamental right of a child to be born as a whole, functional human being ..."[106] or on the grounds that there is no way to compare the state of existence with the state of nonexistence. The exception was *Park* v. *Chessin*. After their first child died of a fatal hereditary kidney disease, a couple asked several physicians if they were likely to conceive another child with the same disease. The physicians assured the couple that the chances for a repeat tragedy were minuscule. The couple proceeded to have a child and the disease struck again. These parents sued the physicians on behalf of their child. The appellate division ruled in the couple's favor, but the court of appeals reversed its ruling. It found two flaws in the child's wrongful life claim: first, the infant did not suffer a "legally cognizable injury" by reason of its birth, and second, it was impossible to compute damages because this calculation depended on the comparison between "life in an impaired state and nonexistence."[107] To these two flaws, we may add a third—namely, that a severely handicapped child cannot sue for wrongful life since she or he is not worse off than she or he would have been otherwise, for she or he would not otherwise have been. Rather, some other child would have been.

Social Dimensions of In Vitro Fertilization and Embryo Transfer

According to philosopher LeRoy Walters, test-tube babies are becoming widely accepted in the United States and many other Western nations. As he sees it, general social responses to GIFT, IVF, and embryo transfer cluster around two sets of issues, which he classifies as first-generation and second-generation.[108] In general, first-generation issues involve the acceptability of ex utero fertilization. With few exceptions, most of the policy-making bodies that have pronounced on IVF have endorsed it as a treatment for infertility but expressed some reservations about its laboratory research applications. However, these reservations are beginning to dissipate with each new discovery IVF researchers make. Increasingly, policymakers are convinced that the fundamental goal of IVF research is to help people have healthy babies and not to create chimeras (half-human, half-animal hybrids) or to clone themselves.

Liberty and Welfare Approaches to IVF

As astute as Walter's comments are about the general acceptability of IVF, of even greater interest are his comments about second-generation IVF issues: (1) the screening of prospective social parents; (2) the sale and purchase of human gametes; (3) elective use of the new reproductive technologies; (4) anonymity versus identification in cases involving third parties; (5) quality control in programs offering the new reproduction technologies; and (6) insurance coverage for the new reproductive technologies. Walters argues that people who have a "liberty-oriented viewpoint that emphasizes privacy rights and resists regulation by third parties" have very different attitudes toward each of these six issues than do people who have a "welfare-oriented viewpoint that advocates external regulation for either paternalistic or nonpaternalistic reasons."[109]

People who stress liberty values over welfare values believe that any individual who wishes to use a reproduction-aiding technology should be free to use one provided that she or he can pay for it and that any individual or commercial sperm (and, in the future, egg) bank that wishes to buy and sell sperm (and, in the future, eggs) should be free to do so, provided that minimum safety standards are met. Liberty-oriented people also believe that any individual who wishes to use a reproduction-aiding technology should be free to use one even if it is not necessary—that is, even if she or he is fertile and genetically sound. Thus, liberty-oriented people affirm the right of fertile individuals to use IVF to produce a baby "better" than the one they think they would produce naturally. When it comes to considerations involving third parties to IVF, liberty-oriented people believe that it is up to prospective IVF parents, egg donors, or sperm donors either to know or not to know one another and that it is up to IVF children either to know or not to know their genetic parents. Finally, liberty-oriented people argue that IVF clinics should be free to operate and advertise for clients, subject only to the standards that govern good businesses, and that people who wish to use reproduction-aiding technologies are free to shop for any insurance plan that is willing to cover such expensive services.[110]

In contrast to liberty-oriented people, welfare-oriented people are very much in favor of screening prospective IVF patients. Many of them wish to exclude from IVF programs child abusers, poor people, single women, nontraditional couples (for example, homosexual couples), and unmarried heterosexual couples. The fact that these infertile people would not be subject to screening if they were fertile does not strike welfare-oriented people as discriminatory. Welfare-oriented people are opposed to the sale and purchase of human eggs and sperm. They favor a voluntary, nonprofit system for donating eggs and sperm. As they see it, nonprofit systems symbolize social solidarity, whereas for-profit systems simply tempt people to sell defective gametes. Welfare-oriented people are also opposed to totally elective use of IVF and embryo transfer. In their opinion, IVF should be limited to infertile or genetically diseased couples in order (1) to conserve a relatively scarce medical resource for those who really need it, (2) to prevent the exploitation of poor women, and (3) to discourage either a designer-baby approach or an animal-breeding approach to human reproduction. When it comes to considerations involving third parties to IVF, welfare-oriented people believe that the less gamete "sellers" and gamete "buyers" know about one another the better. Finally, welfare-oriented people insist that IVF programs should either be certified by a professional organization (for example, the American Fertility Society) or be licensed by a public body (for example DHEW). They also insist that society has a moral obligation to provide infertile people with "infertility insurance" because "infertility seriously disrupts their life plans and diminishes their happiness."[111]

What is interesting about these two approaches to reproduction-aiding technologies is that almost every official group that has studied IVF and embryo transfer has adopted a welfare attitude toward what Walters classifies as second-generation issues. In contrast to these official groups, many private citizens are extremely enthusiastic about IVF and cannot understand why the government wishes to control it. Still, not all private citizens are wholehearted advocates of IVF; in fact, some women's groups and minority organizations have serious reservations about IVF.

Women's, Men's, and Minorities' Attitudes Toward IVF

Among the women who are particularly ambivalent about reproduction-aiding technology are certain feminists. Although liberal feminists, for example, have mostly positive things to say about IVF and also AID, radical feminists have mostly negative things to say about these technologies. As liberal feminists see it, women should be permitted to choose those reproduction-controlling and reproduction-aiding technologies that further their life plans. If a woman has the right to prevent a pregnancy or to terminate it through contraception, abortion, or sterilization, then she also has the right to begin a pregnancy through AID or IVF.

Radical feminists believe that liberal feminists forget that women's choices are rarely autonomous choices. Sometimes husbands pressure their wives to use IVF because it is the only way that they can have a child that is genetically related to them without employing a contracted mother. A woman who cannot conceive a child naturally may be inclined to adopt a child instead, but if her husband is intent on doing all that it takes for him to have a genetic child, she may find herself in line outside an IVF clinic instead of an adoption agency.

The fact that genetic fatherhood may be more important, on average, to men than is genetic motherhood, on average, to women does not mean, for example, that women who adopt children do not in any way miss the good as well as the bad experiences associated with pregnancy. Rather it means that, on average, the most important thing for women is that they have the opportunity to rear a child, whether or not that child is genetically related to them. It also means, say radical feminists that, on average, women are not willing to jeopardize their physical and psychological health substantially in the name of genetic motherhood. Indeed, if more women knew just how costly IVF can be—physically and psychologically as well as financially—fewer women would be inclined to submit to it, spousal pressure notwithstanding.[112]

Radical feminists point out that many women mistakenly believe that IVF is no more difficult than AID when, in fact, there is no real comparison between the two technologies. To become pregnant, a woman has to be willing to go through at least two or three IVF cycles, say radical feminists Gena Corea and Susan Ince. Each IVF cycle lasts approximately 2 weeks. First, the woman is an outpatient. She is monitored for her daily plasma levels and cervical mucus, and she submits to ultrasound examinations to determine ovarian progress. Then the woman is an inpatient. She becomes the object of hormonal assays and the collection of eggs through laparoscopy. Finally, if egg collection and fertilization are successful, she submits to embryo transfer. If egg collection, fertilization, and embryo transfer are unsuccessful, however, the whole process must be reinitiated. Each time the woman goes through a cycle, she is subjected to powerful superovulatory drugs (with the usual unpleasant side effects) and to laparoscopy. Attempts to reduce the risks from general anesthesia associated with laparoscopy have not been particularly felicitous. For example, TUDOR, an alternative to laparoscopy, is purported not to be painful and therefore should not require general anesthesia. Unfortunately, many women find TUDOR very painful in practice. As a result, many physicians resort to general anesthesia during the TUDOR procedure. Comments one physician:

The problem with the ultrasound is that there is no way to grab the ovary. So you stick your needle through the bladder.... The ultrasound can take a long time because you're working with shadows. Before, we were quite optimistic that ultrasound might be the wave of the future, but I have reservations about it now.[113]

In addition to objecting to the ways in which women are not fully informed about just how uncomfortable IVF can be, radical feminists object to the ways in which success rates for IVF are sometimes misrepresented. Robyn Rowland writes that for every 100 women who go into an Australian or British IVF program—probably the most successful programs in the world—only 14 of them will become pregnant. Despite this relatively low 14 percent success rate, IVF clinics around the world continuously announce success rates of 20 to 25 percent.[114] In view of the fact that a recent U.S. survey found that of 54 clinics queried, half had never sent a woman home with a baby, radical feminists are enraged by what they view as an unconscionable manipulation of the facts.

Another, more subtle harm done to women is, according to radical feminists, the way in which her desire to have a genetically related child can blind a woman to the ways in which having her desire fulfilled can put another woman at risk. For example, some variations of IVF such as surrogate embryo transfer or lavage pose special risks. In this flushing technique, a fertile female donor is inseminated with the sperm of an infertile woman's partner. If she conceives, the embryo is flushed from her womb into the womb of the infertile woman. In North America, the results of 29 surrogate embryo transfers were 12 embryos, 2 successful pregnancies, and 1 ectopic pregnancy. In addition, one donor woman had a retained pregnancy that spontaneously aborted.[115]

A desire to have a genetically related child can also blind an infertile woman to the fact that only advantaged infertile women usually use IVF. Should advantaged infertile women respond to the gap that separates them from disadvantaged infertile women by arguing that all infertile women (more properly, infertile couples) should have access to IVF, they may find themselves contributing to health care havoc. Physician Leon Kass points out that the legislative act that required the federal government to pay approximately $25,000 to $30,000 per patient each year for kidney dialysis for everyone in need (cost to the taxpayers in 1978 was nearly $1 billion) is an "impossible precedent."[115] Kass estimates that if only the 500,000 infertile women with blocked oviducts were to demand IVF treatment as their right, the taxpayers would have to foot an estimated bill of $2.5 to $5 billion. Even if Kass's figures are exaggerated, Grobstein, Flower, and Mendelhoff report that a typical test cost to the patient for an initial IVF treatment (screening, laparoscopy, and embryo transfer) is nearly $7,500, with each subsequent attempt (omitting screening) costing approximately $5,000.[117]

Over and above questions of financial cost, society must confront some even harder questions. For example, should infertile people spend thousands of dollars to bring another child into an already overpopulated world—indeed, a world in which orphans abound? As philosopher Peter Singer sees it, if we lived in an ideal world, we would see to it that everyone had enough to eat before we even thought of adding another mouth to the world's population or of increasing our calorie consumption. But we do not live in an ideal world, and each of us who indulges in Haagen-Dazs ice cream while children in Ethiopia go without milk is partially responsible for the ugly realities that we supposedly lament. Thus, says Singer, it is unfair to burden infertile people with more ethical duties than those that burden fertile people: "If fertile couples are free to have large families rather than adopt destitute children, infertile couples must also be free to do whatever they can to have their own children."[118]

Singer also addresses Kass's point concerning the right of infertile couples to community medical resources. Singer believes that it is unfair to single out IVF for tougher evaluation than other medical techniques of similar expense. If surgery to correct blocked fallopian tubes is covered by health insurance, and if couples can obtain free or subsidized psychiatric care to help them come to terms with their infertility, then at least some of society's medical resources should be channeled to IVF users.[119] Surely, society cannot afford to provide every individual with every unneeded, expensive, or extraordinary treatment she or he may desire, but an affluent society certainly can afford more in the way of health care for its citizens than the bare minimum of emergency treatment for life-threatening conditions.

High economic cost is not the social woe that most concerns radical feminists, however. Corea, for example, fears that "the 'missing link' to the assembly-line, brothel approach to human reproduction is being forged in IVF clinics around the world where teams are working intensely to control the cycles of women."[120] IVF contributes, in her view, to society's tendency to regard women as little more than machines for reproduction. To prove her point, Corea recounts the tale of Sabine 2A, a championship cow that died in 1982. After her death, her frozen eggs were fertilized in vitro, producing embryos worth more than $10,000 each. Breeders then had those embryos transferred to less valuable female cows for gestation. As Corea sees it, human breeders will be able to do something similar once it is possible to freeze eggs as well as sperm. They will extract eggs from "valuable" women, freeze them for future IVF, and transfer them into "nonvaluable" women at the appropriate time. In this way, says Corea, "a woman could be used for reproduction long after she is dead."[121] But, we may wonder, why is this such a worrisome state of affairs? After all, some men are very eager to freeze their sperm and to have them used for reproductive purposes after their death. Why is it that sperm freezing makes men godlike in that it enables them to achieve corporeal immortality, whereas egg freezing makes women animallike? Is there anything we can do as a society to make the reproduction-aiding technologies as liberating for women as they seem to be for men? To this query Corea has a number of replies, including that society should regard women as no less "godly" than it regards men.

One concern about IVF that radical feminists share with a wide range of concerned citizens is that it may lead to full-scale genetic manipulation. Corea points out that in the future many IVF researchers will use screening techniques to eliminate defective preimplantation embryos. Although eliminating birth defects may sound like a wonderful advancement, Corea cautions her readers that even if genetic manipulation starts out benevolently, it may not end benevolently if "breeders" decide to select only for certain "genetic types"—for example, white, Anglo-Saxon types. Corea reports that Professor Carl Wood of the Monash IVF team is becoming interested in genetic breeding because, "Already we have had couples come and ask us if a male other than the husband could donate sperm because they were not happy with the husband's appearance or personality. Similarly women have been asking for donor eggs because they're not happy with some aspects of themselves."[122] Once genetic breeding is developed, many concerned citizens speculate that IVF, which offers control over the quality of offspring, will become more common than natural reproduction. Moreover, if the courts accept the concept of fetal rights—including the fetus's right to be born physically and mentally sound—then to knowingly beget defective children will be recognized as a legal wrong and women will not have a right to bring a defective fetus to term.

As Corea sees it, the stage is now being set for laws and medical practices that would not only prohibit women from bearing "defective babies" but also from exposing fetuses to their own "defective intrauterine environment" or using their own eggs to reproduce if those eggs have not met quality standards.[123] Whatever the right to procreate will mean, it will not mean the right for a couple to conceive and bring to term a severely handicapped child for whose support society as a whole will in some measure be responsible. Indeed, philosopher Joseph Fletcher has already asserted that "the right to conceive and bear children has to stop short of knowingly making crippled children."[124] Told that they are victimizing their offspring and the whole of society by using their defective eggs or sperm, a shamed couple will willingly accept a donor's eggs or sperm. However responsible this might sound, there is something very worrisome about it. After all, if people are no longer willing or able to accept unconditionally the imperfect children born to them—to love these children as they are—chances are that the human species will be somewhat worse for this new intolerance.

10 Contracted Motherhood

Contracted motherhood, sometimes called *surrogate motherhood*,[1] is typically undertaken when the female member of a married couple is either unable to produce eggs or unable to carry a pregnancy to term. If she and her husband have a very strong desire to rear a child to whom they are at least 50 percent genetically related, they may decide to seek a woman who is willing, out of generosity or for a monetary fee, to carry a pregnancy to term for them. There are, according to philosopher Peter Singer and physician Deane Wells, two types of contracted mothers: those who gestate an embryo genetically related to them (so-called partial surrogacy) and those who gestate an embryo genetically unrelated to them (so-called full surrogacy).[2]

At present, most cases of contracted motherhood are still cases of partial surrogacy. A woman contracts to be artificially inseminated with the sperm of a man who is not her husband, to carry the subsequent pregnancy to term, and to turn the resulting child over to the man and his wife to rear. Because the child is genetically related to the contracted mother, at the time of transference she must relinquish her parental rights to the child, and because the child is not genetically related to the woman who wishes to rear the child, at the time of transference or some time later she must legally adopt him or her.

In the future, an increasing number of cases of contracted motherhood may be cases of full surrogacy. Full surrogacy, sometimes called *surrogate gestational motherhood*, involves an embryo transfer after in vivo or in vitro fertilization. A woman may be able to produce eggs but unable to carry a pregnancy to term. If she and her husband are able to conceive a genetic child in vivo, physicians can then flush the embryo out of her womb into the womb of a woman who has agreed to gestate it. If she and her husband are not able to conceive a genetic child in vivo, however, physicians may suggest in vitro fertilization (IVF). As was noted in the previous chapter, physicians will remove one or more eggs from the woman's womb and join them with the sperm of her husband ex utero. If fertilization takes place, the physicians will introduce the embryo(s) into the womb of the woman who has agreed to gestate it. Clearly, full surrogacy is technologically more complex than partial surrogacy, a factor that accounts for its current limited use.

Although the process whereby one woman bears a child for another woman may strike us as new, it is, say Singer and Wells, as old as the biblical account of Abraham and Sarah, a couple who had not been able to conceive a child on account of Sarah's infertility.[3] The couple's childlessness was not only a cause of personal sadness for Abraham and Sarah but also a matter of tribal concern. Abraham needed to produce a male heir to found the nation of Israel. Realizing that time was not on their side, Sarah suggested to her husband that he have sexual intercourse with her slave-girl, Hagar. On becoming pregnant, Hagar prematurely arrogated to herself a certain place of pride in Abraham's household. In an effort to show her slave-girl who was the real mistress of Abraham's house and heart, however, Sarah made life so miserable for Hagar that the pregnant slave-girl fled into the desert. Seeing fit to intervene in this all-too-human drama, God promised Hagar that He would bestow considerable blessings on her son. Thereupon, Hagar returned to Abraham's house where she subsequently delivered a son, Ishmael. Contrary to everyone's expectations, however, Ishmael, who was blessed in other ways, was not destined to found the nation of Israel. Remembering His promise to bless Sarah with a son of her own, God worked a miracle and the postmenopausal, 90-year-old Sarah conceived a child, Isaac. When Isaac was born, Sarah insisted that Abraham send away Hagar and her son, Ishmael. It pained Abraham to send away Ishmael, but he gave in to Sarah's demands and Ishmael and Hagar were exiled from his household.

The story of Abraham, Sarah, and Hagar is one that, with considerable variations on its major themes, has been told for centuries. In one of the most recent versions, William Stern, a 40-year-old biochemist, and his pediatrician wife, Elizabeth, also 40, were unable to have a child because Elizabeth was unwilling to assume certain pregnancy risks. Through the Infertility Center of New York, the Sterns contracted Mary Beth Whitehead to be artificially inseminated by William Stern. Mary Beth and her husband, Richard, had 2 children of their own, aged 12 and 10. As a result of the artificial insemination, Mary Beth became pregnant and agreed to carry the fetus to term for $10,000 and to give it up after birth to the Sterns. Nine months later, Mary Beth gave birth to a girl, whom she named Sara. Then the unexpected happened. Mary Beth realized that she could not, in good conscience, deliver the baby to the Sterns. Dismayed by Mary Beth's change of heart, the Sterns swiftly secured a court order for temporary custody of the child, whom they named Melissa. When the Sterns, accompanied by 5 police officers, came to take custody of the infant from the Whiteheads, Mary Beth fled with the baby and the rest of her family to Florida. The Sterns tracked the Whiteheads down and, with the help of Florida police, recovered the baby. Since the Sterns's legal custody of the baby was only temporary, they as well as the Whiteheads appealed to the New Jersey courts to decide on a permanent home for Sara/Melissa, who was by then nearly 1 year old. In granting custody to the Sterns, Judge Harvey R. Sorkow ruled that contracted motherhood arrangements were legally binding, although neither New Jersey nor any other state specifically authorized such contracts.[4] On appeal, the New Jersey Supreme Court voided the contract between Mary Beth Whitehead and the Sterns as being against public policy, holding that such transactions constitute illegal baby selling[5] under New Jersey adoption laws and may be "perhaps criminal and potentially degrading to women."[6]

Clearly, contracted motherhood raises many serious ethical, legal, and social issues, challenging us to determine whether the right to procreate includes a right to procreate children collaboratively. In this chapter, we focus primarily on partial, commercial surrogacy. We present several ethical cases for and against this practice as well as several legal remedies that have been proposed to resolve the problems of surrogate motherhood. Finally, we argue that the basic controversy about contracted motherhood stems from (1) uncertainty about the criteria of parenthood and (2) cultural taboos against treating children as if they were commodities.

The Ethics of Contracted Motherhood

General Ethical Arguments Against Contracted Motherhood

Among the many ethicists who object to contracted motherhood are natural-law theorists and kantians (ethicists who agree with the eighteenth-century philosopher Immanuel Kant that no person should ever be reduced to an object, thing, or instrument for another person's use). As these ethicists see it, contracted motherhood has at least four morally objectionable features.

First, it is unnatural because it involves techniques such as artificial insemination and IVF. Supposedly, what is wrong about these artificial means of procreation is that they transform reproduction into mere production. Comments philosopher Ronald D. Lawler:

When a new human life comes to be out of an act of love between two persons who will forever be parents, and responsible to the child—a child not made but begotten, not a product that its makers may manipulate, but an offspring that is their equal— the entire context suggests an attitude and a moral stance different from that which arises when human life is originated in the context of production, manufacturing, and quality control.[7]

Second, both natural-law ethicists and Kantians argue that contracted motherhood is inconsistent with human dignity, a dignity that supposedly requires persons to perceive themselves as the kind of beings who would never put their bodies on the market.[8] A woman's right to control her own body and to make decisions about its proper use does not, they insist, entitle her to exploit her body willy-nilly.

Third, these ethicists object not only to contracted motherhood but also to artificial insemination by donor (AID) and certain types of IVF on the grounds that these practices introduce a third party into the process of procreation, a process that should be confined to a loving relationship between 2 people. As they see it, a contracted mother substantially threatens a couple's relationship. Compared to an anonymous sperm donor or an anonymous egg donor, the contracted mother is not a peripheral presence in a couple's life; rather, she is a central, unavoidable presence in the couple's life for at least 9 months. As a result, the woman who, together with her husband, has contracted a mother may grow jealous of her. Alternatively, the genetic father may believe he should have more influence on how his child ought to be reared than does his wife, treating his wife as if she were his child's stepmother.[9]

Fourth and finally, natural-law ethicists and Kantians claim that contracted motherhood is not really motherhood but a disguised form of baby selling in which a woman deliberately becomes pregnant with the intention of giving up the child to whom she will give birth.[10] This state of affairs is damaging to the contracted mother since she must continually remind herself that she is merely an incubator, a vessel that has been hired to experience not only physiological but also psychological sensations for someone other than herself. It is also potentially damaging to the child, especially if she or he is born defective. Since the contracting couple presumably contracts for a healthy child, a defective child might find itself an unwanted child: "Like bruised fruit, in the produce bin of a supermarket, this child is likely to become an object of avoidance."[11]

Reading between the lines, these natural-law and Kantian arguments are based on two separate, but nonetheless related, considerations. As we noted in chapter 4, natural-law theorists believe that from the natural fact that humans must produce offspring to continue the species, people are to infer that procreation is a value and that they have an obligation to bear and rear children. Nevertheless, natural-law theorists do not commend infertile contracting couples for contracting mothers and then using AID or IVF technology to help them procreate; rather they condemn them for procreating unnaturally—that is, without engaging in sex. But if contracted motherhood is wrong to the degree that it circumvents the "natural" way of doing things, then perhaps intravenous feeding is also wrong. Yet natural-law theorists do not condemn physicians who feed sick persons intravenously on the grounds that the natural way for people to eat is to ingest their food orally. Just because nourishment is the essential goal of eating does not mean that it is wrong, under all circumstances, for persons to get nourishment without ingesting their food orally. Analogously, just because procreation is the essential goal of sexual intercourse does not mean that it is wrong, under all circumstances, for persons to procreate without sexual intercourse.

Related to these natural-law arguments against contracted motherhood are some Kantian arguments based on the end-in-itself formulation of the categorical imperative.[12] According to Kant, it is always wrong to disrespect a person, including one's own person. To respect persons is to treat them as unconditionally valuable human beings who have their own unique plans of action; to disrespect persons is to treat them merely as conditionally valuable things who have no unique plans of action. When someone treats someone else as a mere means, she or he runs roughshod over the freedom and well-being of that person to secure and enhance her or his own freedom and well-being; and when someone treats himself or herself as a mere means, he or she shows no respect for his or her own freedom and well-being.

As many Kantians see it, a contracting couple disregards the fundamental interests, rights, and needs of the contracted mother—that is, those having to do with her freedom and well-being. They burden the contracted mother with stipulations that threaten her freedom, limiting what she may eat or drink, prescribing with whom she may have sex and when, and forbidding her to abort any normal fetus. In addition, they burden the contracted mother with stipulations that jeopardize her well-being. No matter the cost to her physical and psychological well-being, she must give up the child. However, because the strength of this objection to contracted motherhood rests on the contracting couple's disregard for the fundamental interests, rights, and needs of the contracted mother, it fails to the extent that the contracting couple respects and considers these interests, rights, and needs. If the contracting couple permits the contracted mother to live as she chooses to live during her pregnancy, and if they permit her to keep the child if she is unwilling to relinquish him or her, they treat the contracted mother as much more than a mere means to their own selfish ends.

But even if the contracting couple is able to escape the grip of the categorical imperative, the contracted mother may not be able to weaken its hold on her. Kantians argue that in making herself a "womb for rent," the contracted mother reduces herself to an object either to improve her financial status or to enhance her self-image as a giver. To satisfy one or the other of these inclinations—the former less crass than the latter—she jeopardizes her freedom and well-being as a person. Many Kantians believe that there are certain services persons should never sell—for example, sexual services or reproductive services. As they see it, when persons sell their bodies, they sell more than their bodies. Indeed, they sell their entire selves, entering into a form of slavery in which they are no longer autonomous agents but the passive instruments of other people. Thus, Kantians argue that when the prostitute sells her sexual services to her patron, she becomes his plaything, his instrument of desire fulfillment. Similarly, they argue that when the contracted mother sells her reproductive services to a contracting couple, she becomes the couple's incubator, an instrument of desire fulfillment.

However plausible such an argument is, it has its limits. For every Kantian who makes this argument, someone will object that when the prostitute sells her genitals or when the contracted mother sells her womb, she does not lose control over her person any more than does the athlete who sells his body to a football team or the teacher who sells her mind to a university. Although prostitutes and contracted mothers accept certain limitations on their physical freedom, says the objector, they do so in exchange for money and, provided that they receive fair payment for the sexual or reproductive services they render, they are no more alienated from their persons than millions of other workers who sell their brawn or brain services for money.[13]

Nevertheless, even if people who sell their sexual or reproductive services are not necessarily alienated from their persons, journalist Roger Rosenblatt suggests that people who sell their emotions are so alienated. As he sees it, William and Elizabeth Stern paid contracted mother Mary Beth Whitehead for more than her gestational services. Rather they paid her "to experience maternal love, the forced cessation of that love, and a whole range of feelings in the process that are not ordinarily put up for sale."[14] What the Sterns were buying and what Whitehead was selling was not really Baby M but a very profound set of emotions and, says Rosenblatt, the "transaction fell through because neither buyer nor seller had a grasp of the commodity in the first place".[15]

Although Rosenblatt's argument is rhetorically effective, it is not impervious to criticism. All kinds of workers sell emotional labor, the kind of labor that Arlie Hochschild defines as "the management of feeling to create a publicly observable facial and bodily display."[16] According to Hochschild's definition, flight attendants, development officers, and sympathetic psychiatrists are selling their emotions, and yet society does not fault these professionals for striking some sort of Faustian bargain by which they exchange the essence of their souls for cash. Perhaps Rosenblatt's point is that unlike flight attendants, development officers, and sympathetic psychiatrists, contracted mothers are selling what they really feel, not what they pretend to feel. However, if this is Rosenblatt's argument, some of his assumptions—for example, that every pregnant woman really experiences "maternal love" and "a whole range of feelings ... that are not ordinarily put up for sale."—are false. Even if no pregnant woman can escape certain physiological sensations, she can escape certain emotional reactions by virtue of schooling herself to do so. To this objection, Rosenblatt may reply that the contracted mother cannot possibly appreciate in advance the full nature of the emotional quagmire into which she is descending. But no matter how forcefully this reply is made, the fact is that some contracted mothers insist that they knew what they were getting into when they got into it and that the contracted motherhood experience was, for them, an unemotional one. Thus, it is not clear in what sense the contracted mother treats herself as a mere means.

Regardless of whether the contracted mother treats herself as a mere means, most Kantians believe that when the contracted mother agrees to procreate a child with the intention to abdicate personal responsibility for it, she treats the child as a mere means:

The procreator should desire the child for its own sake, and not as a means to attaining some other end. Even though one of the ends may be stated altruistically as an attempt to bring happiness to an infertile couple, the child is still being used by the surrogate. She creates it not because she desires it, but because she desires something from it.[17]

The fact that the contracting couple desire the child for its own sake does not cancel out the fact that the contracted mother desires it for her own, supposedly ulterior motives. For anyone to procreate a child with no desire for a personal relationship with him or her, says the Kantian, is to change the way everyone looks at children.

Like Rosenblatt's conviction that no woman can possibly appreciate in advance the emotional complications that attend any and all contracted-mother arrangements, the Kantian conviction that everyone will view children as commodities if anyone does strikes critics as exaggerated. These critics concede that society's view of children would change if a majority of people were no longer able to distinguish between dolls and real babies, but they do not concede that society's view of children is going to change because a small minority of people view children as consumer goods. Advances in genetic technology, and not contracted motherhood, are more likely to alter society's attitude toward children, they say. Although couples are still not able to custom-design their children, they soon may be, and then society will have cause for real concern.

General Ethical Arguments for Contracted Motherhood

Invoking both utilitarian reasoning, according to which an action is right if it maximizes the utility (pleasure or happiness) of the aggregate affected by the action, and contractarian reasoning, according to which contracts freely entered into ought to be honored, supporters of contracted motherhood defend this practice. As they see it, it is desirable, useful, and even necessary for society to permit noncoerced women to sell their reproductive services at least to childless, infertile couples but perhaps also to fertile women (married or single) who wish to avoid pregnancy, to single men who wish to avoid marriage, and to homosexual couples.

Since utilitarian advocates of contracted motherhood claim that the aggregate benefits of this practice outweigh its aggregate harms, they must produce evidence that contracted motherhood actually increases the collective utility quotient of contracting couples, contracted mothers, and contracted children. This is a difficult task because researchers have only recently begun to study the causes and effects of contracted motherhood. As a result, utilitarian observations are more likely to be based on common sense than on current scientific data.

That the contracted mother assumes certain physical risks when she agrees to gestate a child is obvious. Pregnant women inevitably experience at least some of the following conditions and events: fatigue, nausea, weight gain, discomfort, skin stretching, insomnia, altered or suspended sexual activity, miscarriage, cesarean section, and labor pains; and the contracted mother will not be immune from these physical risks. Neither will she be immune from certain psychological risks, especially those that are related to traumatic mother-child separations or to forced mother-child unions. Writer Anne Taylor Fleming summarizes a contracted mother's second thoughts about the son she had borne and surrendered shortly after birth as follows:

She had meant to be unfazed, meant to make her parents and friends proud of her generosity, meant to make the couple she had had the baby for like her so much that "afterwards" she would be part of their extended family and could watch her son grow up. But none of it, not one piece of that, came out the right way. Her parents were not particularly proud. The couple did not want her around. And she was not unattached from her son and clearly never would be.[18]

As poignant as this contracted mother's experience was, it is rivaled by the traumatizing experience of a contracted mother who is required to keep or to put up for adoption a child she never intended to rear. Already, several contracting couples have refused to accept the children for whom they contracted. Some of these couples have faulted the contracted mother for producing a defective child; others have accused her of providing them not with a child genetically related to them but with a child genetically related to some unknown third party; and still others have simply reneged on the deal for any number of reasons including divorce, separation, or death. Whatever the reason the contracting couple offers to the contracted mother for nonacceptance of the baby, it is unlikely to alleviate her distress.

The practice of contracted motherhood poses risks to the contracting couple as well as to the contracted mother. For example, a contracted mother may blackmail a contracting couple, threatening to abort the child or to keep it unless they pay her more money than they originally promised to pay her. Should the contracted mother decide to keep the baby, the contracting couple may have no legal remedy other than getting their money back from the contracted mother or collecting damages.[19] The contracting couple also risks prosecution under the criminal law in those states that prohibit payment beyond certain itemized medical and legal expenses of a woman in connection with her giving up her child for adoption.[20] Finally, the contracting couple risks future visits from the contracted mother, the kind of visits that could cause their much-loved child to reject them in favor of his or her birth mother.

Children who are born of contracted mothers are also at physical and psychological risk. If the contracted mother is not screened for genetic defects, she may pass them on to the child, and if she drinks, smokes, or engages in other fetus-threatening behavior during pregnancy, the child may be born less healthy than it would have been born under more ideal circumstances. Along similar lines, a contracted mother may decide to abort the fetus the first time any risk to her health, however small, presents itself. Since she has no vested interest in the child, the contracted mother will tend to overemphasize her interests and underestimate those of the fetus.

Among the psychological harms that a contracted child may experience is the kind of psychological harm that an adopted child sometimes experiences—namely, the desire to know his or her real mother and to understand why his or her mother either would not or could not keep him or her. Even worse than this type of psychological harm are the feelings of rejection experienced by the child who, due to some physical or mental defect, is wanted neither by the contracting couple nor by the contracted mother. To be a child that no one wants is a tragic burden and one that every child should be spared if possible.

Although the possible, probable, and actual harms of contracted motherhood seem serious, harm is only half the utilitarian story. The other half is benefit. Utilitarians observe that the benefits to contracted mothers are clear. Like male sperm vendors, these women get an opportunity to sell their reproductive wares for a good price. They also get an opportunity to do something worthwhile and, indeed, many contracted mothers report that, as far as they are concerned, contracted motherhood is a good practice because there is no greater gift to give than the gift of a child.[21] Even clearer than the benefits to the contracted mother, say the utilitarians, are the benefits to the contracting couples. Anyone who has ever known an infertile couple that has tried virtually everything to have a child can imagine how happy a contracting couple must feel when they finally secure their precious bundle of joy. Clearest of all, insist the utilitarians, are the benefits to the contracted child. Since everyone went through such trouble to bring him or her into the world, the (healthy) contracted child is an "excruciatingly wanted" child,[22] and wanted children are supposedly loved, and therefore happy, children.

In weighing its harms against its benefits, utilitarians who favor contracted motherhood note that most of the harms associated with contracted motherhood can be eliminated or at least substantially ameliorated with clear legal remedies, rigorous medical screening, and sensitive psychological counseling. In contrast, utilitarians who disapprove of contracted motherhood observe that the combined forces of law, medicine, and psychology are unlikely to produce a silken purse of bliss out of a sow's ear of sorrow. Clearly, utilitarian cases for and against contracted motherhood are likely to remain highly speculative until researchers produce more empirical evidence for the relative harms and benefits of this practice.

Since contractarian arguments that favor contracted motherhood do not rely on empirical states of affairs, they tend to be stronger than utilitarian arguments in favor of this practice. Among the main supporters of contracted motherhood is lawyer John A. Robertson who describes it as "collaborative reproduction"—that is, reproduction that requires more than the energies, efforts, and endowments of one married couple.[23] Throughout the ages, collaborative reproduction has, says Robertson, assumed many forms:

Children have often been reared by genetically unrelated stepparents, wet nurses, nannies, babysitters, and other surrogates. Donor insemination has been available for forty years as an accepted treatment for male infertility.[24]

What distinguishes current forms of collaborative reproduction from past forms, says Robertson, is that we now have the possibility of breaking the line not only between bearing and rearing a child (as in adoption) but also between begetting and bearing a child. What also distinguishes between the old and new forms of collaborative reproduction is that the surrogates of the past—at least the wet nurses, nannies, and babysitters —made no legal, and perhaps no moral, claims on their charges. For example, when their charges reached school age, nannies did not insist on their right to remain in relationship with their charges. Perhaps they should have, but the fact is that they did not, and any full-blown defense of contracted motherhood as collaborative reproduction will have to spell out the rights and responsibilities of each and every parental collaborator.

To the objection that he has failed to spell out the terms of collaborative reproduction, Robertson may reply that it is not crucial that he do so immediately because the major moral justification for contracted motherhood depends not on its collaborative nature but on its contractual nature. To the degree that contracted motherhood involves the noncoerced exercise of free choice—more specifically, the noncoerced exercise of economic choice—Robertson believes that it is morally justified. As Robertson sees it, "The morality of surrogate mothering depends on how the duties and responsibilities of the role are carried out, rather than on the mere fact that a couple produces a child with the aid of a collaborator."[25] Provided that the contracting couple and the contracted mother enter into and conclude their negotiations freely, and provided that they fully intend to abide by the terms of their mutual contract, there is no reason to be more morally dubious about their "business" arrangement than about any other professional business arrangement.

Faced with the objection that contracted motherhood is an unjust practice because only a rich, infertile couple can afford to pay a contracted mother her $10,000 fee plus $15,000 worth of associated expenses, Robertson replies that limited accessibility is not unjust to poor, infertile couples because it does not leave them worse off than they were before.[26]

To argue that rich, infertile couples should not be allowed to employ contracted mothers because poor, infertile couples cannot afford them is like arguing that rich, sick people should not be allowed to spend their money on artificial hearts since poor, sick people cannot afford them. Justice, implies Robertson, does not have as one of its axioms the rule that if everyone cannot have something, then no one can. Admittedly, concedes Robertson, a state of affairs in which the parental dreams of the rich but not of the poor can come true is less than ideal. Nonetheless, the solution to this dilemma is not for the state to outlaw contracted motherhood; rather it is for the state to determine whether it has the responsibility to subsidize contracted motherhood so that poor as well as rich infertile couples can make a genuine choice between hiring and not hiring a contracted mother.

Feminist Ethical Arguments For and Against Contracted Motherhood

Liberal Feminist Arguments

Liberal feminists typically argue that (1) women should be permitted to use whatever reproduction-controlling or reproduction-aiding technologies they wish, provided that they do not harm anyone in the process, and (2) if women want to be treated as autonomous persons, then they must act like autonomous persons, living up to the terms of their contracts. For these reasons, lawyer Lori B. Andrews argues that no matter what their reservations about contracted motherhood are, women should be adamantly opposed to a legal ban on it. To support a ban on contracted motherhood, says Andrews, is to let the government dictate "the circumstances under which a woman should be allowed to have a child and under which families may be formed."[27] If such dictation is anathema to women insofar as contraception, abortion, and sterilization are concerned, it should be anathema to them insofar as artificial insemination, IVF, and contracted motherhood are concerned.

Like many feminists with a predominantly liberal perspective, Andrews believes that in the case of contracted motherhood, a pregnant woman's rights to make decisions about herself and the fetus during pregnancy must be reaffirmed. Any contract to which she is a party must be worded in such a way that she, the pregnant contracted mother, is free to engage in whatever activities she wishes, to refuse or accept any medical treatments, and to abort or not abort based on her own judgment. Under no circumstances, says Andrews, should the contracted mother be liable for damages or subject to a court suit in the event that the fetus spontaneously aborts, is delivered stillborn, or is born with defects.[28]

Andrews also believes that informed consent is crucial for contracted motherhood. Physicians and psychologists must clearly outline to potential contracted mothers all the physical and psychological risks that attend the practice of contracted motherhood. However, says Andrews, physicians and psychologists must remember that too much information of the wrong kind, as well as too little information of the right kind, can undermine a woman's reproductive freedom. Andrews notes, for example, that antiabortion forces have already used the doctrine of informed consent to serve their own purposes. Several years ago the city of Akron, Ohio, passed an ordinance that required physicians to inform women seeking abortions that the fetus is sentient (able to feel pain) and that the abortion procedure is often dangerous.[29] This misleading, and arguably false, information, says Andrews, caused several women to change their abortion decision from yes to no. What concerns Andrews is that, fearing liability suits or worse, some physicians and psychologists will exaggerate the risks that attend the practice of contracted motherhood, failing to tell the potential contracted mother that the risks of this practice do not exceed the risks women routinely take in many other areas of life.

Marxist Feminist Arguments

In contrast to liberal feminists, Marxist feminists typically argue that when a woman consents to sell her reproductive services to an infertile couple, her consent is more often the product of economic coercion than of free choice. Marxist feminists note that most contracted mothers, like most prostitutes, are much poorer than their clients. Unable to get a decent job, a woman is driven to sell her body, the only thing she has that anyone seems to want and perhaps even need. To say that a woman chooses to do this, says the Marxist feminist, is to say that when a woman is forced to choose between being poor and being exploited, she may choose being exploited as the lesser of the two evils. Although some agencies refuse to accept indigent women into their program,[30] other agencies prefer poor women, reasoning that poor women on unemployment and with children of their own are unlikely to change their minds and want to keep the babies they are gestating for profit.[31] John Stehura, president of the Bionetics Foundation, Inc., an agency that contracts mothers, has suggested that a contracted mother can never be poor enough. Since the going rate for contracted mothers is high even by middle-class American standards, he is urging the contracted mother industry to move either to poverty-stricken parts of the United States, where women are willing to gestate fetuses for one-half the standard fee, or to the Third World, where women are willing to do so for one-tenth the standard fee.[32]

Since Marxist feminists view contracted motherhood as an exploitative practice, they have urged that commercial surrogacy be banned. As noted previously, liberal feminists including Lori Andrews doubt the wisdom of such a ban. To the contracted mother who asked, "Why is it exploitation to go through a surrogate pregnancy for someone else if I am paid, but *not* if I am not paid?"[33] Andrews responds that if economic exploitation is what makes contracted motherhood wrong, then the legal focus "should not be on banning payment but on making sure the surrogates get paid more."[34] As Andrews sees it, although we can *imagine* situations in which a woman becomes a contracted mother in order to avoid destitution or worse, in fact most contracted mothers are not desperate for such basic necessities as food, clothing, and shelter. Noting that Mary Beth Whitehead became a contracted mother partly to pay for her children's education, that Kim Cotten did so to pay for much-desired home improvements, and that yet another woman did so to pay for a car, Andrews concludes that these women chose as they did not because they had to but because they wanted to.[35]

In response to Andrews' objections, Marxist feminists note that her view of economic exploitation is rather simplistic. Andrews suggests that if commercial contracted motherhood is exploitative, it is exploitative only because contracted mothers are paid too little. For example, for her $10,000 fee Mary Beth Whitehead was required to "assume all risks, including the risk of death, which are incidental to conception, pregnancy, childbirth, including but not limited to postpartum complications," with no compensation whatsoever in the event of a first-trimester miscarriage and a mere $1000 if she aborted on Mr. Stern's demand.[36] But Marxist feminists believe that had Whitehead been offered $1,000,000 and $10,000, respectively, rather than $10,000 and $1000, respectively, her decision to serve as a contracted mother would have been no less coerced. Indeed, as philosopher Mary Gibson has argued, it would probably have been *more* coerced. As she sees it, "undue inducement" is an indirect form of economic exploitation that differs from direct forms of economic exploitation only because it is disguised and even more likely to weaken the wills of poor women than its undisguised counterparts.[37]

Radical Feminist Arguments

Agreeing with Marxist feminists that contracted motherhood ought to be discouraged, radical feminists broaden the Marxist feminist analysis of exploitation to include cases of noneconomic exploitation. Radical feminists observe that even when a well-heeled college graduate decides to work as a high-priced call girl, her choice is not necessarily free. Women, says the radical feminist, are socialized to meet male sexual wants and needs as a matter of duty and pride. In this connection, one feminist prosecutor reported that in her district a man approached several mothers on welfare with the following proposition: If the mothers would permit him to spend time with their daughters, aged 7 to 12, he would give money to the mothers and gifts to the little girls. The mothers agreed, and their daughters spent after-school hours with "Uncle Charlie" who routinely molested them. Gradually, a rivalry developed among the girls, each of them trying to be Uncle Charlie's favorite. Indeed, so attached did the girls become to him that when one of the mothers finally called the police in, the girls were depressed at the thought of not seeing Uncle Charlie anymore. The prosecutor predicted that without first-rate counseling some of the girls would spend their lives trying to "turn men on" sexually.[38]

Just as prostitutes are not born but made by a society that teaches girls that, if all else fails, they can always sell their bodies to men, contracted mothers are not born but made by a society that teaches girls that they are *better* than boys because they are so willing to share all that they have, including their bodies. Although many radical feminists believe that biological motherhood is a highly valuable activity, some radical feminists caution that because *only* women can be mothers, contracted motherhood is a "compassion trap" for women.[39] Frequently, the call for contracted mothers is accompanied by visions of desperately lonely, tragically unfulfilled infertile couples. An appeal is made to generous, loving, altruistic women to step forward to give the gift of life to these unfortunate couples, and the fact that approximately one-third of all the women who answer this appeal have either had an abortion or given up a child for adoption strengthens the radical feminist suspicion that deep and dark forces are driving women to choose contracted motherhood even when it may not be in their best interests to do so.[40]

Whatever force this aspect of the radical feminist case against contracted motherhood has, liberal feminists note that *if* it is true that women are "brainwashed" into being contracted mothers, then they are also "brainwashed" into being mothers. Therefore, if radical feminists wish to be fair, they "should not forbid women to be mothers through alternative reproduction without forbidding them to be mothers through normal reproduction as well."[41]

But even if they are correct to challenge the claim that contracted mothers are victims of brainwashing, liberal feminists may not have a decisive response to the final, and perhaps strongest, objection some radical feminists make against contracted motherhood—namely, that it creates several destructive divisions among women. The first destructive division is the one described earlier, between economically privileged women and economically disadvantaged women. Relatively rich women hire relatively poor women to meet their reproductive needs, adding childbearing services to the childrearing services that economically disadvantaged women have traditionally provided to economically privileged women. The second destructive division is the one that feminist Gena Corea envisions, between childbegetters, childbearers, and childrearers. According to Corea, society is segmenting reproduction as if it were simply a form of production. In the future, no one woman will beget, bear, and rear a child. Rather, genetically superior women will beget embryos in vitro; strong-bodied women will carry these test-tube babies to term; and sweet-tempered women will rear these newborns from infancy to adulthood.[42]

As a result of this undesirable division of labor, Corea fears that the fictional dystopia described by Margaret Atwood in her novel *The Handmaid's Tale* may yet become a reality. What we see in the Republic of Gilead, Atwood's dystopia, are women reduced to their respective functions: There are the Marthas, or domestics; the Wives, or social secretaries and functionaries; the Jezebels, or sex prostitutes; and the Handmaids, or reproductive prostitutes. One of the most degrading Gileadean practices, from a woman's perspective, consists of the Commanders engaging in ritualistic sexual intercourse with their Wives. The Wife, who is infertile, lies down on a bed with her legs spread open. The Handmaid, one of the few fertile women in Gilead, then assumes this same position but with her head cradled between the spread legs of the wife, whereupon the Commander engages in sexual intercourse not with his Wife but with her Handmaid. Should the Handmaid become pregnant, the child she bears will be regarded as that of the Commander and his Wife. Indeed, on the day the Handmaid gives birth to the child, the Wife will simulate labor pains, and all the Wives and Handmaids in Gilead will gather around the fortunate Wife and her blessed Handmaid, experiencing through them an ephemeral moment of female bonding, of women's pride, passion, and power.

After one such birth day, the central character, a woman named Offred, thinks back to better times, and speaks in her mind to her mother, who had been a feminist leader:

Can you hear me? You wanted a woman's culture. Well, now there is one. It isn't what you meant, but it exists. Be thankful for small mercies.[43]

And, of course, they are *very* small mercies, for with the exception of birth days—those rare occasions when a Handmaid manages to produce a child—women have little contact with one another. The Marthas, Wives, Jezebels, and Handmaids are segregated by function, and what contact women do have—even within their own class—is largely silent, for they are permitted to speak to one another only when absolutely necessary.

Despite the chilling effect that Corea's analysis and Atwood's novel have on any wholesale endorsement of reproductive technology, some radical feminists surprisingly agree with lawyer John Robertson that if handled properly (that is, controlled by women), arrangements such as contracted motherhood could bring women closer together rather than further apart. Already there are some reports of contracted mothers living in close proximity to the couples who contracted them and sharing with them the joy of the new life they have together brought into the world.[44] Such reports bolster the claim that contracted motherhood can be viewed not as the male-manipulated specialization and segmentation of the female reproductive process but as women getting together—as in the case of the postmenopausal South African mother who carried her daughter's in vitro fetus to term—to achieve, collaboratively, something that neither of them could do alone.[45]

Nonetheless, if it is plausible that in a nonpatriarchal society, genetic, gestational, and rearing mothers could determine the extent of their interaction with each other and their collective child, radical feminists who oppose contracted motherhood note that in a patriarchal society, what we see is not collaborative reproduction among women but nasty court battles between the child's genetic father and the contracted mother. Far from being viewed as the contracting couple's collaborator, the contracted mother is most typically viewed as someone who must be controlled by as restrictive a contract as possible.

Legal Aspects of Contracted Motherhood

When it comes to limiting a person's liberty in this society, we earlier noted that few people invoke (1) the offense principle (a person's liberty may be restricted to prevent offense to other specific individuals, where *offense* is interpreted as "behavior that causes feelings of embarrassment, shame, outrage, or disgust in those against whom it is directed"); (2) the principle of legal paternalism (a person's liberty may be restricted to protect himself or herself from self-inflicted harm or, in its extreme version, to guide that person, whether or not he or she likes it, toward his or her own good); or (3) the principle of legal moralism (a person's liberty may be restricted to protect other specific individuals, but especially society as a whole, from immoral behavior, where the word *immoral* means neither "harmful" nor "offensive" but something like "against the rule of a higher authority" (God) or "against a societal taboo". Rather, most people invoke the harm principle, according to which a person's liberty may be restricted only to prevent physical or psychological injury to some other person.[46] Keeping this point of political morality in mind, we propose to assess the relative merits and demerits of four possible legal remedies for contracted motherhood: (1) to criminalize contracted motherhood, at least in its commercial form; (2) to refuse to enforce contracted motherhood arrangements, relying on family law model in disputed cases; (3) to enforce contracted motherhood arrangements through either a specific performance or damages approach; and (4) to treat contracted motherhood as a type of adoption.

Contracted Motherhood as a Criminal Offense

Some legal theorists have argued that the best remedy for commercial contracted motherhood is simply to see it for what it is—a disguised form of baby selling—and to forbid it. Already there is some precedent for a law against contracted motherhood. In 1985, the United Kingdom passed the Surrogacy Arrangements Act. Reasoning that it is not in the best interests of a child to be born of parents "subject to the taint of criminality," the House of Lords decided not to impose criminal sanctions on contracting couples and contracted mothers.[47] Rather, this legislative body decided to penalize the people who serve as intermediaries in contracted motherhood negotiations. Lawyers, physicians, and social workers are subject to fines or imprisonment if they (1) initiate or take part in any negotiations with a view to the making of a surrogacy arrangement, (2) offer or agree to negotiate the making of a surrogacy arrangement, or (3) compile any information with a view to its ease in making, or negotiating the making of, surrogacy arrangements.[48] In addition, publishers, directors, and managers of newspapers, periodicals, and telecommunications systems are subject to fines or imprisonment if they accept ads such as "womb for hire" or "couple willing to pay royally for host womb."[49]

The rationale given for the Surrogacy Arrangements Act is largely based on the principle of legal moralism, according to which a person's liberty may be restricted to prevent immoral conduct on his or her part. The authors of the statute do not argue that contracted motherhood always or usually has harmful consequences. On the contrary, they proclaim in the manner of Kant that:

Even in compelling medical circumstances the danger of exploitation of one human being by another appears to the majority of us far to outweigh the potential benefits, in almost every case. That people would treat others as a means to their own ends, however desirable the consequences, must always be liable to moral objection. Such treatment of one person by another becomes positively exploitative when financial interests are involved.[50]

Although, as previously noted, U.S. legal theorists are uncomfortable with the idea of criminalizing something simply because it violates a widely held moral principle, several states are nonetheless contemplating a wholesale ban of a practice they view as horrible.[51] In fact, Michigan has already passed a law making it a felony to serve as a "surrogate broker," the penalty being a maximum $50,000 fine and 5-year imprisonment.[52]

Arguments against following the United Kingdom's lead in the United States are threefold. First, there is the philosophical objection that there is no real difference between treating someone as a *mere means* and treating him or her as a *means*. Students treat their teachers as a means to their end of gaining knowledge, but no one is ready to criminalize the student-teacher relationship. Presumably the student-teacher relationship is morally unobjectionable because teachers willingly contract to instruct students in exchange for pay. The student-teacher relationship would become morally objectionable if, for example, the students demanded that their teacher teach them pulp for a pittance or be detenured. However, if coercion is what transforms a morally permitted means-end relationship into a morally forbidden *mere* means-end relationship, then a contracted motherhood arrangement is morally forbidden only if the parties to it have not freely agreed to its terms.

Second, there is the pragmatic objection that a ban on contracted motherhood is a largely unenforceable ban. Were law enforcement officials to question her, an unmarried contracted mother could simply claim that as a result of a one-night stand she became pregnant and is now most desirous that a couple adopt her child so that he or she can be reared in a proper family environment. To the extent that contracted motherhood arrangements resemble private adoption arrangements, the rule could rapidly become, Where there is a will, there is always a good story to tell.

Third, there is the strictly legal objection that a ban on contracted motherhood may be unconstitutional. If obtaining a genetically related child through the use of a contracted mother is an infertile couple's only way to produce such a child, and if the equal protection clause, the due process clause, and the right to privacy protect all procreative decisions, then a ban on contracted motherhood would seem to constitute unjustified interference with one's freedom.[53]

Even if it is unconstitutional to ban all forms of contracted motherhood, several theorists, including A. M. Capron and M. J. Radin, nonetheless believe that it may be constitutional to ban commercial contracted motherhood. In the first place, as Capron and Radin understand the equal protection clause, its function is to make certain that no group is disadvantaged as compared to other similarly situated groups. Therefore, the question to ask is whether a ban on commercial contracted motherhood would disadvantage infertile couples who suffer from female infertility in ways that it would not disadvantage infertile couples who suffer from male infertility. On the face of it, such a ban would seem to affect the former group of couples in ways that it would not affect the latter group. If a woman is married to an infertile man, she is permitted to be artificially inseminated by donor so that she can bear a child genetically related to her. Why, then, should a man married to an infertile woman not be permitted to artificially inseminate a contracted mother so that he can father a child genetically related to him?

As Capron and Radin see it, this last question is not difficult to answer. The state has good reasons to permit wives of infertile men what it does not permit husbands of fertile women. It is one thing for a woman to use AID and quite another for a man to use a contracted mother. Whereas AID is a very safe procedure for both the donor and the donee, pregnancy can be a physically and psychologically risky experience for a contracted mother. Moreover, sperm donors do not need as much legal protection as contracted mothers.

Paying women to deliver children to genetic fathers may pose a greater risk of commodifying women than paying men for sperm poses of commodifying men because, given the current gender structure, these payments may have different social significance. The desire to carry on the male line through the use of surrogates is more likely to render women fungible than is the desire to carry on the female line through the use of sperm donors likely to render men fungible.[54]

In other words, because men are more socially and economically powerful than are women, they can exploit contracted mothers in ways that women cannot exploit sperm donors.

Second, as Capron and Radin understand the due process clause, its function is to protect fundamental rights such as the right to liberty. Therefore, the question to ask is whether a ban on commercial contracted motherhood would interfere with contractors' liberty rights. Clearly, such a ban would frustrate both the women who want to be hired as contracted mothers and the couples who want to hire them. Nevertheless, this frustration may be justified, for no right is absolute. For example, a state may ban contracted motherhood to prevent the commodification of women and children if there is no less restrictive way for it to accomplish this end.[55]

Finally, as Capron and Radin understand the right to privacy, one of its general functions is to protect procreative freedom. Therefore, the question to ask is whether this right protects an infertile couple's choice to use an artificial rather than a natural mode of procreation. Conceding that the right to privacy does indeed protect this infertile couple's choice, Capron and Radin still caution that the right to privacy is a negative, not a positive, liberty. In recognizing a freedom from state interference in making procreative choices, the Supreme Court did not also recognize a corresponding right to state assistance in implementing those procreative choices. In *Maher* v. *Roe*,[56] for example, the Supreme Court ruled that although the state may not prevent a woman from choosing an abortion,[57] it is not required to fund that abortion. Thus, the Supreme Court could rule that although the state may not ban commercial contracted motherhood, it is not required to pay a contracted mother's fee in the event that an infertile couple were unable to do so. In fact, say Capron and Radin, the Supreme Court could even rule that although an infertile couple has a right to use a contracted mother, it has no right to pay her. To the objection that because few women are willing to gestate other people's children for free, the right to use a contracted mother without the right to also pay her is useless, the Michigan Appellate Court has replied that:

The Constitution does not guarantee that all infertile couples desiring surrogate motherhood will find willing surrogates any more than it guarantees that all infertile couples desiring adoption will find available children to adopt. The wife's infertility, not the state's prohibition against payment to the surrogate, prevents the couple's exercise of their right to bear and beget children.[58]

It is not clear, however, that the Michigan Appellate Court's reasoning is correct. Although it is true that the infertile woman was the original cause of the couple's infertility, the state becomes the sustaining cause of this situation when it bans commercial contracted motherhood. Be this as it may, Capron and Radin are probably correct to argue that the Supreme Court is already inclined to view the right to procreate as a negative rather than as a positive right.

Refusing to Enforce Contracted Motherhood Arrangements

In the original Baby M case, District Judge Harvey R. Sorkow had ruled that it was in Baby M's best interests to enforce the terms of the contract

William and Elizabeth Stern had made with Mary Beth Whitehead. In overturning Judge Sorkow's ruling, the New Jersey Supreme Court proclaimed that contracts for mothers cannot be enforced because they are against public policy for at least two reasons. First, contracts for mothers may lead to the exploitation of financially needy women and, second, contracts for mothers are a disguised form of baby selling.[59]

Not everyone was impressed by the New Jersey Supreme Court's anti-contract rationale, however. Some critics faulted the court for its paternalism toward women. Women, they observed, are the best judges of what is in their own best interest, and offering them money "to do unpleasant tasks is not in itself coercive."[60] Other critics faulted the court for its inability to distinguish between baby selling (in which the people who "buy" the baby are not genetically related to it) and contracted motherhood (in which the person "buying" the baby is its genetic father). Still other critics went further. They challenged the New Jersey Supreme Court to convince them that baby selling is, in fact, intrinsically evil.

In articulating this last challenge, these critics relied on a decade-old article entitled "The Economics of the Baby Shortage," in which economists Elizabeth Landes and Richard Posner argued that because there are not enough babies available for adoption, a free market in babies ought to be permitted. In the course of defending their proposal, these two economists claimed that although abuses such as exorbitant prices, fraud, dishonesty, and undesirable prospective parents characterize the existing black market in babies, they would not characterize a future free market in babies where "prices for children of *equivalent quality* would be much lower."[61]

Not surprisingly, Landes and Posner's proposal met with heavy criticism. Some critics objected that a free market in babies would encourage prospective parents to pay more for perfect babies than for imperfect babies. Rather than denying this distressing consequence of a free market in babies, however, Landes and Posner resolutely insisted that that is just the way a free market in any commodity operates. If the demand for perfect babies exceeds the demand for imperfect babies, for example, the market "will generate incentives to improve the product as well as to optimize the price and quantity of the current level of the product."[62]

Other critics simply charged that a free market in babies is a slave market, but Landes and Posner resisted the analogy. The only point of resemblance between a baby market and a slave market, they said, is the fact that money passes hands. There is, insisted the two economists, no true analogy between buying a baby whom you plan to love and buying a person whom you plan to work to the bone. Moreover, there is no true analogy between the absolute property rights slave owners had over their slaves and the limited property rights purchasing parents would have over their purchased children. Whereas slave owners were permitted to beat and even kill their slaves, purchasing parents would be forbidden from neglecting or abusing their purchased children.[63]

Not particularly impressed by Landes and Posner's handling of the slavery issue, still other critics have complained that the two economists fail to justify what is arguably the worst feature of their proposal: the mere suggestion of the baby market itself. As Philosopher J. R. S. Pritchard has argued, most people are repelled by notions such as getting discounts on babies, setting up prices for them, and buying them "on special" or on the installment plan.[64] As Pritchard sees it, were society to permit a market in babies, it "would commodify something—life—which should not be treated as a commodity."[65] Gradually, people would come to view the purchase of a baby as no more special than the purchase of an equally costly object—say, a new house or a new car. A parent's love for his or her child would no longer be unconditional; rather, it would depend on how good a product the child turned out to be.[66] In a worst-case scenario, parents might trade in defective models for the latest models science and technology had to offer.

The conviction that babies should not be commodified has struck a responsive chord. Already eight states agree with the New Jersey Supreme Court that contracts for mothers are against public policy and therefore unenforceable.[67] To proclaim that a contract for a mother is unenforceable is to say that if the contract is breached by either the contracted mother or the contracting couple, the court will leave the parties as it finds them. Hence, for example, if the contracting couple fails to pay the contracted mother her fee, the courts will not help her collect it, or if the contracting couple refuses to take the child from the contracted mother, the courts will not force the couple to do so. Instead, the courts will require the contracted mother either to assume parental responsibilities for the child or to put the child up for adoption. In the former case, she may be entitled to child support from the genetic father; in the latter case, she may be entitled to financial assistance from the genetic father.[68] Alternatively, if the contracted mother refuses to give the child to the contracting couple, the genetic father will not be able to secure custody based on the contract he and his wife made with her. Neither will he and his wife be able to legally force the contracted mother to waive her abortion rights or to maintain a program of proper diet and exercise during pregnancy.[69]

What this approach to contracted motherhood amounts to, then, is a proceed-at-your-own-risk advisement. Because there is a great deal of social concern for contracted infants, however, the state is unlikely to let them be the objects of an unsupervised tug-of-war between the contracting couple and the contracted mother. Rather, the state will probably resolve these disputes by invoking the best-interests-of-the-child test, the custody test that is employed in divorce cases.[70]

Although a custody test that stresses the best interests of the child sounds eminently enlightened, there are certain drawbacks to it. In assessing what is best for a child, courts are not supposed to be unduly influenced by economic considerations. Just because someone is more wealthy than someone else does not mean that she or he qualifies as a good parent. Nevertheless, theory is not always translated into practice, and courts often give custody to the parent who can provide his or her child with a higher material standard of living. Thus, the fact that a contracted mother is typically poorer than the contracting couple will work to her disadvantage in a custody hearing. Also to her disadvantage is the mere fact that she signed the contract in the first place. Indeed, in the Whitehead-Stern dispute over Baby M, Judge Sorkow observed that the day she signed on the dotted line, Mary Beth Whitehead proved her "unfitness" as a mother.[71]

In an effort to be fair to both the contracting couple and the contracted mother, some commentators recommend joint custody or liberal visitation rights for the noncustodial parent(s) in the event of a custody dispute over a contracted child. As well intentioned as this proposal is, it is not particularly well conceived. Joint custody is difficult even when both parents have been in a relationship with each other and with their child for a long time; it will probably be more difficult when the parents are strangers not only to each other but to the child.

Given that custody disputes almost always traumatize the involved parties, several commentators insist that legislators must decide in advance for all contracted couples and contracted mothers who shall be the child's parent(s) before that child is born. Lawyer George Annas suggests that all states should recognize the contracted mother as the legal custodian of the contracted child because of "her gestational contribution to the child" tainly identifiable, and available" to care for the child.[72] Unless it can be proved that the contracted mother is truly unfit, says Annas, she should be awarded sole custody of the contracted child. In contrast to Annas, lawyer Lori Andrews suggests that all states should recognize the contracting couple as the child's legal custodians. Andrews favors the contracting couple over the contracted mother because "a woman who is uncertain about whether she can give the child up may nonetheless agree to be a surrogate because of the possibility that she will have a second chance at the child after its birth before the adoption procedure."[73]

Enforcing Contracted Motherhood Agreements

Unconvinced of the merits of the custody approach, some commentators have urged that states should view all disputes between contracted mothers and contracting couples as breaches of contract. The contracted mother can breach her agreement with the contracting couple in three ways: (1) failing to abort or not to abort the fetus at their instruction; (2) negligently, recklessly, knowingly, or purposely harming the fetus; or (3) refusing to give the child up at birth. In contrast, the contracting couple can breach its agreement with the contracted mother in one of two ways: (1) failing to pay her the agreed-on fee and (2) refusing to accept the child on its birth.

Over the years, contract lawyers have developed two sorts of remedies for breaches of contract—*specific performance* and *damages*—and it is not immediately clear which, if either, of these two approaches really addresses the grievances that contracted mothers and contracting couples sometimes report.[74]

Specific Performance

Because specific performance forces the parties to a contract to fulfill its terms, it eliminates the kind of uncertainty that characterizes less formal human arrangements. Uncertainty is always difficult for human beings to handle, but it is especially difficult when what is at stake is a person's most precious dreams. To wait 9 months for a child, not knowing whether it will ever be yours to love, is as agonizing as not knowing whether the people who contracted you to bear a child for them will take it from you as they promised.

Significantly, specific performance is not usually the preferred way to enforce personal service contracts. For example, if a comedian refuses to come on stage and perform, no court is going to force him to do his monologue. Under such circumstances, the comedian is not apt to be very funny. Analogously, a contracting couple will achieve less than optimal results if they attempt to force a contracted mother to follow reasonable medical instruction during her pregnancy; to carry the fetus to term unless doing so endangers her life; or to surrender the child to them no matter how much she loves it. Similarly, a contracted mother will achieve less than optimal results if she attempts to force a contracting couple to take the child she has borne for them but whom they no longer want.

Nevertheless, because a contract for a mother is for such a unique personal service, some legal theorists believe that specific performance may be the only remedy that is truly effective, for example, when the contracted mother refuses to surrender the child.

The surrogate's services—the conceiving and bearing of a child and the terminating of her parental rights to and responsibilities for the child—cannot be compared to any other services that person might perform. The desire to reproduce and to create a family is one of the strongest human longings and needs. Expectations based on the promises of parties to cooperate in reproductive activity are particularly intense. No other expectations that serve as a basis for contractual remedies compare to the expectations that develop when the parties begin to undertake their obligations in a surrogate parenthood arrangement.[75]

Even if it is correct to argue that some aspects of a contract for a mother beg for specific enforcement, it is unlikely that all of them do. Most legal theorists observe that it is one thing to force a contracted mother to give up her child and quite another to force her to waive her abortion rights or even to submit to unwanted medical treatment.

Arguments for forcing the contracted mother to relinquish the child to the genetic father are based on the intuition that "denying enforcement of the surrogate mother's promise to give up the child threatens the father's personhood in much the same way as specific performance ... threaten(s) the [surrogate] mother's."[76] In other words, genetic fathers, "unwillingly deprived of access to their children" suffer from "feelings of regret and self-betrayal" similar to those that contracted mothers feel when similarly deprived.[77] Thus, if the contracted mother has given her informed consent to the contract, she should be forced to hand over the child to the genetic father. Although she and he have contributed equal genetic material to the child, what breaks this equilibrium is presumably the promises the contracted mother made to the contracting couple.

Arguments against forcing the contracted mother to have an abortion, or to carry the pregnancy to term, or simply to take care of herself during pregnancy (eating properly, exercising moderately, not drinking or smoking) are based on widely accepted interpretations of constitutional law.[78] Because of equal protection, due process, and privacy considerations, it is unlikely that courts would enforce a contracted mother's waiver of her abortion rights or other rights related to her bodily integrity. Past judicial decisions have given the genetic father's interest in the abortion decision short shrift, even though the child might represent the genetic father's only hope of natural reproduction.[79] Even assuming that a genetic father's paternal rights are stronger than usual in cases where he and a contracted mother have deliberately arranged to bring into existence a child genetically related to him, and recalling that it is not impossible to waive a constitutional right (consider the Fourth Fifth, and Sixth Amendments), it is still unlikely that courts would enforce a contracted mother's waiver of her abortion rights.

When it comes to the contracting couple, the weaknesses as well as the strengths of a specific performance approach again become apparent. It is one matter to require a contracting couple to pay the contracted mother whether the child is delivered stillborn, impaired, or perfectly healthy; however, it is quite another matter to require a contracting couple to assume full parental responsibilities for the child whether or not they want him or her. Obviously, a child's best interests are ill served when she or he is handed over to parents who do not want her or him. Of course, if the contracted mother does not want the child either, then, according to a modified version of the specific performance approach, the contracting couple and not the contracted mother must put the child up for adoption.

Damages Approach

Unconvinced that specific performance is the appropriate remedy for breach of a personal service contract, some legal commentators have stressed the advantages of the remedy termed *damages*. In this circumstance, these commentators borrow from the work of legal theorists such as Anthony Kronman, who has argued that a damages remedy lets people depersonalize their mistakes in a way that keeps their sense of personal integrity intact.[80]

To understand this, let us look at the example of a porn queen who "gets religion." As a result of her newfound faith, she refuses to honor her contract to star in what had promised to be a quadruple-X-rated pornographic film, a real money-maker. When a woman such as this changes her mind about the contract she signed, she will probably view her earlier decision to sign the contract as a foreign and irrational act. She will view her earlier self as a false self—an unborn Christian, say, who caused her true self to act against her best interests. She will want to disassociate herself from the false self who led her true self astray. Since specific performance of her promise to star in the pornographic film would violate her born-again Christian self by forcing her, physically and psychologically, to confront her former unredeemed self repeatedly, courts permit her an *impersonal* way to make good on her contract without doing violence to her new, true self—namely, the paying of damages.

If it is wrong to force a reformed porn queen to go through with the making of an XXXX-rated movie, then, say these commentators, it is also wrong to force a contracted mother to continue her pregnancy if she wakes up one morning and wonders, "What was I ever thinking when I agreed to be artificially inseminated? I can't possibly be a party to this arrangement. I want out." To force the contracted mother to continue her pregnancy under these circumstances is, they say, to impose on her a constant, sometimes painful, and always invasive physical reminder of her mistake; it is to compel her labor in a particularly person-negating way.[81]

What the supporters of the damages approach offer the parties to a contract for motherhood, then, is a choice when they are unwilling to fulfill its terms. They may choose either to honor the contract but do violence to their persons or to breach the contract and pay damages but emerge with their persons relatively intact. Presumably, the fact that they will have to pay considerable damages will deter contracted mothers and contracting couples from breaching a contract unless it is crucial for them to do so. To avoid tort claims for intentional emotional distress, outrageous conduct, or wrongful death, for example,[82] a contracted mother will think twice before she aborts or fails to surrender the child to the contracting couple. Similarly, to avoid punitive damage or child-support claims, for example, a contracting couple will think twice before it fails to pay the contracted mother her due or to accept parental responsibility at the birth of the child.

Whatever the theoretical merits of the damages approach, however, it lacks several practical advantages. Since contracted mothers are generally less well off than the couples who contract them, they will have difficulty paying the damages assessed against them and, even if they are able to pay the assessed damages, the money will not adequately compensate the childless contracting couple. After all, money is no substitute for a baby. Likewise, money will not adequately compensate a contracted mother who is left holding a baby in her arms whom she never intended to parent. What is more, it is not clear just how theoretically sound the damages approaches really is. If pregnant women have the right to bodily integrity, including the right to engage in a wide range of activities, to seek or refuse medical treatments, and to abort or not abort their fetuses, then contracting couples may lose more suits than they win against contracted mothers.

Treating Contracted Motherhood as a Form of Adoption

Because they find both the specific performance and damages approaches to contracted motherhood wanting, some legal commentators have urged that this practice be assimilated into adoption law. As these commentators see it, contracted motherhood is best considered prenatal adoption because there is very little difference between making arrangements to adopt a teenager's baby as soon as she knows she is pregnant and making arrangements to adopt a contracted mother's child before she has even conceived it. However, as feminist Phyllis Chesler sees it, adoption is a child-centered practice whereby already existing children are embraced by adults willing to give them the kind of love they need. It is not an adult-centered practice whereby children are deliberately brought into existence so that "unfulfilled" adults can be fulfilled, nor should it become one.[83]

Chesler's admonition is one on which we should all reflect, but the fact remains that many adults deliberately bring children into existence because they think that parenting a child will contribute to their overall happiness. Thus, it is probably unfair to fault contracting couples for doing something that fertile couples do without hesitation.

In what definitely represents a modification of traditional adoption law, Peter Singer and Deane Wells envision a future in which couples wanting a mother's services as well as women wishing to serve as mothers would contact a non-profit-making state surrogacy board. If few women were willing to serve as mothers for free, the board would offer women a fair fee for their services. Because the board would be non-profit-making, its overhead costs would be minimal. As a result, it would be able to charge its clients several thousand dollars less than would its profit-making competitors. The board would also require medical evaluation and psychiatric counseling for all parties and would supervise whatever agreements the parties made. Indeed, preventing some of the unfortunate occurrences associated with current contracted motherhood arrangements would be a major goal of a non-profit-making state surrogacy board. Unlike a profit-making agency, a non-profit-making board would not be tempted to employ slipshod or bogus medical evaluations and psychiatric counseling.[84] That no one at the profit-making Infertility Center of New York bothered to question Mary Beth Whitehead about her ability to relinquish a baby suggests that the center may have been overly eager to supply the well-to-do Sterns with a "compatible surrogate" (the physical resemblance between Elizabeth Stern and Mary Beth Whitehead has not gone unnoticed).[85]

Lawyers A. M. Capron and M. J. Radin also favor an adoption paradigm, but they do not believe that contracted mothers should be paid a fee. As they see it, as soon as a woman accepts a fee for her gestational services, she becomes a baby seller. Capron and Radin wish to bring contracted motherhood within the standard rules of adoption. These rules permit payment but only for the pregnant woman's reasonable medical expenses. They also provide for a change-of-heart period: After the woman gives birth to the child, she has several days to decide whether she really wants to relinquish it.[86]

Other supporters of the adoption paradigm are even more solicitous about the contracted mother than are Capron and Radin. For example, lawyer Martha Field argues that if a woman agrees to become pregnant in order to carry a child to term for a contracting couple, that agreement is voidable but *only* at her option.[87] The reason Field gives this advantage to the contracted mother is that, as she sees it, had it not been for the contracting couple's desire to have a child, the contracted mother would never have signed the contract and become pregnant. Since the surrogacy arrangement is more the idea of the contracting couple than of the contracted mother, she probably has less of a commitment to its terms than does the couple. Therefore, the contracted mother is the one who should be permitted to renege on the contract because it is not the fundamental and direct product of her most treasured goals. In contrast, the contracting couple should not be permitted to renege on the contract because it is the expression of the couple's deepest wishes. Not everyone is persuaded by Field's line of reasoning, however. As the critics see it, had it not been for the contracted mother's voluntary agreement to serve as the couple's incubator, she would never have signed the contract and become pregnant. There is, therefore, no reason to accord the contracted mother any privilege not accorded to the contracting couple. The contract is the collective product of their separate wishes, and the contracted mother as well as the contracting couple must live up to its terms.

Philosopher Sara Ann Ketchum, an opponent of contracted motherhood, believes that even if Field's arguments for privileging the contracted mother over the contracting couple fail, there are other arguments that support this position. First, since the genetic father in a contracted motherhood arrangement is generally, though not always, distanced from a number of the connections that a genetic father can ordinarily make with his developing child—following gestational development, attending birthing classes, participating at delivery, caring for the child immediately at birth—the genetic father in a contracted motherhood arrangement will have a harder time forging bonds with his child than the genetic father in a traditional arrangement. Second, there is a prima facie case that the kinds of bonds a genetic father can forge with his child are simply less deep and intense than the bonds a genetic or gestational mother can form with her child as she carries it to term. It is the genetic or gestational mother, not the genetic father, who stands in direct relationship to the child at the moment of his or her birth. Given this male-female asymmetry, says Ketchum, it seems appropriate to weight contracted motherhood arrangements in the direction of the genetic or gestational mother rather than the genetic father.[88]

To the objection that to give custodial advantage to the contracted mother is unfair to the contracting couple, supporters of the adoption approach argue that it is no more unfair to the contracting couple than the kind of disappointment a couple sustains when an attempt to secure a child through a traditional adoption fails. From the very beginning of their negotiations, would-be adoptive parents know that the adoption negotiations may fall through if the natural mother decides not to give up her child for adoption after all. Thus, provided that a contracting couple understands that the contracted mother may void the contract at any time, no injustice is done in the event that the contracted mother decides to keep her baby.

To the further objection that the adoption and contracted motherhood cases are not analogous because, in the case of contracted motherhood, the man who wishes to adopt the child is also the genetic father of the child, supporters of the adoption approach argue that genetic linkage is not the determining criterion for parenthood. What genetic linkage to a child gives a man or a woman is a right to establish a relationship with a child, whereby *relationship* is defined as "any mode of nurturance from the most physical to the most psychological." In other words, the fact that a man's sperm constitute 50 percent of the genetic material necessary for conception does not make him 50 percent owner of any resultant child. Likewise, the fact that a woman's egg constitutes 50 percent of the genetic material necessary for conception does not make her 50 percent owner of any resultant child. Children are not possessions; rather they are the kind of beings with whom relationships can be forged and, at birth, the only direct relationship a child has is with the woman who has carried him or her for 9 months. To be sure, this biological relationship is not an interpersonal one, but it is one that shows that the contracted mother was committed enough to the fetus to bring it to term.

Social Dimensions of Contracted Motherhood

The nurture-versus-nature argument as it relates to parenting is controversial. Among the arguments Ketchum raises against the genetic criterion for parenthood, five are especially salient. First, as soon as scientists develop gene-splicing and chromosome-combining techniques, it will be possible to procreate IVF children with enormously complex genetic backgrounds. Who, then, says Ketchum, will count as the genetic parents of these children? Will only the donors who contributed the *most* genes or chromosomes to the child count as his or her parents? Or will the donors who contributed only one less gene or chromosome than the highest donors also count as his or her parents? Or will all the donors count as the child's parents, no matter how many or how few genes or chromosomes they contributed to him or her? After all, had even one gene or chromosome been different, the child of whom we speak would not have been the same child. Second, insists Ketchum, our intuitions suggest that at least in the case of rape, it is implausible to regard genetic connection as conferring parental rights. Third, as some radical feminists (for example, Mary O'Brien) see it, men valorize genetic fatherhood because there is no such experience as gestational fatherhood. O'Brien points out that men's experience of reproduction is indirect for at least three reasons:

1. Because the physical and temporal continuity between the sperm and the resulting child takes place outside the man's body, the seed is "alienated."

2. Because the basic labor of reproduction—pregnancy and birth—is necessarily performed by a woman, when a man appropriates a child (even his genetic child), he is appropriating the product of someone else's labor.

3. Whereas a woman's connection to a particular child is proved in the act of birth, a man's connection to a particular child is always arguable since the child he wishes to call *his* may be the product of a liaison between another man and his wife or girlfriend.[89]

Fourth, says Ketchum, to identify genetic connection as the essential criterion for parenthood is to suggest that this abstract relationship with a child is more important than such concrete relationships as gestation and child care. Fifth, and finally, observes Ketchum, to stress genetic connection as the essential criterion for parenthood is to imply that adoptive parents are not real parents.[90]

Nonetheless, even if the negative case against the genetic criterion for parenthood is fairly strong, some positive argument needs to be made on behalf of treating nurture as the primary criterion for parenthood. Ketchum provides this argument when she observes that parents who nurture—be it the kind of nurturing that occurs during gestation, or at the moment of birth, or throughout the childrearing process—are, by virtue of that nurturing, showing their commitment to their children.

Because they have invested so much of themselves in their children's lives, they have a right to maintain their relationships to their children unless these relationships are in some way harmful or wrong. What makes a parent a parent, therefore, is the fact that the parent is living (or, as in the case of an adult child, has lived) a relationship with his or her child.[91]

Although the arguments against nature and for nurture as the determining criterion of parenthood seem strong, a variety of critics are reluctant to downplay the genetic criterion. Among these critics are those who refuse to look at gestation or childbirth as lived relationships, as active encounters between a woman and a child. As these critics see it, pregnancy and childbirth are events that simply happen to a woman; she has little, if any, control over them.

But surely this view of pregnancy is rather "male." Although male gynecologists and obstetricians did not conspire to take charge of the birthing process, they did take over the work of female midwives, replacing their hands of flesh (female hands sensitive to female anatomy) with hands of iron (e.g., obstetrical forceps). In addition, these male gynecologists and obstetricians wrote the official rules not only for giving birth but also for being pregnant: when to eat, sleep, exercise, have sex, and feel pain. Arguing against these rules, feminist poet Adrienne Rich writes that when they clash with a woman's lived experience—and they do so frequently—a woman does not know whether to trust the rules of the doctors or the sensations of her own body. Such self-doubting experiences can transform a pregnancy into a profoundly alienating experience. Indeed, Rich writes that this is precisely what happened in her own case:

When I try to return to the body of the young woman of twenty-six, pregnant for the first time, who fled from the physical knowledge of her pregnancy and at the same time from her intellect and vocation, I realize that I was effectively alienated from my real body and my real spirit by the institution—not the fact—of motherhood. This institution—the foundation of human society as we know it—allowed me only certain views, certain expectations, whether embodied in the booklet in my obstetrician's waiting room, the novels I had read, my mother-in-law's approval, my memories of my own mother, the Sistine Madonna or she of the Michelangelo Pietà, the floating notion that a woman pregnant is a woman calm in her fulfillment or, simply, a woman waiting.[92]

Were women in charge of pregnancy and childbirth, suggests Rich, these experiences would have active rather than passive meanings for them. Women would no longer sit passively, waiting for the birth event to seize them. Rather, they would actively direct the birthing of their children, regaining control of the pleasures as well as the pains of the experience.

As convincing as Rich's view of pregnancy and childbirth may be, there still are reasons not to stress nurture over nature as the determining criterion of parenthood. Concerned about identifying gestation as *the* relationship that makes a woman a mother, some feminists point out that women's reproductive role has traditionally been the major source of women's oppression. Since this point is one that is not easily dismissed, it is important to consider the debate between both those feminists who wish to de-emphasize the parental significance of gestation and those who wish to emphasize it.

The Early Radical Feminist Position on Begetting, Bearing, and Rearing Children

In the late 1960s and early to middle 1970s, many radical feminists responded positively to the new reproductive technologies, seeing in them liberating opportunities for women. In contrast to liberal feminists who tend to believe that the causes of and solutions for women's oppression are legal, political, occupational, and educational, radical feminists tend to believe that the ultimate causes of women's oppression are biological and that the only way for women to liberate themselves is to somehow overcome or control their own female biology. Among the radical feminists who have written forcefully about the liberating potential of the new reproductive technologies are Shulamith Firestone and Marge Piercy.

Convinced that the roots of women's oppression are biological, Firestone argues that women's liberation requires a biological revolution in much the same way that workers' liberation requires an economic revolution. Firestone insists that until artificial reproduction is just as socially acceptable as is natural reproduction, women will remain slaves to their reproductive role. No matter how much educational, legal, and political equality women achieve, and no matter how many women enter public industry, nothing fundamental will change for them as long as they continue to bear children. Women must convince themselves that biological reproduction is neither in their own best interests nor in those of the children so reproduced. The joy of giving birth, invoked so frequently in our society, is a patriarchal myth. In fact, Firestone insists that pregnancy is "barbaric," and that natural childbirth is, at best, "necessary and tolerable" and, at worst, "like shitting a pumpkin."[93] Moreover, biological motherhood is the root of further evils. Not only does it force women to play a passive second fiddle to men; it accounts for the awful feelings of possessiveness that generate hostility among human beings. As Firestone sees it, this feeling of possessiveness—this favoring of one child over another on account of its being the product of one's own egg or sperm—is precisely what must be overcome if human beings are to destroy divisive hierarchies. Firestone believes reproductive technology is providing human beings with the condition of possibility of this overcoming.

This last point of Firestone's is one that radical feminist Marge Piercy develops in her science fiction novel, *Woman on the Edge of Time*.[94] Piercy sets the story of her utopia within the tale of a multiply disadvantaged woman. Connie Ramos is a middle-aged, lower-class Chicana with a history of what society describes as mental illness and violent behavior. She has been trying desperately to support herself and her daughter, Angelina, on a pittance. One day, when Connie is near the point of exhaustion, she loses her temper and hits Angelina too hard. As a result of this one outburst, Connie is judged an unfit mother and her daughter is taken away from her. Depressed and despondent, angry and agitated, Connie is committed by her family to a mental hospital, where she is selected as a human research subject for brain-control experiments. Just when things could get no worse, Connie is transported by a woman named Luciente to a future world called Mattapoisett, a world in which women are not defined in terms of their reproductive functions and in which both men and women delight in rearing children.

What makes Piercy's future world plausible is artificial reproduction. In Mattapoisett, babies are born from what is termed the *brooder*. Female eggs are fertilized in vitro with male sperm in a way that preserves a full range of racial, ethnic, and personality types, and then gestated within an artificial placenta. Unable to comprehend why Mattapoisett women have rejected the experience that meant the most to her—physically gestating, birthing, and nursing a child—Connie is initially repelled by the brooder. She sees the embryos "all in a sluggish row … like fish in the aquarium."[95] Not only does she regard these embryos as less than human; she pities them, for no woman loves them enough to carry them in her own womb and, bleeding and sweating, to bring them into the world.

Eventually, Connie learns from Luciente that the people of Mattapoisett did not easily give up biological reproduction for technological reproduction. They did so only when they realized that the loss of biological reproduction was the price to pay for the elimination of not only sexism but also racism and classism:

It was part of women's long revolution. When we were breaking all the old hierarchies. Finally there was that one thing we had to give up too, the only power we ever had, in return for no power for anyone. The original production: the power to give birth. Cause as long as we were biologically enchained, we'd never be equal.

And males never would be humanized to be loving and tender. So we all became mothers. Every child has three. To break the nuclear bonding.[96]

Thus, as a result of women giving up their exclusive power to give birth, the original paradigm for power relations is destroyed and everyone in Mattapoisett is in a position to reconstitute human relationships in ways that defy the hierarchical ideas of better-worse, higher-lower, stronger-weaker and, especially, dominant-submissive.

In Mattapoisett individuals possess neither private property nor private children. No one has his or her own genetic child. Children are not the possessions of their biological mothers and fathers to be brought into this world in their parents' image and likeness and reared according to their idiosyncratic values. Rather, children are precious human resources for the entire community, to be treasured on account of their uniqueness. Each child is reared by three comothers (one man and two women, or two men and one woman) who are assisted by "kidbinders," a group of individuals who excel at mothering.[97] Childrearing is a communal effort, with each child moving between large-group experiences at child-care centers and small-group experiences in the separate dwellings of each of his or her comothers.

Initially, Connie doubts that Mattapoisett's system for begetting, bearing, and rearing children is all it claims to be. She wonders whether comothers and kidbinders really love the children they are rearing, but eventually she decides that technological reproduction is superior to biological reproduction because this kind of comothering is truly nurturing and unselfish.

A More Recent Radical Feminist Position on Begetting, Bearing, and Rearing Children

As beautifully as Piercy expresses and modifies some of Firestone's more controversial ideas, she, like Firestone, has been challenged by a new generation of radical feminists who believe that women should not give up biological motherhood for ex utero child gestation. Empathizing with Connie's initial reaction of disgust at ex utero gestation and her initial reaction of bewilderment at Luciente's explanation for why women had to give up the only power they ever had, feminist philosopher Ann Donchin observes that, from the point of view of women who are currently living with patriarchy, Mattapoisett is both implausible and unintelligible.[98]

Mattapoisett is implausible because women's oppression is not likely to end if, as feminist philosopher Azizah al-Hibri observes, women give up the only source of men's dependence on them:

Technological reproduction does not equalize the natural reproductive power structure —it inverts *it. It appropriates the reproductive power from women and places it in the hands of men who now control both the sperm and the reproductive technology that could make it indispensable ... it 'liberates' them from their 'humiliating dependency' on women in order to propagate.*[99]

And Mattapoisett is unintelligible—at least its notions of who counts as a mother are—because what patriarchal society means by a mother is a woman who is defined and defines herself in terms of a 9-month pregnancy, a 24-hour or so delivery, and 18 years or so of childrearing. On account of this implausibility and unintelligibility, there is, insists Donchin, no way that a woman can imagine what it would be like to be a comother or a kidbinder instead of the kind of mother she is—namely, a woman who, as Connie says, knows what it means to carry a child 9 months "heavy under her heart," to bear a baby "in blood and pain," and to suckle a child.[100]

To the degree that Piercy's utopian vision has been criticized as implausible and unintelligible, Firestone's analysis has been criticized as being a blueprint not for women's ultimate liberation but for women's permanent enslavement. Firestone's critics argue that the cause of women's oppression is not women's biology per se. Rather, the cause of women's oppression is men's control of women's biology, a control that could become total depending on how reproductive technology is developed.

Gena Corea and Robyn Rowland are two of the radical feminists most critical of Firestone. As Corea sees it, because men currently control the new reproductive technologies, they will use these technologies not to empower women but to further consolidate men's control over women. Corea describes Dr. Robert Edwards of IVF fame as if he were Count Dracula: Just as Dracula never had enough blood to drink, she exclaims, Dr. Edwards never had enough eggs on which to experiment. As a result, he would routinely appear at the hysterectomies his colleagues were performing so that he could secure enough eggs for his experiments.[101] Toward the end of her essay entitled "Egg Snatchers," Corea asks:

Why are men focusing all this technology on woman's generative organs—the source of her procreative power? Why are they collecting our eggs? Why do they seek to freeze them?

Why do men want to control the production of human beings? Why do they talk so often about producing "perfect" babies?

Why are they splitting the functions of motherhood into smaller parts? Does that reduce the power of the mother and her claim to the child? ("I only gave the egg. I am not the real mother." "I only loaned my uterus. I am not the real mother." "I only raised the child. I am not the real mother.")[102]

Robyn Rowland agrees with Corea that biological motherhood is a power base for women and that the new reproductive technologies will simply increase men's control over women. Rowland points to the work of John Postgate, a British professor of microbiology, as an example of the forms this new power over women may take. Postgate suggests that the best way to curb overpopulation is to develop a pill—the "manchild pill"—that would ensure the conception of male children, eventually creating a scarcity of women and a decline in birth rates. He blithely forecasts that restrictions on women's freedom would, of course, be necessary in order to curb women's indiscriminate breeding and to control men's access to women (unlucky men could resort, he says, to homosexuality or to autoeroticism).[103]

As if visions of future worlds in which women are more tightly controlled by men than ever before are not bad enough, Rowland imagines an even worse scenario: a world in which only a few superovulating women are permitted to exist, a world in which eggs are taken from women, frozen, and fertilized in vitro for transfer into artificial placentas. The replacement of women's childbearing capacity by male-controlled technology would, concedes Rowland, remove women's biological burden, but it would also leave women without their traditional ace in the hole. Rowland worries that if women no longer are the ones who give birth, they may find themselves without a product with which to bargain:

For the history of "mankind" women have been seen in terms of their value as childbearers. We have to ask, if that last power is taken and controlled by men, what role is envisaged for women in the new world?[104]

Clearly, Rowland could not disagree more with the moral of Piercy's novel which, we will recall, urged women to give up freely their ultimate power, their power over life, so that the paradigm for power, of one person's (group's) control over another, would be destroyed. As Rowland sees it, Piercy may have failed to see the difference between the kind of power that women exert in bringing new life into the world and the kind of power that men exert in their efforts to control nature and also women through technology.

To be sure, Corea's and Rowland's speculations are not pleasant ones. They are also ones to which not only many men but also many women take exception. As these critics see it, no matter who developed reproductive technology initially, it is gradually becoming the equal responsibility of both men and women. The kinds of questions we should be asking ourselves about contracted motherhood, for example, should be far less focused on the rights of the contracted mother and the contracting couple and far more focused on the responsibilities of all the adults to the children they wish to contract into existence. It is not the mere existence of the reproduction-aiding technologies that is the source of our problems; rather, it is our needs, wants, and desires that have produced this complex social arrangement. Whether technology will liberate or enslave us, make us better or worse, is for us to decide.

Appendix: Basic Biochemistry

If we wish to understand the old and new reproductive technologies fully, we must be familiar with not only the human reproductive system but also a number of the biochemical molecules and biological structures that play a general role in our life processes. In this appendix, we provide needed information about the nature and function of cells. In particular, we focus on cellular reproduction, especially the two modes of cell division, mitosis and meiosis. Only if we understand how cells divide can we speak authoritatively about the human reproductive process.

Important Biochemical Molecules

Of the more than 100 chemical elements known, just 6 are the major components of all living things: carbon, hydrogen, oxygen, sulfur, nitrogen, and phosphorus.[1-4] Arranged in multiple different ways, atoms of these six elements form the basic structures of the myriad organic compounds found in nature. Among these organic compounds, carbohydrates, proteins, lipids, and nucleic acids are the most important for our purposes. Living systems such as our own use these compounds to constitute their structural frameworks, to secure the energy they need for their life processes, to serve as messengers in their communications network, and to act as modulators in the regulation of their cellular functions.

As we look at the chemical structures for these compounds we must keep in mind the shorthand notation that chemists have devised to represent the molecules. The common elements are represented by the normal chemical abbreviation such as hydrogen, H, carbon, C, nitrogen, N, and oxygen, O. The bonds that link the atoms together are represented with a straight line; two parallel lines represent a double bond between two atoms. While many molecules have linear structures, there are also molecules with structures in the form of a ring. The ring is usually either five or six membered and frequently consists of carbon atoms. In some cases, other atoms such as nitrogen or oxygen are members of the ring structure. As a shorthand notation, the carbon atoms are left out of the ring structure (but oxygen and nitrogen are always indicated). That means that a structure such as that in figure A.6 for cholesterol should be interpreted to mean that carbon atoms exit at each of the "corners" where there is no other atom specified. In addition, chemists frequently leave off the hydrogen atoms when they are attached to carbon atoms. Keep in mind that carbon always has four bonds to other atoms; if it has less than four, the implication is that the other bonds are to hydrogens which are not shown in the shorthand notation.

Carbohydrates

When we use the term *carbohydrates*, we are usually referring to breads, cereals, cookies, and cakes, but when biochemists use this same term, they are referring to a class of organic compounds in which the usual ratio of hydrogen to oxygen is 2:1 and the general formula is $C_nH_{2n}O_n$. Biochemists categorize carbohydrates according to the complexity of their structure (figure A.1). The simplest are *monosaccharides*, or simple sugars such as glucose, fructose, and ribose. More complex are the *disaccharides*, composed of two monosaccharides linked together in a specific way. Sucrose, or common table sugar, is a disaccharide made up of one glucose and one fructose. Most complex are the *polysaccharides*, composed of more than two monosaccharides. Plant starch (amylose) and glycogen are both polysaccharides made of glucose, but the glucose molecules in their chains are linked together in different ways.

Carbohydrates are important biologically as energy sources: Glucose is a primary cellular fuel. In the reproductive process, the sperm rely exclusively on fructose for the energy to propel them in the female reproductive tract. Carbohydrates associated with proteins—glycoproteins—present in the cell membrane, facilitate intercellular communication and recognition such as that between the egg and the sperm just before fertilization.

Proteins

Compared to carbohydrates, proteins, the most common organic compound in living systems, are very complex and large. Yet all proteins are made up of relatively simple and small molecules called *amino acids* (figure A.2). Although amino acids share a common structure, different R groups

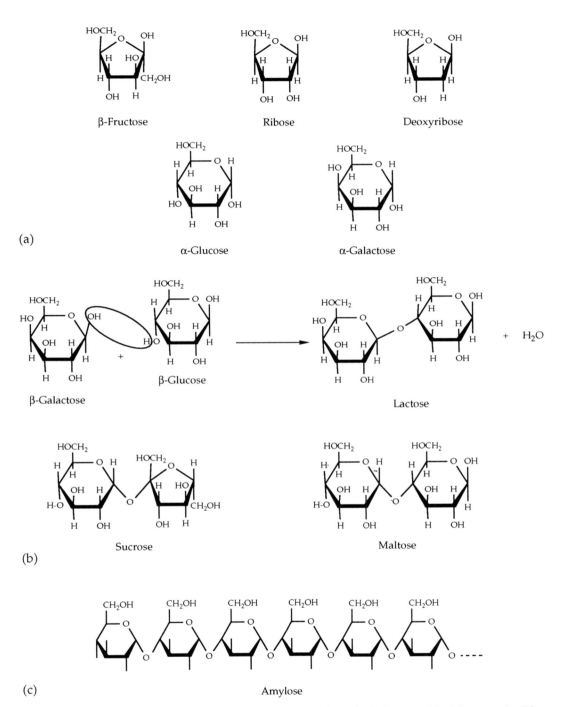

Figure A.1 The chemical structure of carbohydrates. (a) Monosaccharides; ribose is the sugar present in RNA and deoxyribose is present in DNA. (b) The formation of a disaccharide by the condensation of two monosaccharides with the loss of a molecule of water; representative disaccharides. (c) The polysaccharide amylose, which is present in starch.

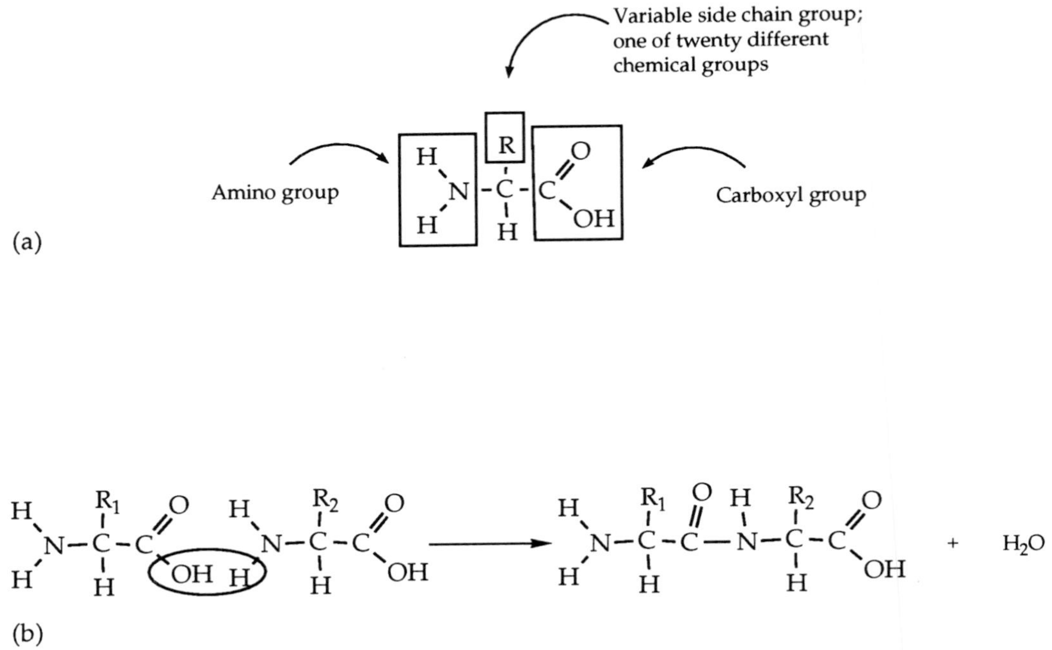

(a)

(b)

Figure A.2 (a) A generalized chemical structure of the amino acids. (b) The formation of the peptide bond between two amino acids with the loss of a molecule of water.

(different chemical groups) attached to their basic backbone differentiate one from another. Peptide bonds link into *polypeptides* the 20 different amino acids found in living systems.

Proteins consist of long polypeptides, sometimes just one chain, sometimes several chains bound together. There are four levels of protein structure (figure A.3). The *primary* structure is the sequence of amino acids in the polypeptide chain. This sequence essentially determines the *secondary* level of protein structure, in which various sections of the polypeptide are coiled and pleated together by the hydrogen bonds that arise between amino acids in close proximity to one another. The *tertiary* level of protein structure is the overall shape of the protein as determined by the folding of the coiled or pleated sections of the polypeptide. Covalent, ionic, and hydrogen bonds between the different R groups of the contiguous amino acids determine the particular folding pattern. Finally, the *quaternary* level of protein structure is the association of two or more polypeptide chains, each with its own primary, secondary, and tertiary structures. Each such polypeptide chain is called a *subunit*

Although the role of proteins as structural components in living systems is vital, so too is their role as enzymes, the biological catalysts necessary

(a)
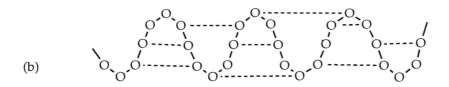

(b)
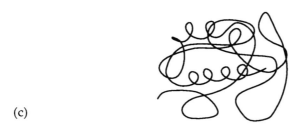

(c)
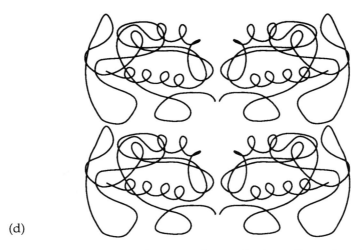

(d)

Figure A.3 The levels of structural organization of proteins: (a) the primary structure, showing the linear string of amino acids (represented by the circles); (b) the secondary structure, showing the coiling of the polypeptide; (c) the tertiary structure, showing the three-dimensional folding of proteins and the interaction of various regions of the molecule with other regions; and (d) the quaternary structure of proteins, showing the interaction of four globular units with one another.

for virtually all cell processes. Most of us are probably familiar with the role enzymes play in the digestion of food, but we may not be familiar with the role they play in the reproductive process. A crucial step in the fertilization process occurs when the sperm releases enzymes that digest part of the egg. Were these enzymes not released, the nucleus of the sperm would not be able to enter the egg. Because proteins must maintain their shape to function properly, it is somewhat of a miracle that fertilization occurs as often as it does. Heat, physical damage, or change in the chemical environment can destroy (denature) the shape of a protein, and the possibility for such destruction would seem to loom large during the reproductive process.

Lipids

In contrast to carbohydrates and proteins, it is difficult for us to characterize lipids. If lipids such as fats and oils have any common attribute, it is that they are not readily soluble in water. A fat is the combination of a glycerol molecule and one, two, or three fatty acid chains linked to this backbone (figure A.4). When double bonds exist between certain carbons in a fatty acid, we call it *unsaturated*, but when only single bonds exist between certain carbons in a fatty acid, we call it *saturated*. Unsaturated fats tend to be more liquid than saturated fats, and those fats that are liquid at room temperature are called *oils*.

Breaking the bonds of fats releases more than twice the energy released by breaking the bonds of an equivalent mass of carbohydrates or proteins; thus, the primary role of fats is energy storage. The body also uses fat for insulation, for cushioning vital organs, and for protecting the developing embryo and fetus.

Less well recognized than fats and oils, but just as biologically essential, are the lipids known as *phospholipids* and *steroids*. The importance of phospholipids, which are composed of glycerol, fatty acids, and a negatively charged phosphate group, derives from their structure and the charge distribution that results from this structure (figure A.5). The hydrocarbon (hydrogen and carbon) portion of the fatty acids is hydrophobic ("water-fearing"), whereas the phosphate portion is hydrophilic ("water-loving"). When phospholipid molecules are placed in water, they will automatically tend to orient themselves so that their hydrophilic "heads" are in the water and their hydrophobic "tails" are out of the water. This forms the basic structure of the cell membrane (see below.).

Steroids are lipids that do not contain glycerol or fatty acids. Sharing a common four-ring structure (three of the rings are cyclohexanes [six-sided]

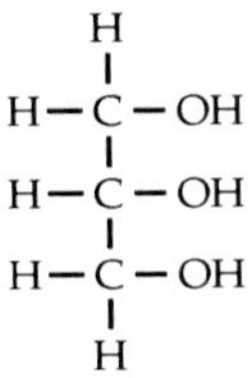

(a)

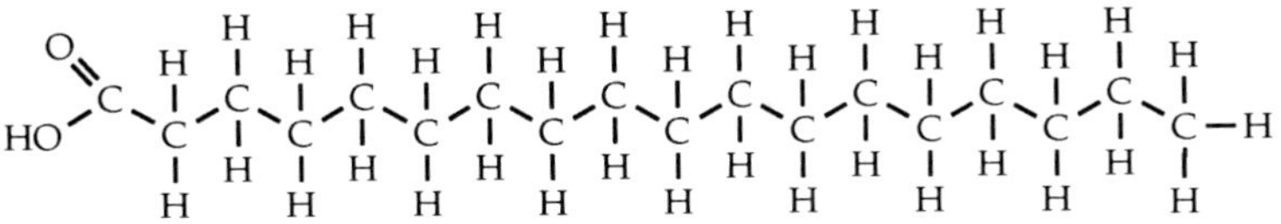

(b)

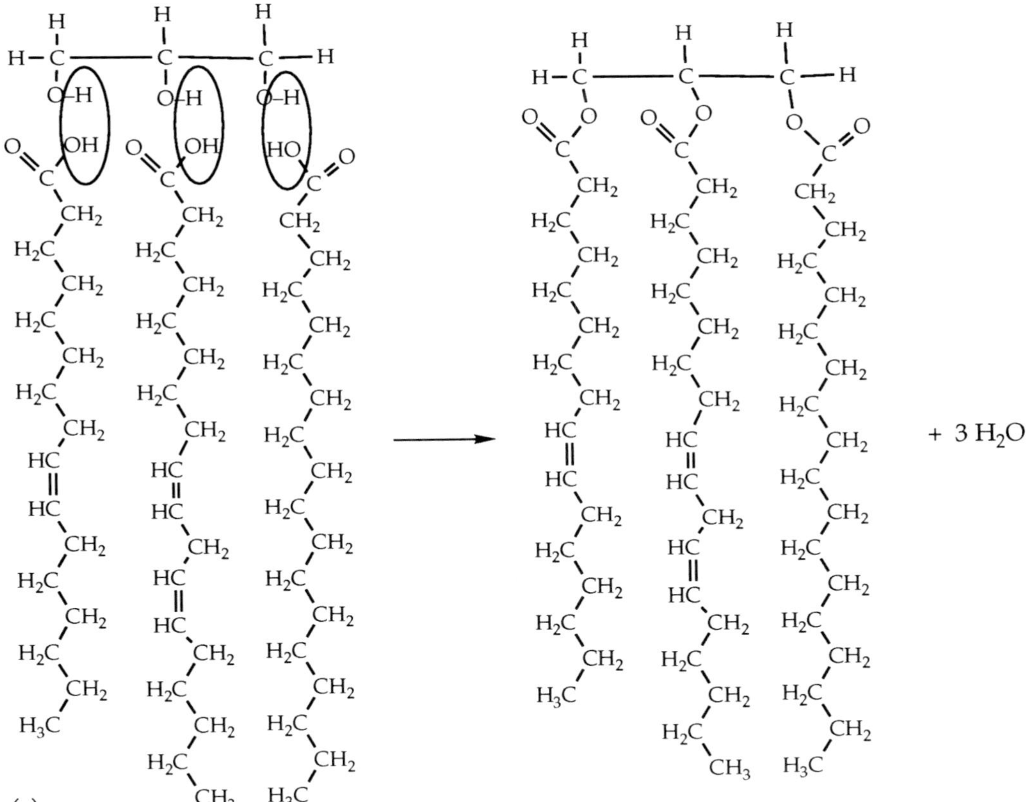

(c)

+ 3 H₂O

Figure A.4 The chemical structure of fatty acids and lipids: (a) glycerol; (b) the fatty acid, stearic acid; (c) the formation of a triglyceride from three fatty acid and glycerol with the loss of three molecules of water.

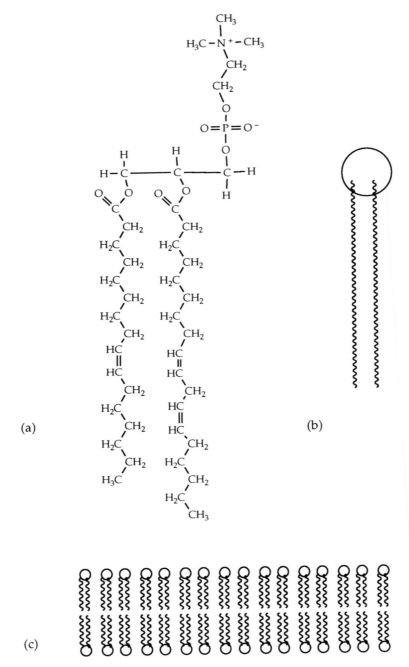

(a)

(b)

(c)

Figure A.5 The chemical structure of complex lipid. (a) A phospholipid. (b) A representation of a phospholipid with the circle representing the polar, charged head and the wavy line representing the nonpolar tails. (c) A lipid bilayer showing the heads on the outside in contact with water and the tails inside away from water.

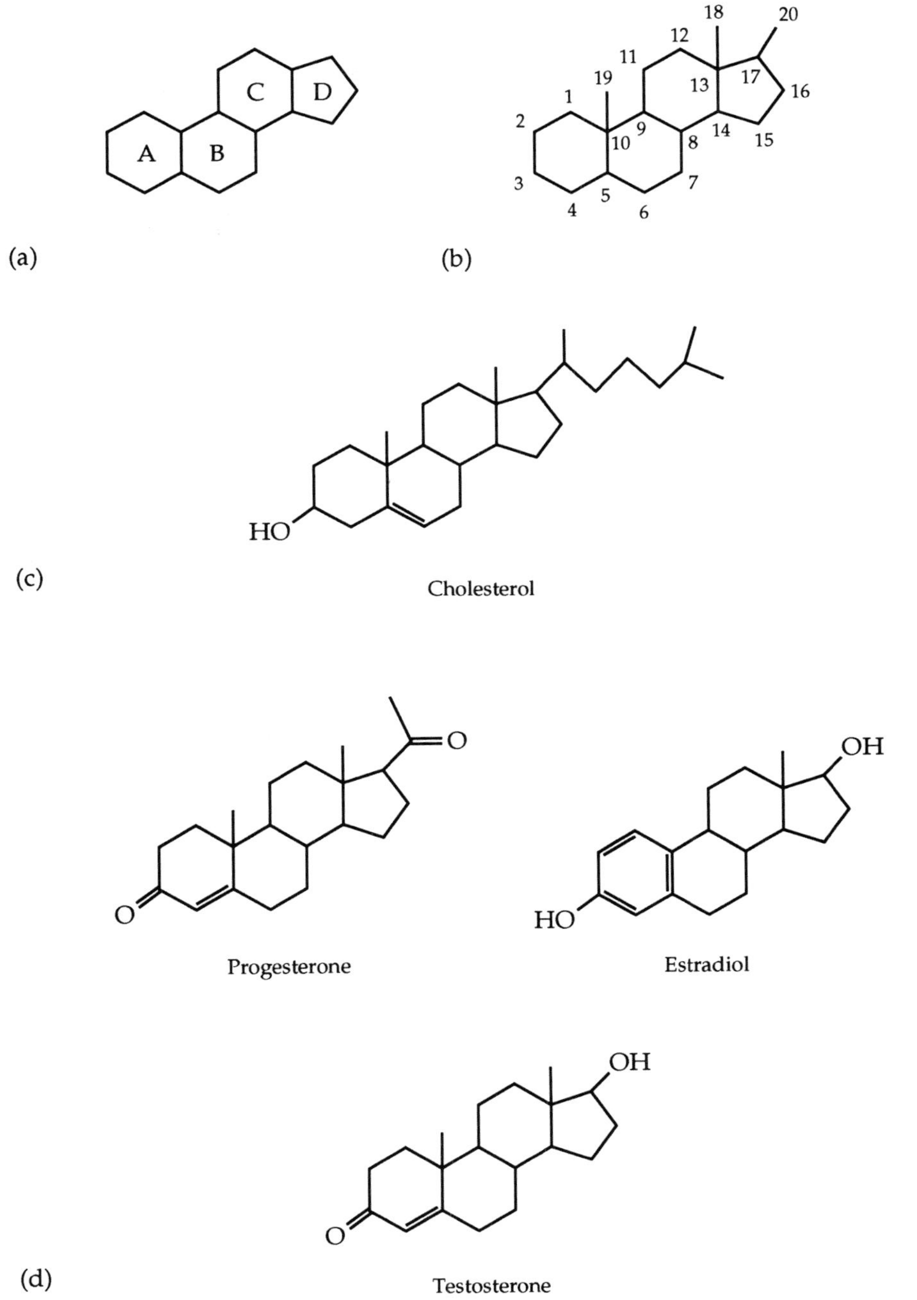

(a)

(b)

(c)   Cholesterol

Progesterone   Estradiol

(d)   Testosterone

Figure A.6   The structure of steroids. (a) The basic steroid nucleus with the fused three six membered rings and one five membered ring. (b) The numbering system for the identification of the individual carbon atoms (note that carbon atoms are actually present at each vertex although in this shorthand notation they are not shown). (c) Cholesterol. (d) The primary sex hormones.

and one of the rings is cyclopentane [five-sided], steroids differ one from another in the side chains that are attached to their common structure (figure A.6). Cholesterol and many hormones, including the sex hormones estrogen and testosterone, are steroids. Because many of the synthetic hormones used in both reproduction-aiding and reproduction-controlling treatments require structural knowledge of natural steroids, we need to have a good understanding of the nature and function of all lipids but especially of phospholipids and steroids.

Nucleic Acids

Largest of the four major organic compounds, nucleic acids are nonetheless composed of long chains of repeating smaller units called *nucleotides*. In turn, nucleotides consist of three components: a sugar (ribose or deoxyribose), a phosphate group, and a nitrogen base. Depending on whether it has one nitrogen-carbon ring or two, a nitrogen base is called a *pyrimidine* or a *purine*, respectively. Thymine, cytosine, and uracil are pyrimidines; adenine and guanine are purines.

There are two main types of nucleic acids, differentiated by the sugar used in the nucleotides: Ribonucleic acids (RNA) have ribose and deoxyribonucleic acids (DNA) have deoxyribose, a ribose with one less oxygen. RNA and DNA are each made up of four different types of nucleotides, each type containing a different nitrogen base (figure A.7). RNA nucleotides have the nitrogen bases cytosine, guanine, adenine, and uracil, whereas DNA nucleotides have the bases cytosine, guanine, adenine, and thymine.

RNA and DNA also differ in that RNA is most often a single-stranded structure, whereas DNA is most often double-stranded. Held together by many intermolecular interactions called *hydrogen bonds*, in DNA cytosine pairs up with guanine, and adenine pairs up with thymine (figure A.8). In the normal structure the two polynucleotide chains coil around each other in a structure called the double helix.

Because it is the principal component of the genes that direct all cell processes and that give each individual organism its unique identity, DNA's importance cannot be overemphasized. The sequence of bases in this nucleic acid is very precisely specified; even minute changes in this sequence prove disastrous for a cell or an entire organism. Essential to DNA's proper functioning is RNA's proper functioning, which largely consists of acting as an intermediary between DNA and the production of the proteins DNA dictates.

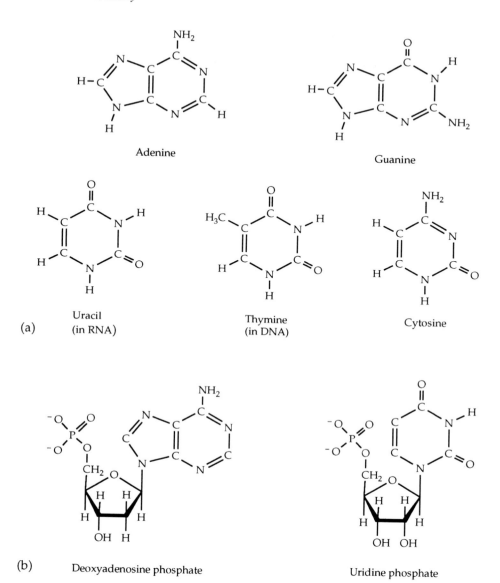

Adenine

Guanine

Uracil
(in RNA)

(a)

Thymine
(in DNA)

Cytosine

(b)   Deoxyadenosine phosphate

Uridine phosphate

Figure A.7 The structure of the chemical units that make up nucleic acids. (a) The nitrogen-containing bases present in both DNA and RNA. (b) Examples of nucleotides present in DNA and RNA. (c) A representation of a polynucleotide present in RNA. (d) A representation of a polynucleotide present in DNA.

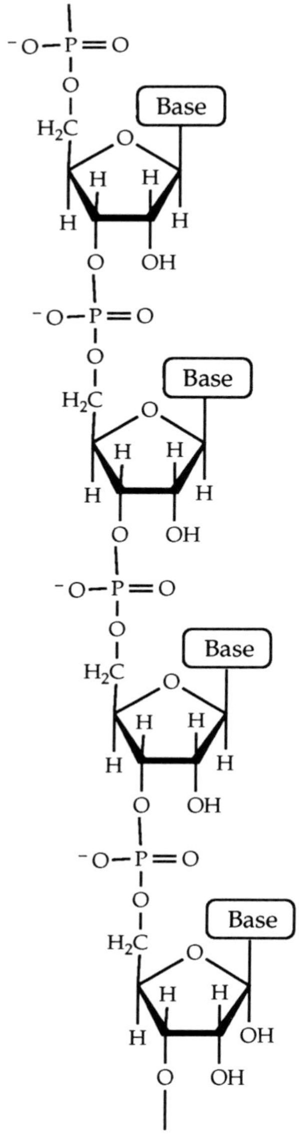

(c)

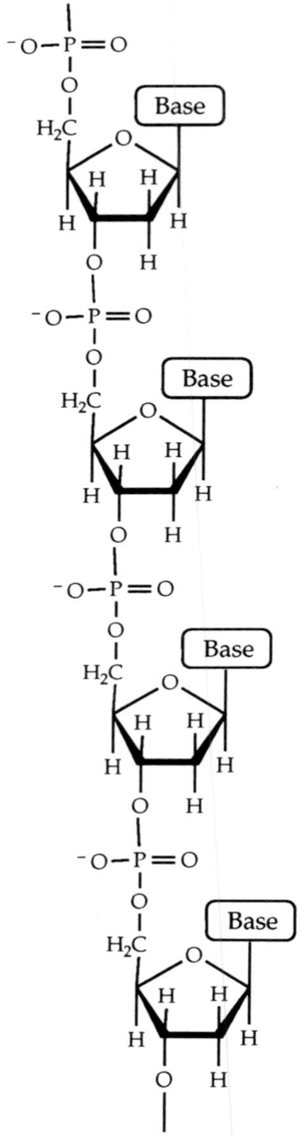

(d)

Figure A.7 (cont.)

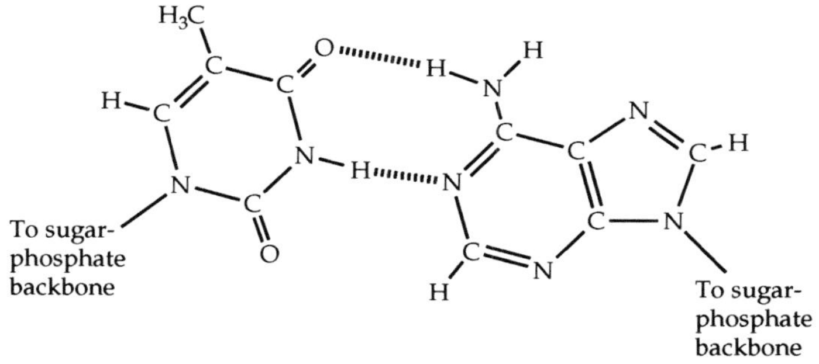

Figure A.8 The base pairing in DNA (a) between thymine and adenine; (b) between cytosine and guanine; (c) the two-dimensional structure of DNA showing the pairing of the bases and the antiparallel orientation of the two polynucleotides; (d) the double helix formed by two polynucletides twisted around one another. (From D. D. Ritchie and R. Carola, *Biology*, 2nd edition. Reading, MA: Addison-Wesley, 1983, p. 105; used with permission.)

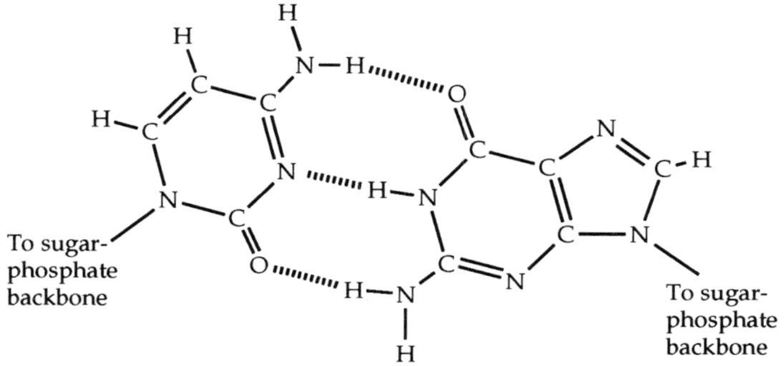

General Characteristics of the Cell

Each of us begins life as a single cell, a microscopic package containing directions for all our identifying features. Although cells are the basic building blocks of all organisms, they are far from simple. Ever since cells were first observed microscopically by the seventeenth-century Dutch merchant Anton van Leeuwenhoek and the English physicist Robert Hooke, who reported seeing "pores" or "cells" in thin slices of cork, scientists have been studying cellular structures. Although they have learned much about cells, scientists are the first to admit that much more remains to be uncovered.

Not only are the processes that take place inside and between the cells of a given species innumerable and complex, but each species has its own unique kind of cells.[5-8] Yet despite the overwhelming diversity we observe in cells, some fundamental structures and processes are common

(c)

Figure A.8 (cont.)

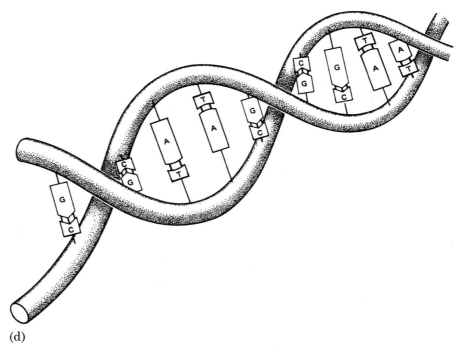

(d)

Figure A.8 (cont.)

to all of them, a fact first recognized by the nineteenth-century botanist Matthias Schleiden and zoologist Theodor Schwann. As a result of Schleiden's and Schwann's work and that of many subsequent scientists, what was common to all cells was articulated as the *cell theory* according to which:

1. All organisms are made of one or more cells.

2. Cells are alike in their structure and composition.

3. All cells carry out similar functions that keep them alive.

4. New cells arise only from old cells, usually by dividing into two equal parts at regular intervals.

That all cells share certain characteristics is reassuring because it suggests that all organisms have a common origin.

To say that cells (be they sex cells, muscle cells, liver cells, bone cells, or nerve cells) are alike in their structure and composition is not to say that they do not differ, for example, with respect to size and shape. It is to say, however, that virtually all cells have, for example, a *cell membrane* and *nucleus*. The cell (or plasma) membrane keeps the internal cellular components separate from the external environment. By permitting transportation of only certain substances into and out of the cell in a very regulated, systematic fashion, the cell membrane maintains the integrity of the cell, including the nucleus or nuclear region, in which DNA is concentrated.

In addition to a cell membrane and a nucleus, virtually all cells have a number of small organelles that move in the fluid environment called the *cytoplasm* (figure A.9). Their number, kind, and size depend on the cell's function. If the cell is involved in strenuous activity, it will have many *mitochondria*, which are involved in the production of large quantities of energy. If the cell produces large quantities of protein, either for use or for secretion, then it will have many *ribosomes*, or factories for protein synthesis. If the cell breaks down large quantities of waste, it will contain many *lysosomes*.

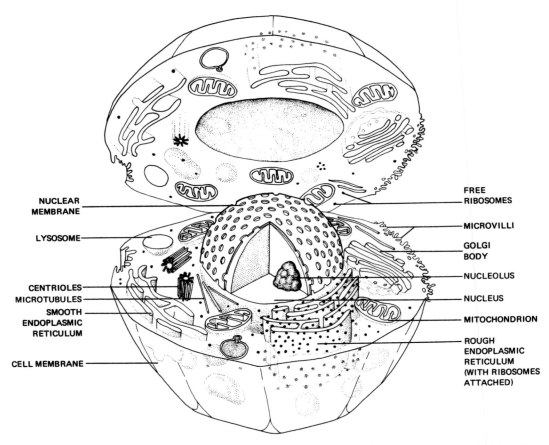

Figure A.9 Cross-section of an animal cell showing the organelles inside. This diagram is more of a theoretical cell than an actual one, which may vary in its constituents. (From D. D. Ritchie and R. Carola, *Biology*, 2nd edition. Reading, MA: Addison-Wesley, 1983, p. 52; used with permission.)

Because the cell membrane, the nucleus, and certain organelles play key roles in the reproductive process, we need to discuss at some length these common characteristics of the cell. To the degree that we understand this much of cell theory, we will deepen our appreciation of the procreative process's complexity.

Cell (Plasma) Membrane

According to the most widely accepted model, called the *fluid mosaic model*, the cell membrane is made up of a lipid bilayer of phospholipid molecules with hydrophobic tails in its interior and hydrophilic heads on its two exterior surfaces. Inside the bilayer float proteins, some of which span its entire interior but others of which are merely associated with one of its two exterior surfaces. Many of the proteins have carbohydrate branches attached and are called *glycoproteins*. Because these proteins and

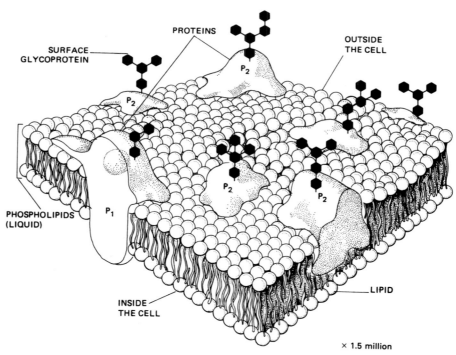

Figure A.10 Sketch of a model of a biological membrane. The phospholipids form the fundamental bilayer structure with the polar heads outside in contact with water and the nonpolar tails inside away from the water; proteins and glycoproteins are seen spanning the bilayer as integral proteins and on one surface as peripheral proteins. (From D. D. Ritchie and R. Carola, *Biology*, 2nd edition. Reading, MA: Addison-Wesley, 1983, p. 54; used with permission.)

glycoproteins engage in hormonal communication within the body, they play an essential role in the process of human reproduction as well as in many other human biological processes. A model of a cell membrane is shown in figure A.10.

Nucleus

The nucleus is usually the most visible component of a cell. (Some cells have more than one nucleus.) Except in bacteria and some blue-green algae, the nucleus is clearly delimited by a boundary that consists of not one but two double-layered membranes. Whereas organisms with membrane-bound nuclei are called *eukaryotic*, those without membrane-bound nuclei are called *prokaryotic*. There are visible pores in the nuclear membranes, allowing for the exchange of materials between the nucleus and the cytoplasm. When nuclear division takes place in the process of cell division, the membranes surrounding the nucleus are dissolved only to be reformed when nuclear division is completed.

Within the nucleus, *chromatin* is the material responsible for the nucleus's role as the cellular command center. Made up of DNA and associated specialized proteins, chromatin is coiled into bundles called *chromosomes*. These chromosomes are clearly distinguishable during nuclear division but, between nuclear divisions, the chromosomes are in a loosely coiled state and are not easily identifiable. It is during this state that the genes, the sequences of DNA coding for specific proteins, are being transcribed into RNA for subsequent translation by the ribosomes in the cytoplasm.

All higher organisms have a certain number of chromosomes characteristic of the particular species. Sexually reproducing species have paired chromosomes; human beings, for example, have 23 pairs of homologous chromosomes (the so-called haploid number) or 46 total chromosomes (the so-called diploid number). One of the chromosomes from each pair comes from the mother and the other from the father.

Over and beyond chromatin, the nucleus also contains one or more visible, rounded bodies called *nucleoli*. Composed of protein and ribosomal RNA, nucleoli are responsible for the preliminary assembly of ribosomes, which are then transported out of the nucleus into the cytoplasm.

Mitochondria

Although most of the organelles are delimited by membranes similar in structure to the cell membrane, one organelle, the mitochondria, which is principally responsible for the production of the energy-storage molecule adenosine triphosphate (ATP), has an additional inner membrane with many folds. On this inner membrane, the mitochondria's primary enzymatic activity takes place. Depending on its particular energy needs, a cell may have anywhere from two or three to hundreds of mitochondria. This can be dramatically seen in sperm that contain many mitochondria to power their movement in the female reproductive tract. Another feature that differentiates the relatively large kidney bean–shaped mitochondria from other organelles is that they contain some of their own DNA and thus are able to carry on some genetic activity by themselves.

Endoplasmic Reticulum

Another structure readily apparent in the cytoplasm is the *endoplasmic reticulum*. The endoplasmic reticulum is composed of branched and folded double membranes that are attached to its cell membrane at various points. The functions of the endoplasmic reticulum are threefold: (1) It serves to transport certain substances within the cell and to the plasma membrane for exit from the cell; (2) it helps produce membranes for the entire cell as well as for the structures within it; and (3) it serves as a site for the attachment of ribosomes, the tiny, rounded structures necessary for the synthesis of proteins.

Golgi Apparatus

Associated with the endoplasmic reticulum are membranous sacs called *Golgi bodies*, which look like stacks of disks when examined under a microscope. Apparently, cellular products caught between the folds of the endoplasmic reticulum bud off to form Golgi bodies. In turn, the Golgi bodies bud off vesicles that contain molecules formed within the cell but are destined for transportation to the outside of the cell. As the vesicles migrate through the cytoplasm to the periphery of the cell, they fuse with the cell membrane, releasing their cargo of molecules to the outside of the cell.

Ribosomes

Ribosomes, tiny particles of half protein and half RNA, float freely in the cytoplasm as well as on the endoplasmic reticulum. Containing two subunits, ribosomes are the site of the translation process whereby amino acids are lined up and bonded together to form proteins. A piece of RNA that has copied a message from the nuclear DNA supplies directions for this translation process. (During the process of transcription, the double-stranded nuclear DNA is "unzipped" and used as a template for the construction of a specifically sequenced RNA molecule from individual RNA nucleotides. After some processing, the RNA strand is transported out of the nucleus into the cytoplasm, where it becomes associated with ribosomes.)

Lysosomes

Lysosomes, containing a single membrane, are organelles in which hydrolytic enzymes are encased. In most cases, digestion occurs when the lysosomes ingest the substance to be degraded (e.g., old, unneeded cell

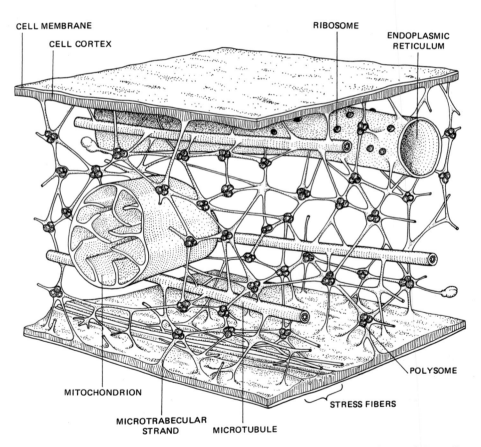

Figure A.11 A diagram of the filamentous structures in the cytoplasm of the cell. The microtrabeculae support other components in the cytoplasm. (From D. D. Ritchie and R. Carola, *Biology*, 2nd edition. Reading MA: Addison-Wesley, 1983, p. 65; used with permission.)

parts or foreign material), but in some cases, whole lysosomes burst and the very cell they inhabit is digested, as when a tadpole's tail is degraded during its development into a frog.

Microtubules

Using today's electron microscopes, cell biologists have established that organelles do not float freely in the liquid of the cytoplasm. Indeed, far from free-floating, organelles are actually surrounded and supported by a network of tiny filaments called *microtrabeculae*.

The microtrabeculae not only hold the organelles in place but also give shape to the cell (figure A.11). In addition, they are flexible enough to adjust when changes in cell shape are necessary or when organelles must change positions within the cell. Intimately connected with the microtrabeculae are the *microtubules*, straight tubular structures made of a protein called *tubulin*. Microtubules are associated with movement in amebic pseudopods, in flagella, and in cilia, which help sweep the egg along the fallopian tubes. During cell division, microtubules play a critical role by forming a network along which the chromosomes migrate as they are pulled apart. Microtubules may also play a critical role in nuclear division, but biochemists are not yet certain how best to describe this role except to say that it is played out when various microtubules arrange themselves in precise patterns of nine triplets each, called *centrioles*.

Cellular Reproduction

At any moment in the human body, millions of cells are reproducing.[9-12] The body needs a constant supply of new cells to replace dead cells, to grow, and simply to meet changing environmental demands. Biochemists differentiate between *nuclear division*, which refers only to division of the nucleus, and *cell division*, which includes cytoplasmic division as well. There are two types of nuclear division: that which takes place in the somatic (body) cells and that which takes place in the sex cells. The former is called *mitosis*, and the latter, *meiosis*. Although these processes are very similar, they are crucially different in some respects (see figure A.12).

Mitosis

The aim of mitosis is to produce two identical complements of genetic material (DNA) that are exactly the same as the parent cell's genetic

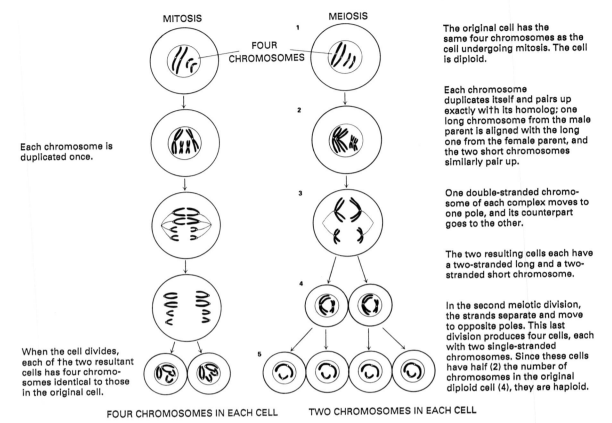

MITOSIS

MEIOSIS

FOUR CHROMOSOMES

The original cell has the same four chromosomes as the cell undergoing mitosis. The cell is diploid.

Each chromosome duplicates itself and pairs up exactly with its homolog; one long chromosome from the male parent is aligned with the long one from the female parent, and the two short chromosomes similarly pair up.

Each chromosome is duplicated once.

One double-stranded chromosome of each complex moves to one pole, and its counterpart goes to the other.

The two resulting cells each have a two-stranded long and a two-stranded short chromosome.

In the second meiotic division, the strands separate and move to opposite poles. This last division produces four cells, each with two single-stranded chromosomes. Since these cells have half (2) the number of chromosomes in the original diploid cell (4), they are haploid.

When the cell divides, each of the two resultant cells has four chromosomes identical to those in the original cell.

FOUR CHROMOSOMES IN EACH CELL   TWO CHROMOSOMES IN EACH CELL

Figure A.12 A comparison of the stages of mitosis and meiosis. (a) The result of the stages of mitosis is the production of two daughter cells containing the same amount of DNA. (b) The result of the stages of meiosis is the production of four daughter cells containing half the amount of DNA; the pictures are only discrete representative stages of the smooth transition from the initial cell to the resulting diploid (mitosis) or haploid (meiosis) cells. (From D. D. Ritchie and R. Carola, *Biology*, 2nd edition. Reading, MA: Addison-Wesley, 1983, p. 290; used with permission.)

material (DNA). Although mitosis is a smooth, continuous process, it is artificially divided into stages so that it can be explained.

Strictly speaking, stage one of mitosis, *interphase*, is not really a part of mitosis. It is a time when cellular processes other than cellular reproduction are taking place; nevertheless, the cast of characters for mitosis is assembling. Although the nucleolus is clearly visible, and although several microtubules have arranged themselves into two pair of centrioles, the chromatin is still a tangle of fine threads, the DNA of the chromosomes is very loosely coiled, and the individual chromosomes are scarcely perceptible. Only much later in interphase does DNA replication take place. As the double-stranded DNA unwinds, individual DNA nucleotides line up, match with the original DNA, and bond together to form a new strand, which is then hydrogen-bonded to its template. The end result is duplex DNA—two complete, identical sets of chromosomes (each member of a homologous pair is replicated), still very filamentous and not easily distinguishable.

When the cell is ready for nuclear division, it enters stage two, *prophase*. As the chromosomes become shorter and thicker, a light microscope shows that they are indeed doubled, their halves (chromatids) connected by a centromere. Meanwhile, the nuclear membrane disintegrates and the two pairs of centrioles start to move apart to opposite sides of the cell, a spindle of microtubules forming between them.

In stage three, *metaphase*, the now fully shortened and fully thickened chromosomes line up across the middle of the cell on the equator between the centrioles. Although some spindle fibers span all the way across the cell, others become attached only to the centromeres of the aligned chromosomes. By this time, the centromeres themselves have doubled so that each chromatid, by now a full-fledged chromosome, has its own centromere.

In stage four, *anaphase*, the chromosome pairs begin splitting up, each member of a pair moving to opposite poles of the spindle. The microtubules attached to centromeres shorten, while the poles themselves move farther apart.

When the chromosomes reach the poles of the spindle, the mitotic division is in stage five, *telophase*. The spindle begins to break down, and the chromosomes become looser and less defined again. The endoplasmic reticulum surrounds the two chromosomal masses, and two new nuclear membranes are created. Nucleoli reform and the centrioles double, so that each new cell will have two pairs of centrioles just like the parent cell. Nuclear division is now complete.

In most cells, nuclear division is followed by cytoplasm division or *cytokinesis*. In animal cells, the cell membrane pinches in between the two new nuclei, forming a *cleavage furrow*. Eventually, the furrow completely divides the cell into two separate diploid cells, each of which has identical genetic material.

Meiosis

In sexual reproduction, the offspring receive genetic information from both parents. A male gamete fuses with a female gamete to produce a cell that will develop into a new individual, with its own unique combination of genetic information. Obviously, gametes cannot have the same number of chromosomes as normal cells; otherwise, the offspring of two individuals would have double the species number of chromosomes, and successive generations would continue the doubling.

Meiosis is the mechanism employed by sexually reproducing organisms to avoid an increase in chromosome number. The end result of meiosis is the production of cells with half the number of chromosomes of normal body cells; just one member of each homologous pair ends up in a gamete. Meiosis further differs from mitosis in that in the end, four cells are produced from the original parent cell. There are two sequences of division in meiosis, meiosis I and meiosis II.

Both sequences of meiosis include the same stages as mitosis—namely, prophase, metaphase, anaphase, and telophase. In prophase I, the chromosomes double into sister chromatids connected by a centromere, and these chromosomes align themselves with their homologues. The resulting four-stranded groups are called *bivalents*. At this point, a process called *crossing over* occurs. The four chromatids become entangled, and breaks occur in the DNA stands at corresponding points. In the course of healing these breaks, a chromatid frequently exchanges a segment with another chromatid instead of reattaching its own DNA. When the exchange occurs between chromatids that are not sisters, new gene combinations on the chromosome result. After the opportunity passes for crossing over, the chromosomes shorten and thicken, and the regions of crossing over (chiasms) can be seen under a light microscope. The centrioles move to opposite sides of the cell, the nuclear membrane and nucleoli break down, and a spindle begins to form. In metaphase I, the homologous pairs line up along the equator, and spindle fibers attach to the centromeres. Then, in anaphase I, homologous chromosomes (actually still pairs of chromatids) move to opposite ends of the cell. Finally, in telophase I the migration ends, and a new nuclear membrane forms at each pole. Cytokinesis occurs, and two new cells are the result.

In meiosis II, the analogue phases of prophase, metaphase, anaphase, and telophase occur in each of the cells, the difference being that there is no further doubling of the chromosomes and no crossing over. Four haploid nuclei are the result. Cytokinesis then divides the cytoplasm evenly, producing four haploid gametes, or unevenly, favoring just one haploid cell and leaving the others to die. The former case is characteristic of spermatogenesis, and the latter of oogenesis.

Notes

Chapter 1

1. N. Tuana, "The Weaker Seed: The Sexist Bias of Reproductive Theory," *Hypatia* 3, no. 1 (Spring 1988): 36–37.

2. Ibid., 41–44.

3. W. Pagel, *William Harvey's Biological Ideas* (New York: Hafner Publishing, 1967), 314.

4. Ibid., 316.

5. Tuana, "The Weaker Seed," 52.

6. Ibid., 53.

7. Ibid., 53.

8. R. A. Hatcher, F. Guest, F. Stewart, G. K. Stewart, J. Trussell, and E. Frank, *Contraceptive Technology: 1986–1987* (New York: Irvington Publishers, 1986).

9. A. L. Wisot and D. R. Meldrum, *New Options for Fertility: A Guide to In Vitro Fertilization and Other Assisted Reproduction Methods* (New York: Pharos Books, 1990).

Chapter 2

1. R. Lacayo, "Abortion's Hardest Cases," *Time* (July 9, 1990): 23.

2. Aristotle, *The Nicomachean Ethics*, commentary by H. H. Joachim (London: Clarendon Press, 1951), 26.

3. Ibid., 38–39.

4. For a fuller discussion, see Immanuel Kant, *The Groundwork of the Metaphysics of Morals*, trans. H. J. Paton (New York: Harper & Row, 1964), 88–89.

5. A. C. MacIntyre, *After Virtue* (Notre Dame, IN: University of Notre Dame Press, 1981), 6–7.

6. Ibid., 9.

7. Ibid., 10.

8. For a complete explanation of these four liberty-limiting principles, see Joel Feinberg, *Social Philosophy* (Englewood Cliffs, NJ: Prentice-Hall, 1973), 36–55.

9. J. S. Mill, *On Liberty* (Indianapolis: Hackett Publishing Company, 1978), 9.

10. J. Elster, *Ulysses and the Sirens* (Cambridge, MA: The University Press, 1979), 36ff.

11. G. Hardin, "The Tragedy of the Commons," in *Managing the Commons*, eds. G. Hardin and J. Baden (San Francisco: W. H. Freeman and Company, 1977), 20.

12. "Wolfenden Committee Report," in *Law Liberty, and Morality*, ed. H. L. A. Hart (Stanford, CA: Stanford University Press, 1963), 14.

13. Ibid., 48–52.

14. Ibid., 19.

15. K. Vonnegut, *Welcome to the Monkey House: A Collection of Short Works* (New York: Delacorte Press, 1968).

16. Feinberg, *Social Philosophy*, 44.

17. M. Piercy, *Woman on the Edge of Time* (New York: Fawcett Crest Books, 1976), 102.

Chapter 3

1. B. Alberts, D. Bray, J. Lewis, M. Raff, K. Roberts, and J. D. Watson, *Molecular Biology of the Cell*, 2nd ed. (New York: Garland, 1989), 85.

2. B. John and K. R. Lewis, "The Meiotic Mechanism," in *Oxford Biology Readers*, ed. J. J. Head (Oxford, Eng.: Oxford University Press, 1976).

3. G. C. Williams, *Sex and Evolution* (Princeton, NJ: Princeton University Press, 1978).

4. B. Lewin, *Gene Expression: Eucaryotic Chromosomes*, vol. 2, 2nd ed. (New York: Wiley, 1980), 102–141.

5. L. Browder, *Developmental Biology* (Philadelphia: Saunders, 1980), 146–172.

6. G. C. Karp and N. J. Berrill, *Development*, 2nd ed. (New York: McGraw-Hill, 1981), 110–116.

7. J. G. Creager, *Human Anatomy and Physiology* (Belmont, CA: Wadsworth, 1983), 735–736.

8. G. Fink, "Feedback Actions of Target Hormones on Hypothalamus and Pituitary with Special Reference to Gonadal Steroids," *Annual Review of Physiology* 41 (1979): 579.

9. Karp and Berrill, *Development*, 116–138.

10. P. Grant, *Biology of Developing Systems* (New York: Holt, Rinehart & Winston, 1978), 265–282.

11. Y. Masui and H. J. Clarke, "Oocyte Maturation," *International Review of Cytology* 57 (1979): 185–282.

12. H. Peters and K. P. McNatty, *The Ovary: A Correlation of Structure and Function in Mammals* (Berkeley, CA: University of California Press, 1980), 98–106.

13. Ibid., 11–22, 60–84.

14. Creager, *Human Anatomy and Physiology*, 737–741.

15. J. S. Richards, "Hormonal Control of Ovarian Follicular Development," *Recent Progress in Hormone Research* 35 (1979): 343–373.

16. E. R. Simpson and P. C. MacDonald, "Endocrine Physiology of the Placenta," *Annual Review of Physiology* 43 (1981): 172–174.

17. D. Epel, "The Program of Fertilization," *Scientific American* 237, no. 5 (November 1977): 128–138.

18. D. Epel, "Fertilization," *Endeavour* (New Series) 4 (1980): 26–31.

19. B. M. Shapiro, R. W. Schackmann, and C. A. Gabel, "Molecular Approaches to the Study of Fertilization," *Annual Review of Biochemistry* 50 (1981): 815–843.

20. J. L. Marx, "The Mating Game: What Happens When Sperm Meets Egg," *Science* 200 (1978): 1256.

21. C. B. Metz, "Sperm and Egg Receptors Involved in Fertilization," *Current Topics in Developmental Biology* 12 (1978): 107–147.

22. J. D. Bleil and P. M. Wassarman, "Mammalian Sperm-Egg Interaction: Identification of a Glycoprotein in Mouse Egg Zonae Pellucidae Possessing Receptor Activity for Sperm," *Cell* 20 (1980): 873–882.

23. B. M. Shapiro and E. M. Eddy, "When Sperm Meets Egg: Biochemical Mechanisms of Gamete Interaction," *International Review of Cytology* 66 (1980): 257–302.

24. J. M. Bedford and G. W. Cooper, "Membrane Fusion Events in the Fertilization of Vertebrate Eggs," in *Membrane Fusion, Cell Surface Reviews*, eds. G. Poste and G. G. Nicholson (Amsterdam: Elsevier, 1978), 65–127.

25. S. Hagiwaraand and L. A. Jaffe, "Electrical Properties of Egg Cell Membranes," *Annual Review of Biophysics and Bioengineering* 8 (1979): 385–416.

26. H. Schuel, "Secretory Functions of Egg Cortical Granules in Fertilization and Development: A Critical Review," *Gamete Research* (1978): 294–382.

27. V. D. Vacquier, "Dynamic Changes of the Egg Cortex: A Review," *Developmental Biology* 84 (1981): 1–26.

28. E. G. Ridgway, J. C. Gilkey, and L. F. Jaffe, "Free Calcium Increases Explosively in Activating Medaka Eggs," *Proceedings of the National Academy of Sciences of the United States of America* 74 (1977): 623–627.

29. J. D. Johnson, D. Epel, and M. Paul, "Intracellular pH and Activation of Sea Urchin Eggs After Fertilization," *Nature* 262 (1976): 661–664.

30. Creager, *Human Anatomy and Physiology*, 758–762.

31. Z. Dickmann, J. Sen Gupta, and S. K. Dey, "Does 'Blastocyst Estrogen' Initiate Implantation?" *Science* 195 (February 18, 1977): 687.

32. P. Beaconsfield et al., "The Placenta," *Scientific American* 243, no. 2 (1980): 95.

Chapter 4

1. *Webster's New Twentieth Century Dictionary*, 2nd ed., 396.

2. *The Depo-Provera Debate: A Report by the National Women's Health Network* (Washington, DC: National Women's Health Network, 1985), 3.

3. A. Lake, "The New French Pill," *McCall's* (March 1990): 58.

4. R. A. Hatcher, F. Guest, F. Stewart, G. K. Stewart, J. Trussell, S. C. Bowen, and W. Cates, *Contraceptive Technology: 1988–1989* (New York: Irvington Publishers, 1988), 368.

5. M. J. Free and N. J. Alexander, "Male Contraception Without Prescription: A Reevaluation of the Condom and Coitus Interruptus," *Public Health Reports* 91, no. 5 (1976): 437–445.

6. World Health Organization, *Special Programme of Research, Development and Research Training in Human Reproduction*, Seventh Annual Report (Geneva: World Health Organization, 1978).

7. E. E. N. Draper, ed., "Birth Control," *The New Encyclopaedia Britannica* 15 (1985): 115.

8. Hatcher et al., *Contraceptive Technology: 1988–1989*, 308–310.

9. S. Findlay, "Birth Control," *U.S. News and World Report* 109, no. 25 (December 24, 1990): 63.

10. B. D. Geis and M. Gerrard, "Predicting Male and Female Contraceptive Behavior: A Discriminate Analysis of Groups High, Moderate, & Low in Contraceptive Effectiveness," *Journal of Personality and Social Psychology* 46, no. 3 (1984): 673.

11. Findlay, "Birth Control," 63.

12. N. B. Ryder, "Contraceptive Failure in the United States," *Family Planning Perspectives* 5, no. 133 (1973): 142.

13. Findlay, "Birth Control," 63.

14. A. Toufexis, "Comeback of a Contraceptive," *Time* 131, no. 23 (June 6, 1988): 67.

15. Findlay, "Birth Control," 63.

16. Toufexis, "Comeback of a Contraceptive," 67.

17. Findlay, "Birth Control," 63.

18. Ibid.

19. *Federal Register* 45, no. 241 (December 12, 1980).

20. R. A. Hatcher, D. Kowal, F. Guest, J. Trussell, F. Stewart, G. K. Stewart, S. C. Bowen, and W. Cates, Jr., *Contraceptive Technology: International Edition* (Atlanta: Printed Matter, 1989), 346.

21. "Plague of Problems," *Forbes* 114, no. 4 (August 15, 1974): 35

22. S. C. Huber, "IUDs Reassessed—A Decade of Experience," *Population Reports [B]* no. 2 (January 1975).

23. R. A. Hatcher, F. Guest, F. Stewart, G. K. Stewart, J. Trussell, S. Cerel, and W. Cates, *Contraceptive Technology: 1986–1987*, ed. N. B. Williams (New York: Irvington Publishers, 1986), 191–192.

24. Ibid., 192.

25. Ibid., 207.

26. N. C. Lee, G. L. Rubin, H. W. Ory, and R. T. Burkman, "Type of Intrauterine Device and the Risk of Pelvic Inflammatory Disease," *Obstetrics and Gynecology* 62, no. 1 (1983): 1–10.

27. J. Shiver, Jr., "Dalkon Shield Company Files for Bankruptcy," *Los Angeles Times* (August 22, 1985): sec. 1, 20.

28. G. Kolata, "For Those Concerned with Pill's Risk, a Look at the Choices," *The New York Times* (January 12, 1989): B10.

29. Hatcher et al., *Contraceptive Technology: 1986–1987*, 194, 197.

30. R. A. Hatcher, F. Stewart, J. Trussell, D. Kowal, F. Guest, G. K. Stewart, and W. Cates, *Contraceptive Technology: 1990–1992* (New York: Irvington Publishers, 1990).

31. E. B. Stockham, "Steroids and Birth Control," in *Applied Chemistry*, 2nd ed., ed. William R. Stine (Boston: Allyn and Bacon, 1981), 536.

32. Ibid, 537.

33. B. L. Xiao, S. Q. Shi, M. C. Jia, S. Xiao, S. L. Huang, and W. Q. Yen, "Effects of Steroid Contraceptives on Follicular Function," *Annals of the New York Academy of Sciences* 626 (June 28, 1991): 50.

34. Stockham, "Steroids and Birth Control," 537.

35. H. B. Croxatto, S. Diaz, and I. Sivin, "Contraceptive Implants," *Annals of the New York Academy of Sciences* 626 (June 28, 1991): 22–29.

36. Ibid.

37. G. Kolata, "U.S. Experts Applaud Growth in Options for Contraception," *The New York Times* (January 12, 1989): B17.

38. Hatcher et al., *Contraceptive Technology: 1990–1992*, 424.

39. Findlay, "Birth Control," 63.

40. Ibid., 60.

41. Ibid.

42. *The Depo-Provera Debate*, 16.

43. Ibid., 3.

44. Ibid., 4.

45. Ibid., 5.

46. R. Stone, "Depo-Provera. Controversial Contraceptive Wins Approval from FDA Panel," *Science* 256 (1992): 1754.

47. S. Koetsawang, "The Injectable Contraceptive: Present and Future Trends," *Annals of the New York Academy of Sciences* 626 (June 28, 1991): 30–41.

48. A. Ulmann, G. Teutsch, and D. Philibert, "RU-486," *Scientific American* 262, no. 6 (June 1990): 42–48.

49. Ibid., 47.

50. R. Peyron, E. Aubeny, V. Targosz, L. Silvestre, M. Renault, F. Elkik, P. Leclerc, A. Ulmann, and E. E. Baulieu, "Early Termination of Pregnancy with Mifepristone (RU 486) and the Orally Active Prostaglandin Misoprostol," *The New England Journal of Medicine* 328 (1993): 1509.

51. Lake, "The New French Pill," 58–59.

52. D. A. Grimes, "Reversible Contraception for the 1980s," *Journal of the American Medical Association* 225 (1986): 69–75.

53. Ibid.

54. A. E. Wilbur, "Woman's Contraceptives: Technologies of the Future," *McCall's* 114 (August 1987): 88.

55. "Appendix B: Human Reproduction and Prospective Means of Fertility Control," in *Reproduction and Human Welfare: A Challenge to Research*, R. O. Greep, M. A. Koblinsky, and F. S. Jaffe (Cambridge, MA: MIT Press, 1976), 480.

56. "New Methods for Fertility Regulation: A Status Report," in *Reproduction and Human Welfare: A Challenge to Research*, R. O. Greep, M. A. Koblinsky, and F. S. Jaffe (Cambridge, MA: MIT Press, 1976), 289–290.

57. T. H. Maugh II, "Male 'Pill' Blocks Sperm Enzyme," *Science* 212 (April 17, 1981): 314.

58. C. Ezzell, "Hormone Blockers May Yield Male 'Pill'," *Science News* 139 (1991): 407.

59. C. L. Chng, "The Male Role in Contraception: Implications for Health Education," *The Journal of School Health* 3 (March 1983): 197–201.

60. M. Fox, "New-Tech Contraception," *Health* (February 1987): 32.

61. R. Kanigel, "Lord, But It's Hard to Sell a Male Contraceptive," *John Hopkins Magazine* (August 1984): 16–20.

62. Ibid.

63. Ibid.

64. M. D. Bayles, *Reproductive Ethics* (Englewood Cliffs, NJ: Prentice-Hall, 1984), 8.

65. "Birth Control: The Pill and the Church," *Newsweek* 64 (July 6, 1964): 51.

66. N. St. John-Stevas, *Life, Death and the Law* (Bloomington: Indiana University Press, 1961), 84.

67. M. Novak, "Frequent, Even Daily, Communion," in *The Catholic Case for Contraception*, ed. Callahan, D. (New York: Macmillan, 1969), 94.

68. T. M. Shapiro, *Population Control Politics: Women, Sterilization, and Reproductive Choics* (Philadelphia: Temple University Press, 1985), 31.

69. E. R. Chasteen, *The Case for Compulsory Birth Control* (Englewood Cliffs, N.J.: Prentice-Hall, 1971), 27.

70. T. A. Mappes and J. S. Zembaty, eds., *Social Ethics: Morality and Social Policy* (New York: McGraw-Hill, 1977), 335.

71. G. Becker, *A Treatise on the Family* (Cambridge, MA: Harvard University Press, 1981), 93.

72. G. J. Stigler and G. S. Becker, "De Gustibus Non Est Disputandum," *American Economic Review* (March 1977): 76–90.

73. T. J. Samuel, "Culture and Human Fertility in India," in *Population Studies: Selected Essays and Research*, ed. K. C. W. Kammeyer (Chicago: Rand McNally 1969), 354.

74. J. Nachtuey, "Romania's Lost Children," *New York Times Magazine* (June 24, 1990): 29.

75. R. M. Veatch, "'Experimental' Pregnancy," *Hastings Center Report* no. 1 (June 1971): 2.

76. Hatcher et al., *Contraceptive Technology: 1986–1987*, p. 116.

77. Ibid., 232.

78. Ibid., 118.

79. 17 Stat. 598–600 (42nd Cong.).

80. *Tileston* v. *Ullman*, 129 Conn. 84; 26A 3d 582 (1942).

81. *Griswold* v. *Connecticut*, 381 US 480 (1965).

82. *Griswold* v. *Connecticut*, 381 US 480 (1965); *Buxton* v. *Connecticut*, 381 U.S. 479 (1965).

83. "Birth Curb Backer Gets 3-Month Term in Boston U. Case," *New York Times* 118, no. 40 (May 20, 1969): 49.

84. *Eisenstadt* v. *Baird*, 334 U.S. 438 (1972).

85. Ibid.

86. *Carey* v. *Population Services International*, 431 U.S. 678 (1977).

87. A. M. Kenney, J. D. Forest, and A. Torres, "Storm over Washington: The Parental Notification Proposal," *Family Planning Perspectives* 14, no. 4 (July/August 1982): 185.

88. Ibid., 189.

89. L. Brown and K. Garloch, "From Cradle to Grave," *The Charlotte Observer* (November 27, 1989).

90. E. R. McAnarney and W. R. Hendee, "Adolescent Pregnancy and Its Consequences," *Journal of the American Medical Association* 262, no. 1 (July 7, 1989): 74.

91. J. Leo, "Sex and Schools," *Time* 128 (November 24, 1986): 58–63.

92. Ibid., 59.

93. Ibid., 63.

94. H. Jones, "Clinic a Good, Cautious Step," *The Boston Globe* (May 31, 1987): A25.

95. W. J. Bennett, "Sex and the Education of Our Children," *America* 156 (February 14, 1987): 122.

96. W. J. Bremner and D. M. de Kretser, "Contraceptives for Males," *Signs: Journal of Women in Culture and Society* (Winter 1975): 387.

97. L. Gordon, *Woman's Body, Woman's Right: A Social History of Birth Control in America* (New York: Penguin Books, 1976), 106.

98. Ibid., 98.

99. Ibid., 42.

100. Ibid.

101. R. Petchesky, "Reproductive Choice in the Contemporary United States: A Social Analysis of Female Sterilization," in *And the Poor Get Children: Radical Perspectives on Population Dynamics*, ed. K. Michaelson (New York: Monthly Review Press, 1984), 93.

102. T. M. Shapiro, *Population Control Politics*, 44.

103. R. Arditti and S. Minden, "An Interview with Martha Quintanales, from the Third World Women's Archives," in *Test-Tube Women: What Future for Motherhood?* eds. R. Arditti, R. D. Klein, and S. Minden (London: Pandora Press, 1984), 119–128.

104. J. Fischer, "The Birth of Control," *The Charlotte Observer* (January 23, 1990): D1.

105. Toufexis, "Comeback of a Contraceptive," 67.

106. P. Bunkle, "Calling the Shots? The International Politics of Depo-Provera," in *Test-Tube Women: What Future for Motherhood?* eds. R. Arditti, R. D. Klein, and S. Minden (London: Pandora Press, 1984), 169–182.

107. Findlay, "Birth Control," 58.

108. A. Woodhouse, "Sexuality, Femininity and Fertility Control," *Women's Studies International Forum* 5, no. 1 (1982): 11.

Chapter 5

1. M. Morain, "Population Update," *The Humanist* 47 (May/June 1987): 33.

2. R. A. Hatcher, F. Guest, F. Stewart, G. K. Stewart, J. Trussell, S. C. Bomen and W. Cates, Jr., *Contraceptive Technology: 1988–1989* (New York: Irvington Publishers, 1988), 400.

3. P. McCarthy, "Sterilization and Its Discontents," *Psychology Today* 21, no. 10 (October 1987): 10.

4. G. Tailly, R. L. Vereecken, and H. Verduyn, "A Review of 357 Bilateral Vasectomies for Male Sterilization," *Fertility and Sterility* 3, no. 41 (March 1984): 425.

5. R. A. Hatcher, D. Kowal, F. Guest, J. Trussell, F. Stewart, G. K. Stewart, S. C. Bowen, and W. Cates, Jr., *Contraceptive Technology: International Edition* (Atlanta: Printed Matter, 1989): 230.

6. B. B. Errey and I. S. Edwards, "Open-ended Vasectomy: An Assessment," *Fertility and Sterility* 49, no. 2 (February 1988): 380.

7. Ibid.

8. E. Ogg, "Voluntary Sterilization," *Public Affairs* 507 (The Public Affairs Committee, 1974): 5–7.

9. Tailly, Vereecken, and Verduyn, "A Review of 357 Bilateral Vasectomies," 426.

10. E. S. Yarbro and S. A. Howards, "Vasovasostomy," *The Urologic Clinics of North America* 14, no. 3 (1987): 515–523.

11. Ibid.

12. Ogg, "Voluntary Sterilization," 5–7.

13. Ibid.

14. G. R. Huggins and S. J. Sondheimer, "Complications of Female Sterilization: Immediate and Delayed," *Fertility and Sterility* 41, no. 3 (March 1984): 338.

15. Ogg, "Voluntary Sterilization," 9–11.

16. J. E. Rioux and R. M. Soderstrom, "Sterilization Revisited," *Contemporary OB/GYN* 30, no. 2 (August 1987): 80.

17. Ibid., 81.

18. Ibid., 84–88.

19. Ibid., 90.

20. Ibid., 94.

21. Ogg, "Voluntary Sterilization," 9–11.

22. Ibid.

23. Rioux and Soderstrom, "Sterilization Revisited," 94.

24. Ibid., 97.

25. Ibid., 97,101.

26. Ibid., 103–104.

27. Huggins and Sondheimer, "Complications of Female Sterilization," 341–342.

28. Ibid.

29. Ibid., 343.

30. McCarthy, "Sterilization and Its Discontents," 10–12.

31. Huggins and Sondheimer, "Complications of Female Sterilization," 352.

32. Ibid., 353.

33. J. Feinberg, *Social Philosophy* (Englewood Cliffs, NJ: Prentice-Hall, 1973), 48.

34. A. Clarke, "Subtle Forms of Sterilization Abuse: A Reproductive Rights Analysis," in *Test-Tube Women: What Future for Motherhood?* eds. R. Arditti, R. D. Klein, and S. Minden (London: Pandora Press, 1984), 189.

35. R. G. Weisbord, *Genocide? Birth Control and the Black American* (Westport, CT: Greenwood Press, 1975), 159.

36. Ibid., 160.

37. Clarke, "Subtle Forms of Sterilization Abuse," 188.

38. Ibid., 192–202.

39. Weisbord, *Genocide? Birth Control and the Black American*, 163.

40. D. Davin, "The Single-Child Family Policy in the Countryside," in *China's One-Child Family Policy* eds. Croll, D. Davin, and P. Kane (New York: St. Martin's Press, 1985), 48–49.

41. Y. W. F. Francis, "Sickle Cell Disease," in D. Halsey and B. Johnston, eds., *Collier's Encyclopedia* 21 (1988): 8–9.

42. D. P. Warwick, "Ethics and Population Control in Developing Countries," *The Hastings Center Report* 4, no. 3 (June 1974): 3.

43. R. H. Blank, *Redefining Human Life: Reproductive Technologies and Social Policy* (Boulder, CO: Westview Press, 1984), 83.

44. R. Neville, "The Philosophical Argument," *The Hastings Center Report* 8, no. 3 (June 1978): 34.

45. H. F. Pilpel, "Know Your Rights About Voluntary Sterilization," in *Foolproof Birth Control*, ed. L. Lader (Boston: Beacon Press, 1972), 227.

46. *Hathaway* v. *Worcester City Hospital*, 475 F.2d 701 (1973).

47. T. M. Shapiro, *Population Control Politics: Women, Sterilization, and Reproductive Choice* (Philadelphia: Temple University Press, 1985), 138.

48. H. Rodriguez-Trias, *Women and the Health Care System: Sterilization Abuse* (New York: Barnard College, 1978), 26.

49. Sir Francis Galton coined the word *eugenics* in 1882, defining it as "the study of agencies under social control that may improve or impair ... future generations either physically or mentally." El. Z. Ferster, "Eliminating the Unfit—Is Sterilization the Answer," *Ohio Law Journal* 27 (1966): 591.

50. Ibid., 592.

51. Ibid., 593.

52. *Buck* v. *Bell*, 274 U.S. (1927).

53. *Buck v Bell*, 47 Sup. Ct. Rep. 584 (1927).

54. *Buck* v. *Bell*, 274 U.S. (1927) at 207.

55. Ferster, "Eliminating the Unfit," 603.

56. G. T. Felkenes, "Sterilization and the Law," in *New Dimensions in Criminal Justice*, eds. H. K. Becker, G. T. Felkenes, and P. M. Whisenand (Metuchen, N.J.: The Scarecrow Press, 1968), 132.

57. 189 Okla. 235;115 P.2d 123 (1941).

58. 62 Sup. Ct. Rep. 1110 (1942).

59. Ibid., 1660. Quoted in Felkenes, "Sterilization and the Law," 137.

60. Ibid., 1110.

61. Blank, *Redefining Human Life*, 86.

62. G. J. Annas, "Sterilization of the Mentally Retarded: A Decision for the Courts," *The Hastings Center Report* 11, no. 4 (August 1981): 18.

63. In the Matter of Lee Ann Grady, 426A 2d 467, NJ (1981).

64. Annas, "Sterilization of the Mentally Retarded," 18.

65. Warwick, "Ethics and Population Control in Developing Countries," 3.

66. M. D. Bayles, "Limits to a Right to Procreate," in *Having Children: Philosophical and Legal Reflections on Parenthood*, eds. O. O'Neill and W. Ruddick (New York: Oxford University Press, 1979), 14.

67. The Simon Population Trust, "Vasectomy: Follow-up of a Thousand Cases," in *Foolproof Birth Control*, ed. L. Lader (Boston: Beacon Press, 1972), 131–140.

68. S. Findlay, "Birth Control," *U.S. News and World Report* 109, no. 25 (December 24, 1990): 58.

69. Ibid., 62–63.

70. H. B. Presser, "Voluntary Sterilization—A World View," in *Foolproof Birth Control*, ed. L. Lader (Boston: Beacon Press, 1972), 185.

71. J. A. Rogue, "Operation Lawsuit," in *Foolproof Birth Control*, ed. L. Lader (Boston: Beacon Press, 1972), 241.

72. E. Campbell, *The Childless Marriage: An Exploratory Study of Couples Who Do Not Want Children* (London: Tavistock, 1985), 133.

73. Ad Hoc Women's Studies Committee Against Sterilization Abuse, *Workbook on Sterilization* (New York: Sarah Lawrence College, 1978), 16.

74. Clarke, "Subtle Forms of Sterilization Abuse," 193.

75. G. Bock, "Racism and Sexism in Nazi Germany: Motherhood, Compulsory Sterilization and the State," in *When Biology Became Destiny: Women in Weimar and Nazi Germany*, eds. R. Brindenthal, A. Grossmann, and M. Kaplan (New York: Monthly Review Press, 1984), 271–296.

76. Clarke, "Subtle Forms of Sterilization Abuse," 196–202.

Chapter 6

1. H. D. Swanson, *Human Reproduction: Biology and Social Change* (New York: Oxford University Press, 1974), 244.

2. M. Dixon, *The Future of Women* (San Francisco: Synthesis Publications, 1983), 129.

3. D. Callahan, *Abortion: Law, Choice and Morality* (New York: Macmillan, 1972), 34.

4. R. A. Hatcher, F. Guest, F. Stewart, G. K. Stewart, J. Trussell, and E. Frank, *Contraceptive Technology: 1986–1987* (New York: Irvington Publishers, 1986), 265–266.

5. Ibid., 270.

6. F. Stewart, F. Guest, G. Stewart, and R. Hatcher, *Understanding Your Body* (New York: Bantam, 1987), 398.

7. Ibid., 191.

8. Ibid., 30.

9. I. W. Sherman and V. G. Sherman, *Biology: A Human Approach*, 3rd ed. (New York: Oxford University Press, 1983), 205.

10. Hatcher et al., *Contraceptive Technology: 1986–1987*, 268.

11. C. Tietze, "Somatic Consequences of Abortion," in *Abortion: Obtained and Denied*, eds. S. H. Newman, M. B. Beck, and S. Lewit (Bridgeport, CT: Key Book Service, 1971).

12. I. M. Cushner, "Outcomes of Induced Abortion: Medical-Clinical View," in *Abortion: Obtained and Denied*, eds. S. H. Newman, M. B. Beck, and S. Lewit (Bridgeport, CT: Key Book Service, 1971), 24–26.

13. Ibid., 26–28.

14. Ibid., 28–29.

15. Hatcher et al., *Contraceptive Technology: 1986–1987*, 274.

16. D. M. Horstmann, "Viral Infections," in *Medical Complications During Pregnancy*, eds. G. N. Burrow and T. F. Ferris (Philadelphia: Saunders, 1975), 415–416.

17. R. V. Lee, "Parasitic Infections," in *Medical Complications During Pregnancy*, eds. G. N. Burrow and T. F. Ferris (Philadelphia: Saunders, 1975), 446–449.

18. Rev. A. S. Moraczewski, "Genetic Diagnosis," in *Genetic Medicine and Engineering*, ed. A. S. Moraczewski (St. Louis: The Catholic Health Association of the U.S. and the Pope John XXIII Medical-Moral Research and Education Center, 1983), 15.

19. R. H. Blank, *Redefining Human Life: Reproductive Technologies and Social Policy* (Boulder, CO: Westview Press, 1984), 59.

20. W. Isaacson, "The Battle Over Abortion," *Time* 117 (April 6,1981): 20.

21. C. Curran, "Abortion: Contemporary Debate in Philosophical and Religious Ethics," in *Encyclopedia of Bioethics*, ed. W. Reich (New York: Free Press, 1978), 17.

22. F. S. Jaffe, "Enacting Religious Beliefs in a Pluralistic Society," *The Hastings Center Report* 8, no. 4 (August, 1978): 14.

23. J. F. Donceel, "Immediate Animation and Delayed Hominization," *Theological Studies* 31 (1970): 76–105.

24. W. Ruff, "Individualität und Personalität in Embryonalen Werden," *Theologie und Philosophie* 45 (1970): 24–59.

25. J. T. Noonan, Jr., "An Almost Absolute Value in History," in *Today's Moral Problems*, 3rd. ed., ed. R. Wasserstrom (New York: Macmillan, 1985), 416–417.

26. Ibid, 416.

27. M. Tooley, "Abortion and Infanticide," *Philosophy and Public Affairs* 2 (1972): 37–65.

28. H. T. Engelhardt, Jr., "The Ontology of Abortion," *Ethics* 84 (1974): 217–234.

29. R. B. Brandt, "The Morality of Abortion," *Monist* 56 (1972): 503–526.

30. Callahan, *Abortion: Law, Choice and Morality*, 349–404, 493–501.

31. L. R. Churchill and J. J. Simón, "Abortion and the Rhetoric of Individual Rights," *Hastings Center Report* 12, no. 1 (February 1982): 10.

32. Ibid., 12.

33. E. A. Langerak, "Abortion: Listening to the Middle," *The Hastings Center Report* 9, no. 5 (October 1979): 25.

34. Ibid., 28.

35. B. Brody, *Ethics and Its Applications* (New York: Harcourt, Brace, Jovanovich, 1983), 138.

36. Ibid.

37. J. J. Thomson, "A Defense of Abortion," in *Today's Moral Problems*, 3rd ed., ed. Richard Wasserstrom, (New York: Macmillan, 1985), 425.

38. Ibid., 421–423.

39. Ibid., 423.

40. Ibid., 420–421.

41. Ibid., 426.

42. Brody, *Ethics and Its Applications*, 152.

43. Ibid.

44. Ibid., 153.

45. Isaacson, "The Battle Over Abortion," 23.

46. J. M. Finnis, "Abortion: Legal Aspects," in *Encyclopedia of Bioethics*, ed. W. Reich, (New York: Free Press, 1978), 27.

47. *Roe* v. *Wade*, 410 U.S., 113, 93 S.Ct. 705, 35 L. ed. 2D. 147 (1973); in *Congressional Record*, Vol. 119, no. 29, February 26,1973, 3.

48. Finnis, "Abortion: Legal Aspects," 27–28.

49. D. Hevesi, "How Debate Over Abortion Evolved with Changes in Science and Society," *The New York Times* (July 4,1989): 11.

50. *Roe* v. *Wade*, 5.

51. Hevesi, "How Debate Over Abortion Evolved," 9.

52. Ibid.

53. *Roe* v. *Wade*, 5.

54. J. H. Ely, "The Wages of Crying Wolf: A Comment on *Roe* v. *Wade*," *The Yale Law Journal* 82 (1973): 932.

55. Ibid., 933.

56. G. Kolata, "Early Tests on Viability of a Fetus Are Limited," *The New York Times* (July 4,1989): 10.

57. *Doe* v. *Bolton*, 410 U.S. 179 (1973).

58. Ibid.

59. L. Fox, "The 1983 Abortion Decisions: Clarification of the Permissible Limits of Abortion Regulation," *University of Richmond Law Review* 18, no. 137 (1983): 137.

60. *Maher* v. *Roe*, 432 U.S. (1977).

61. *Beal* v. *Doe*, 432 U.S. (1977).

62. Hyde Amendment, 1977, Pub. L. No. 95-130, 91 Stat. 1153; Pub. L. No. 95-165, 91 Stat. 1323.

63. American Civil Liberties Union, New York, Report, *The Impact of the Hyde Amendment on Medically Necessary Abortions* (October 1978), 2.

64. From a discussion of this suit, in M. Steinfels, "Is Abortion a Religious Issue?" *Hastings Center Report* 8, no. 4 (August 1978): 12.

65. *Harris* v. *McRae*, in *The United States Law Week*, Vol. 48, no. 50, June 29, 1980, 4943.

66. Ibid., 4946.

67. ACLU Report (October 1987), 5.

68. Ibid., 20.

69. Ibid., 25–49.

70. Ibid., 8–9.

71. M. Steinfels, "Is Abortion a Religious Issue?"; B. Brody, "Religious, Moral & Sociological Issues: Some Basic Distinctions;" F. S. Jaffe, "Enacting Religious Beliefs in a Pluralistic Society"; and L. Newton, "The Irrelevance of Religion in the Abortion Debate," *The Hastings Center Report* 8, no. 4 (August 1978): 12–17.

72. *Harris* v. *McRae*, 4946.

73. Ibid., 4947.

74. Ibid., 4949.

75. Ibid., 4950.

76. Ibid., 4951.

77. *Planned Parenthood of Central Missouri* v. *Danforth*, 428 U.S. 52 (1976).

78. *Bellotti* v. *Baird*, 443 U.S. 622 (1979).

79. *Poe* v. *Gerstein*, 517 F.2d 787, 793 (1975).

80. *H. L.* v. *Matheson*, 450 U.S. 398 (1981).

81. M. Carlson, "Abortlon's Hardest Cases," *Time* (July 9, 1990): 26–27.

82. *Akron, Ohio, Codified Ordinances* Ch. 1879,1870.03 (1978).

83. *Thornburgh* v. *American College of Obstetricians and Gynecologists* 106 S.Ct. 2196 (1986).

84. *City of Akron* v. *Akron Center for Reproductive Health*, 106 S.Ct. 1517 (1983).

85. *Planned Parenthood Association of Kansas City* v. *Asberoft*, 103 S.Ct. 1532 (1983).

86. *Simopoulos* v. *Virginia*, 1035.Ct. (1983).

87. L. Greenhouse, "Change in Course: A Right Is Challenged—Justices Accept More Cases on the Issue," *The New York Times* (July 4,1989): 1,10.

88. *Hallmark Clinic* v. *North Carolina Department of Human Resources*, 380F., Supp. 1153, D.N.C. 1979, 1157–1158.

89. Greenhouse, "Change in Course," 1.

90. *Turnock v. Ragsdale* 112 S.Ct. 1309 (1992).

91. "The Court vs. Abortion" [editorial], *Charlotte Observer* (May 28,1991).

92. E. Goodman, "Court Says the Government that Pays Your Rent Can Buy Your Speech" *Charlotte Observer* (May 27, 1991): 11A.

93. Greenhouse, "Change in Course," 1A.

94. Ibid.

95. Carlson, "Abortion's Hardest Cases," 26.

96. Jaffe, "Enacting Religious Beliefs in a Pluralistic Society," 15.

97. A. Lacy, "A Presumption Against Killing," *The Chronicle Review* (March 5, 1979): R8.

98. R. A. Lake, "The Metaethical Framework of Anti-Abortion Rhetoric," *Signs: Journal of Women in Culture and Society* 11, no. 3 (1986): 480.

99. Ibid., 481.

100. F. Kissling, "Ending the Abortion War: A Modest Proposal," *The Christian Century* (February 21,1990): 183.

101. Carlson, "Abortion's Hardest Cases," 26.

102. C. H. Baron, "Fetal Research: The Question in the States," *The Hastings Center Reports* 15, no. 2 (April 1985): 13.

103. J. A. Robertson, "Rights, Symbolism, and Public Policy in Fetal Tissue Transplants," *The Hastings Center Report* 18, no. 6 (December 1988): 6.

104. E. Willis, "Putting Women Back into the Abortion Debate," *Village Voice* (July 16, 1985): 15.

105. Ibid.

106. "The Scarlet A," *Time* (September 11, 1978): 22.

107. L. S. Cahill, "'Abortion Pill' RU 486: Ethics, Rhetoric, and Social Practice," *The Hastings Center Report* 17, no. 5 (October/November 1987): 7.

108. W. Brown, "Reproductive Freedom and the Right to Privacy: A Paradox for Feminists," in *Families, Politics, and Public Policy: A Feminist Dialogue on Women and the State*, ed. I. Diamond (New York: Longman, 1983), 335.

109. C. Gilligan, *In a Different Voice: Psychological Theory and Women's Development* (Cambridge, MA: Harvard University Press, 1982), 26.

110. Ibid., 28–29.

111. L. Kohlberg, "From Is to Ought: How to Commit the Naturalistic Fallacy and Get Away With It in the Study of Moral Development," in *Cognitive Development and Epistemology* ed. T. Mischel (New York: Academic, 1971), 164–165.

112. Gilligan, *In a Different Voice*, 92.

113. Brown, "Reproductive Freedom and the Right to Privacy," 335.

114. Carlson, "Abortion's Hardest Cases," 24.

Chapter 7

1. C. M. March, "Recurrent Abortion," in *Infertility, Contraception and Reproductive Endocrinology*, eds. D. R. Mishell, Jr., and V. Davajan (Oradell, NJ: Medical Economics, 1986), 539.

2. V. Davajan and D. R. Mishell, Jr., "Evaluation of the Infertile Couple," in *Infertility, Contraception and Reproductive Endocrinology*, eds. D. R. Mishell, Jr., and V. Davajan (Oradell, NJ: Medical Economics, 1986), 381.

3. Office of Technological Assessment, *Infertility: Medical and Social Choices* (Washington, DC: U. S. Government Printing Office, May 1988), 55.

4. Ibid., 56.

5. Davajan and Mishell, Jr., "Evaluation of the Infertile Couple," 381.

6. Office of Technological Assessment, *Infertility*, 51.

7. Ibid., 64.

8. M. Perloe, *Miracle Babies and Other Happy Endings for Couples with Fertility Problems* (New York: Rawson Associates, 1986), 126.

9. R. H. Glass and R. J. Ericsson, *Getting Pregnant in the 1980s* (Berkeley, CA: University of California Press, 1989), 21.

10. Perloe, *Miracle Babies and Other Happy Endings*, 158.

11. Ibid., 158.

12. Ibid., 163.

13. Ibid., 161.

14. Ibid., 162.

15. Ibid., 163.

16. Ibid., 192.

17. Glass and Ericsson, *Getting Pregnant in the 1980s*, 19.

18. March, "Recurrent Abortion," 539.

19. Perloe, *Miracle Babies and Other Happy Endings*, 200.

20. Ibid., 200–201.

21. March, "Recurrent Abortion," 540.

22. Ibid., 541.

23. Ibid., 541.

24. Perloe, *Miracle Babies and Other Happy Endings*, 203.

25. C. M. March, "Hysteroscopy and the Uterine Factor in Infertility," in *Infertility, Contraception and Reproductive Endocrinology*, eds. D. R. Mishell, Jr., and V. Davajan (Oradell, NJ: Medical Economics, 1986), 473.

26. Perloe, *Miracle Babies and Other Happy Endings*, 205.

27. March, "Hysteroscopy and the Uterine Factor in Infertility," 479.

28. March, "Recurrent Abortion," 543.

29. Perloe, *Miracle Babies and Other Happy Endings*, 206.

30. Ibid., 206.

31. Glass and Ericsson, *Getting Pregnant in the 1980s*, 62.

32. March, "Recurrent Abortion," 546.

33. Glass and Ericsson, *Getting Pregnant in the 1980s*, 64.

34. Ibid., 64.

35. Perloe, *Miracle Babies and Other Happy Endings*, 208.

36. Ibid., 209.

37. Glass and Ericsson, *Getting Pregnant in the 1980s*, 67.

38. B. B. Goldberg, *Diagnostic Uses of Ultrasound* (New York: Grune & Stratton, 1975).

39. F. Fuchs, "Genetic Amniocentesis," *Scientific American* 242, no. 6 (June 1980): 47–53.

40. F. Stewart, F. Guest, G. Stewart, and R. Hatcher, *Understanding Your Body: Every Woman's Guide to Gynecology and Health* (New York: Bantam Books, 1987), 156.

41. Ibid., 157.

42. Glass and Ericsson, *Getting Pregnant in the 1980s*, 37.

43. Ibid., 44.

44. Perloe, *Miracle Babies and Other Happy Endings*, 80.

45. Glass and Ericsson, *Getting Pregnant in the 1980s*, 45.

46. Perloe, *Miracle Babies and Other Happy Endings*, 83.

47. Ibid., 84.

48. Ibid., 84.

49. Ibid., 58.

Chapter 8

1. "The Birthpangs of a New Science," *The Economist* 292, no. 7350 (July 14, 1984): 79–83.

2. R. H. Blank, "Making Babies: The State of the Art," *The Futurist* 19, no. 1 (1985): 11–17.

3. H. Brotman, "In Search of a Baby," *Consumers Digest* (1985): 47–50.

4. C. Wallis, "The New Origins of Life," *Time* 124, no. 11 (September 10, 1984): 46–53.

5. "Clearplan Easy Clinical Profile," Whitehall Laboratories, New York, 1993.

6. G. Corea, *The Mother Machine* (New York: Harper & Row, 1985), 12.

7. B. J. Jensen, "Artificial Insemination and the Law," *Brigham Young University Law Review* (1982): 938.

8. R. H. Asch and S. J. Silber, "Microsurgical Epididymal Sperm Aspiration and Assisted Reproductive Techniques," *Annals of the New York Academy of Sciences*, 626 (June 28, 1991): 101–109.

9. Ibid.

10. R. Iizuka, "Artificial Insemination: Progress and Clinical Applications," *Annals of the New York Academy of Sciences*, 626 (June 28, 1991): 399–413.

11. J. A. Kahn, A. Sunde, V. von Düring, T. Sordal, and K. Molne, "Intrauterine Insemination," *Annals of the New York Academy of Sciences*, 626 (June 28, 1991): 452–459.

12. Iizuka, "Artificial Insemination," 405.

13. Ibid.

14. U.S. Congress, Office of Technological Assessment, *Artificial Insemination Practice in the United States* (Washington, DC: U.S. Government Printing Office, 1988), 64–67.

15. G. Annas, "Fathers Anonymous: Beyond the Best Interests of the Sperm Donor," *Family Law Quarterly* 14, no. 1 (Spring, 1980): 1.

16. N. St. John-Stevas, *Life, Death and the Law* (Bloomington: Indiana University Press, 1961), 123, note 3.

17. Ibid., 122–123.

18. Ibid., 124.

19. G. Kelly, "Artificial Insemination: Theological and Natural Law Aspects," *University of Detroit Law Journal* 33 (1955–56): 135.

20. P. Singer and D. Wells, *Making Babies: The New Science and Ethics of Conception* (New York: Charles Scribner's Sons, 1985), 38.

21. St. John-Stevas, *Life, Death and the Law*, 127.

22. Singer and Wells, *Making Babies*, 57.

23. R. Snowden and G. D. Mitchell, *The Artificial Family* (London: Unwin Paperbacks, 1983), 121.

24. S. Bok, *Lying: Moral Choice in Public and Private Life* (New York: Pantheon Books, 1978), 204–219.

25. G. Annas, "Beyond the Best Interests of the Sperm Donor," *Child Welfare* 15, no. 13 (March 1981): 1969.

26. K. Venturatos Lorio, "Alternative Means of Reproduction: Virgin Territory for Legislation," *Louisiana Law Review* 44 (1984): 1649.

27. St. John-Stevas, *Life, Death and the Law*, 144.

28. Annas, "Fathers Anonymous," 7.

29. L. T. Styron, "Artificial Insemination: A New Frontier for Medical Malpractice and Medical Products Liability," *Loyola Law Review* 32 (1986): 414.

30. Singer and Wells, *Making Babies*, 42–46.

31. Corea, *The Mother Machine*, 22.

32. C. L. Allen, "Making Birth Conceivable Through Artificial Means," *Insight* 4, no. 8 (July 11, 1988): 15.

33. B. Menning, "Donor Insemination: The Psychosocial Issues," *American College of Gynecology and Obstetrics* 18 (1981): 155–171.

34. P. Creighton, *Artificial Insemination by Donor: A Study of Ethics, Medicine, and Law in our Technological Society* (Toronto, Canada: The Anglican Book Centre, 1977), 20.

35. R. Rowland, "The Social and Psychological Consequences of Secrecy in Artificial Insemination by Donor (AID) Programmers," *Social Science Medicine* 21, no. 4 (1985): 395.

36. Corea, *The Mother Machine*, 54–55.

37. Styron, "Artificial Insemination," 411–446.

38. Rowland, "The Social and Psychological Consequences of Secrecy," 395.

39. *L.* v. *L.*, (1949) 1 All E.R. 141, 146.

40. Singer and Wells, *Making Babies*, 57.

41. *Oxford* v. *Oxford*, 58 D.L.R. 251 (Ontario Supreme Court, 1921) at 258.

42. *Doornbus* v. *Doornbus*, No. 54-5-14981 (Illinois Superior CT., Dec. 13, 1954), appeal dismissed, 12 Ill. App. 2d 473,139 N.E. 2d 844 (1956).

43. 1958 Sess. Cas. 105 (Scot) at 113.

44. *Strnad* v. *Strnad*, 78 N.Y. Supplement, 2nd Ser. (1948) at 391–392.

45. *People* v. *Sorenson*, 68 Cal. 2d 280, 66 Cal. Rpt. (1968), 437P.

46. Jensen, "Artificial Insemination and the Law," 955–956.

47. Corea, *The Mother Machine*, 49.

48. *C.M.* v. *C.C.*, 170 N.J. Superior Ct. 586, 407 A. 2d 849, 852 (Juv. & Dom. Rel. Ct. 1979).

49. G. Williams, *The Sanctity of Life and the Criminal Law* (New York: Alfred A. Knopf, 1970), 120.

50. Creighton, *Artificial Insemination by Donor*, 50.

51. R. M. Titmuss, *The Gift Relationship: From Human Blood to Social Policy* (New York: Pantheon Books, 1971), 113–115.

52. Snowden and Mitchell, *The Artificial Family* 67.

53. Allen, "Making Birth Conceivable Through Artificial Means," 15.

54. Singer and Wells, *Making Babies*, 53–54.

55. F. Hornstein, "Children by Donor Insemination: A New Choice for Lesbians," in *Test-Tube Women: What Future for Motherhood?* eds. R. Arditti, R. D. Klein, and S. Minden (London: Pandora Press, 1984), 373–379.

56. R. Levine, "My Body, My Life, My Baby, My Rights," *Human Rights* 12 (Spring 1984): 27.

57. Ibid.

58. Ibid.

59. Ibid., 48–50.

60. R. D. Klein, "Doing It Ourselves: Self Insemination," in *Test-Tube Women: What Future for Motherhood?* eds. R. Arditti, R. D. Klein, and S. Minden (London: Pandora Press, 1984), 388.

61. Ibid.

62. Annas, "Beyond the Best Interests of the Sperm Donor," 71.

63. M. Curie-Cohen, " Current Practice of Artificial Insemination by Donor in the United States," *New England Journal of Medicine* 300 (March 1979): 585–590.

64. G. J. Annas, "Artificial Insemination: Beyond the Best Interests of the Donor," *Hastings Center Report* 9 (August 1979): 15.

65. AATB Reproductive Council, *Guidelines for the Banking of Human Sperm.* Approved at the Third Annual Meeting of the AATB, New Orleans, Louisiana (May 1979).

66. M. S. Frankel, "Artificial Insemination and Semen Cryobanking: Health Concerns and the Roles of the Professional," in *The Public Policy Dimensions of Artificial Insemination and Human Cryobanking*, ed. M. S. Frankel (Washington: Program of Policy Studies in Science and Technology, George Washington University, 1973).

67. *Ravenis* v. *Detroit General Hospital*, 234 NW 2d 411 (Michigan Court of Appeals, August 11, 1975).

68. Annas, "Artificial Insemination: Beyond the Best Interests of the Donor," 15.

69. J. Huxley, "Eugenics: Evolutionary Perspective," *Perspectives in Biology and in Medicine* 6 (Winter 1963): 178.

70. Reilly, *Genetics, Law and Social Policy*, 204.

71. R. T. Hull, ed., *Ethical Issues in the New Reproductive Technologies* (Belmont, CA: Wadsworth, 1990), 51–52.

72. M. Curie-Cohen, L. Luttrell, and S. Shapiro, "Current Practice of Artificial Insemination by Donor in the United States," *New England Journal of Medicine* 300, no. 11 (March 1979): 588.

73. Hull, *Ethical Issues in the New Reproductive Technologies*, 52.

74. Corea, The Mother Machine, 34.

75. Ibid., 35.

76. Ibid.

77. Ibid., 41.

78. R. Scott, *The Body as Property* (New York: The Viking Press, 1986), 213–214.

79. S. R. Leiblum and C. Barbrack, "Artificial Insemination by Donor: A Survey of Attitudes and Knowledge in Medical Students and Infertile Couples," *Journal of Biosocial Science* 15 (1983): 169.

80. Ibid., 170.

81. Williams, *The Sanctity of Life and the Criminal Law*, 126–127.

82. G. Hanscombe, "The Right to Lesbian Parenthood," *Journal of Medical Ethics* 9 (1983): 133.

83. Hull, *Ethical Issues in the New Reproductive Technologies*, 52.

84. Hanscombe, "The Right to Lesbian Parenthood," 133.

85. M. O'Brien Steinfels, "AID and the Single Welfare Mother," *Hastings Center Report* 13 (February 1983): 23.

86. Corea, *The Mother Machine*, 21.

87. Ibid., 25

88. Ibid., 25–26.

89. M. Piercy, *Woman on the Edge of Time* (New York: Fawcett Crest Books, 1976).

Chapter 9

1. A. Rosenfeld, "The Case for Test-Tube Babies," *Saturday Review* (October 28, 1978): 10–14.

2. Ibid.

3. Ethics Advisory Board, Department of Health, Education, and Welfare, "Report and Conclusions: HEW Support of Research Involving Human *In Vitro* Fertilization and Embryo Transfer," (May 4, 1979).

4. J. A. Treichel, "Embryo Transfer Achieved in Humans," *Science News* (July 30, 1983): 69.

5. A. Bass, "A Barren Time for Infertility Research," *Technology Review* 87, no. 6 (August/September 1984): 75.

6. Ibid.

7. C. Grobstein, "External Human Fertilization," *Scientific American* 240, no. 6 (June 1979): 57–67.

8. M. I. Evans, A. B. Mukherjee, and J. D. Schulman, "Human *In Vitro* Fertilization," *Obstetrical and Gynecological Survey* 35 (1980): 71–81.

9. G. B. Kolata, "*In Vitro* Fertilization: Is It Safe and Repeatable?" *Science* 201, no. 4356 (1978): 698–699.

10. L. J. DeCrespigny, C. O'Herlihy, I. J. Hoult, and H. P. Robinson, "Ultrasound in an In Vitro Fertilization Program," *Fertility and Sterility*, 35 (1981): 25.

11. R. G. Edwards, and P. C. Steptoe, "Induction of Follicular Growth, Ovulation and Luteinization in the Human Ovary," *Journal of Reproduction and Fertility, Supplement* 22 (1975): 121.

12. R. G. Edwards, P. C. Steptoe, and J. M. Purdy, "Establishing Fullterm Human Pregnancies using Cleaving Embryos Grown In Vitro," *British Journal of Obstetrics and Gynaecology* 87 (1980): 737.

13. P.C. Steptoe, R. G. Edwards, and J. M. Purdy, "Clinical Aspects of Pregnancies Established with Cleaving Embryos Grown In Vitro," *British Journal of Obstetrics and Gynaecology* 87 (1980): 757.

14. R. G. Edwards, P. C. Steptoe, G. E. Abraham, E. Walter, J. M. Purdy, and K. Fotherby, "Steroid Assays and Preovulating Follicular Development in Human Ovaries Primed with Gonadotropins," *Lancet* 2 (1972): 611.

15. P. C. Steptoe and R. G. Edwards, "Laparoscopic Recovery of Preovulatory Human Oocytes after Priming of Ovaries with Gonadotropins, *Lancet* 1 (1970): 683.

16. R. G. Edwards, "Test-Tube Babies," *Nature* 293 (1981): 253–256.

17. Edwards and Steptoe, "Induction of Follicular Growth, Ovulation and Luteinization," 121.

18. A. L. Wisot, and D. R. Meldrum, *New Options for Fertility: A Guide to in vitro Fertilization and Other Assisted Reproduction Methods* (New York: Pharos Books, 1990), 102.

19. A. Lopata, I. W. Johnston, I. J. Houalt, and A. L. Speirs, "Pregnancy Following Intra Uterine Implantation of an Embryo Obtained by in vitro Fertilization of a Preovulatory Egg," *Fertility and Sterility* 33 (1980): 117.

20. C. R. Austin, "Scientific and Clinical Aspects of Fertilization and Implantation," *Proceedings of the Royal Society of Medicine* 67 (1974): 23.

21. P. Soupart and L. L. Morgenstern, "Human Sperm Capacitation and *In Vitro* Fertilization," *Fertility and Sterility* 24 (1973): 462–478.

22. Robert G. Edwards, B. D. Bavister, and Paul C. Steptoe, "Early Stages of Fertilization *In Vitro* of Human Oocytes Matured *In Vitro*," *Nature* 221 (1969): 632.

23. Edwards, "Test-Tube Babies," 253–256.

24. C. B. Jacobson, J. G. Sites, and L. F. Arias-Bernal, "*In Vitro* Maturation and Fertilization of Human Follicular Oocytes," *International Journal of Fertility* 15 (1970): 103.

25. S. Oehninger, D. Franken, T. Kruger, J. P. Toner, A. A. Acosta, and G. D. Hodgen, "Hemizona Assay Sperm Defect Analysis: A Diagnostic Method for Assessment of Human Sperm-Oocyte Interactions, and the Predictive

Value for Fertilization Outcome," *Annals of the New York Academy of Sciences* 626 (June 28, 1991): 111–123.

26. Ibid., 121.

27. Ibid., 122.

28. H. M. Seitz, Jr., G. Rocha, B. G. Brackett, and L. Mastroianni, "Cleavage of Human Ova *In Vitro*," *Fertility and Sterility* 22 (1971): 255.

29. R. G. Edwards, "Studies on Human Conception," *American Journal of Obstetrics and Gynecology* 117 (1973): 587.

30. A. Bongso, S. C. Ng, C. Y. Fong, H. Mok, P. L. Ng, and S. S. Ratnam, "Cocultures in Human Assisted Reproduction: Support of Embryos *In Vitro* and Their Specificity," *Annals of the New York Academy of Sciences* 626 (June 28, 1991): 438–443.

31. P. C. Steptoe, R. G. Edwards, and J. M. Purdy, "Human Blastocysts Grown in Culture," *Nature* (1971): 132.

32. Ibid.

33. D. DeKretzer, P. Dennis, B. Hudson, J. Leeton, A. Lopata, K. Outch, J. Talbot, and C. Wood, "Transfer of a Human Zygote," *Lancet* 2 (1973): 728.

34. O. Bauer, K. Dieddrich, H. van der Ven, S. al-Hassani, and D. Krebs, "The Transvaginal Intratubal Transfer: A New Method in Male Infertility," *Annals of the New York Academy of Sciences* 626 (June 28, 1991): 467–477.

35. Bongso et al., "Cocultures in Human Assisted Reproduction," 438.

36. Treichel, "Embryo Transfer Achieved in Humans," 69.

37. A. E. Beer and R. E. Billingham, "The Embryo as a Transplant," *Scientific American* 230, no. 4 (1974): 36–46.

38. R. M. L. Winston and A. H. Handyside, "New Challenges in Human In Vitro Fertilization," *Science* 260 (1993): 932–936.

39. O. Friedrich, "A Legal, Moral, Social Nightmare," *Time* (September 10, 1984): 55.

40. P. Singer, "Technology and Procreation: How Far Should We Go?" *Technology Review* 88, no. 2 (February/March 1985): 27.

41. C. Grobstein, "Statement to the Ethics Advisory Board," Transcript of Meeting III, September 15, 1978 Washington, DC. (National Technical Information Service, PB-288 764, 1978), 229.

42. L. Kass, "'Making Babies' Revisited," *The Public Interest* no. 54 (Winter 1979): 33.

43. Ethics Advisory Board, "Report and Conclusions: HEW Support of Research Involving Human *In Vitro* Fertilization and Embryo Transfer," 101.

44. J. Fletcher, *Humanhood: Essays in Biomedical Ethics* (Buffalo, N.Y., Prometheus Books, 1979), 82.

45. M. Tooley, "Abortion and Infanticide," *Philosophy and Public Affairs* 2 (1972): 37–65.

46. B. Winters, "Engineered Conception: The New Parenthood," in *The Technological Woman: Interfacing with Tomorrow*, ed. J. Zimmerman (New York: Praeger, 1983), 225.

47. J. A. Robertson, "Embryos, Families, and Procreative Liberty: The Legal Structure of the New Reproduction," *Southern California Law Review* 59, no. 5 (July 1986): 977.

48. F. H. Marsh and D. J. Self, "*In Vitro* Fertilization: Moving from Theory to Therapy," *Hastings Center Report* (June 1980): 6.

49. "The Birthpangs of a New Science," *The Economist* (July 14, 1984): 80.

50. Australian scientists, for example, have announced the world's first "donor-egg baby" ["Amazing Births," *Time* 123, no. 4 (January 23, 1984): 30], and California scientists have announced the world's first two apparently successful transfers of an embryo from the womb of one woman into that of another (Treichel, "Embryo Transfer Achieved in Humans," 67).

51. Robertson, "Embryos, Families, and Procreative Liberty," 977.

52. D. T. Ozar, "The Case Against Thawing Unused Frozen Embryos," *Hastings Center Report* (August 1985): 8–11.

53. Robertson, "Embryos, Families, and Procreative Liberty," 977.

54. Ozar, "The Case Against Thawing Unused Frozen Embryos," 7.

55. Ibid., 8.

56. Kass, "'Making Babies' Revisited," 36.

57. Ibid., 38.

58. Ozar, "The Case Against Thawing Unused Frozen Embryos," 10.

59. T. M. Garrett, H. W. Baillie, and R. M. Garrett, *Health Care Ethics: Principles and Problems* (Englewood Cliffs, NJ: Prentice Hall, 1989), 245.

60. Ibid., 246.

61. Ibid.

62. P. Singer, *Practical Ethics* (New York: Cambridge University Press, 1979).

63. Robertson, "Embryos, Families, and Procreative Liberty," 983.

64. Ibid., 984–985.

65. M. Gold, "The Baby Makers," *Science* 85 (April 1985): 36.

66. L. R. Kass, "Making Babies—The New Biology and the 'Old' Morality," no. 26, *The Public Interest* (Winter 1972): 49.

67. Ibid.

68. Kass "'Making Babies' Revisited," 44.

69. "Breakthrough Test Checks Three-Day-Old Embryos," *Woman's World* 10, no. 34 (August, 1989): 13.

70. P. Singer and D. Wells, *Making Babies: The New Science and Ethics of Conception* (New York: Charles Scribner's Sons, 1985), 25–26.

71. *The Collected Dialogues of Plato*, eds. E. Hamilton and H. Cairns (Princeton, NJ: Princeton University Press, 1961), 699.

72. D. G. Jones, *Brave New People: Ethical Issues at the Commencement of Life* (Grands Rapids, MI: Ferdsman, 1985), 109.

73. R. T. Hull, ed., *Ethical Issues in the New Reproductive Technologies* (Belmont, CA: Wadsworth, 1990), 92.

74. L. Walters, "Human *In Vitro* Fertilization: A Review of the Ethical Literature," *Hastings Center Report* (August 1979): 28.

75. J. Feinberg, *Social Philosophy* (Englewood Cliffs, NJ: Prentice Hall, 1973), 47.

76. Hull, *Ethical Issues in the New Reproductive Technologies*, 91.

77. Ibid., 92.

78. Feinberg, *Social Philosophy*, 48.

79. L. Brown and J. Brown with S. Freeman, *Our Miracle Called Louise: A Parents' Story* (New York: Paddington Press, 1979).

80. W. A. W. Walters and P. Singer, "Conclusions—and Costs," in *Test-Tube Babies: A Guide to Moral Questions, Present Techniques and Future Possibilities*, eds. W. A. W. Walters and P. Singer (Melbourne: Oxford University Press, 1982), 130.

81. Paul Ramsey, "Shall We 'Reproduce'?" *Journal of the American Medical Association* 220, no. 10 (1972): 1346–1350; 220, no. 11 (1972): 1480–1485.

82. Robertson, "Embryos, Families, and Procreative Liberty," 987.

83. Ibid.

84. C. Grobstein, M. Flower, and J. Mendelhoff, "External Human Fertilization: An Evaluation of Policy," *Science* 222 (Oct. 14, 1983): 130.

85. Robertson, "Embryos, Families, and Procreative Liberty," 995.

86. Friedrich, "A Legal, Moral, Social Nightmare," 55.

87. D. M. Flannery et al., "Legal Issues Concerning *In Vitro* Fertilization," in *Appendix: HEW Support of In Vitro Fertilization* (Washington: DHEW, Ethics Advisory Board, 1979).

88. *Maher* v. *Roe*, 432 U.S. 464, 478 (1977).

89. *Skinner* v. *Oklahoma*, 316 U.S. 541 (1942).

90. *Griswold* v. *Connecticut*, U.S. 480 (1965).

91. *Eisenstadt* v. *Baird* 405 U.S. 438 (1972).

92. *Carey* v. *Population Services International*, 431 U.S. 453 (1977).

93. National Commission for the Protection of Human Subjects of Biomedical and Behavioral Research, "Institutional Review Board: Report and Recommendations," DHEW Publication No. (05) 78-0008 (Washington, DC: U.S. Government Printing Office, 1978): 78–79.

94. Ibid.

95. D. M. Flannery, C. D. Weisman, C. R. Lipsett, and A. N. Braverman, "Test Tube Babies: Legal Issues Raised by *In Vitro* Fertilization," *Georgetown Law Journal* 67 (1979): 1328–1329.

96. Flannery et al., "Legal Issues Concerning *In Vitro* Fertilization," 61.

97. Ibid., 61–63.

98. C. C. Hubble, "Liability of the Physicia for the Defects of a Child Caused by *In Vitro* Fertilization," *Journal of Legal Medicine* 2, no. 4 (December 1981): 501–521.

99. Flannery et al. "Legal Issues Concerning *In Vitro* Fertilization," 87–89.

100. Singer and Wells, *Making Babies*, 34.

101. Hubble, "Liability of the Physician for the Defects of a Child Caused by *In Vitro* Fertilization," 512–516.

102. See, for example, *Wolfe* v. *Isbell*, 291 Ala 327, 280 So. 2d 758 (1973); *Berger* v. *Weber*, 82 Mich. App. 199, 267 N.W. 2d 124 (1978); *Simon* v. *Mullin*, 34 Comm. Supp. 139, 380 A. 2d 1353 (1977).

103. *Renslaw* v. *Mennonite Hospital*, 67 Ill. 2d 348, 367 N.E. 2d 1250 (1977).

104. Ibid.

105. Hubble, "Liability of the Physician for the Defects of a Child Caused by *In Vitro* Fertilization," 516.

106. *Becher* v. *Schwartz*, 1978.

107. *Park* v. *Chessin*, 60 App. Div. 2d 80, 400 N.Y.S. 2d 110 (1978).

108. L. Walters, "Test-Tube Babies: Ethical Considerations," in *Ethical Issues in the New Reproductive Technologies*, ed. R. T. Hull (Belmont, CA: Wadsworth Publishing, 1990), 110–111.

109. Ibid., 114.

110. Ibid., 114–117.

111. Ibid.

112. R. Rowland, "A Child at Any Price," *Women's Studies International Forum* 8, no. 6 (1985): 540.

113. G. Corea and S. Ince, "Report of a Survey of IVF Clinics in the U.S.," in *Made to Order: The Myth of Reproductive and Genetic Progress* eds. P. Spallone and D. L. Steinberg (Oxford: Pergamon Press, 1987), 142–143.

114. Thirteen percent is the figure cited by Professor Carl Wood in his paper on factors affecting pregnancy rates (Annual Conference, St. Vincent's Bioethics Center, Melbourne, May 1984). David Davies, a member of the Warnock Committee cited success rates in Britain at 10 to 15 percent [YMCA Conference, "A Child at Any Price?" *Exeter* (Nov. 17, 1984)].

115. Rowland, "A Child at Any Price," 540.

116. Kass, "'Making Babies' Revisited," 50.

117. Grobstein, Flower, and Mendelhoff, "External Human Fertilization: An Evaluation of Policy," 130.

118. Singer and Wells, *Making Babies*, 46.

119. Singer, "Technology and Procreation: How Far Should We Go?," 25.

120. G. Corea, "The Reproductive Brothel," in *Man-Made Women: How New Reproductive Technologies Affect Women*, eds. G. Corea et al. (Bloomington: Indian University Press, 1987), 46.

121. Ibid., 303.

122. G. Corea, "Effects of NRAs on All Women," (unpublished paper), 8.

123. Dr. Margery Shaw has written that once a pregnant woman decides to carry her fetus to term, she insures a "conditional prospective liability" for negligent acts toward her fetus should it be born alive: "These acts could be

considered negligent fetal abuse resulting in an injured child. A decision to carry a genetically defective fetus to term would be an example. Abuse of alcohol or drugs during pregnancy ... [w]ithholding of necessary prenatal care, improper nutrition, exposure to mutagens or teratogens, or even exposure to the mother's defective intrauterine environment caused by her genotype ... could all result in an injured infant who might claim that his right to be born physically and mentally sound had been invaded." In M. S. Henifin, R. Hubbard, and J. Norsigian, "Prenatal Screening," *Reproductive Laws for the 1990s*, eds. S. Cohen and N. Tamb. Clifton, NJ: Humana Press, 1989, p. 167.

124. Fletcher, *Humanhood: Essays in Biomedical Ethics*, p. 90.

Chapter 10

1. R. D. Kempers, ed., "Surrogate Mothers," *Fertility and Sterility* (September 1986): 62S.

2. P. Singer and D. Wells, *Making Babies: The New Science and Ethics of Conception* (New York: Scribners, 1985), 96.

3. Ibid., 93–94.

4. P. Chesler, *Sacred Bond: The Legacy of Baby M* (New York: Times Books, 1988), 187.

5. For a full discussion of arguable distinction between baby-selling and surrogate-parenting contracts, see note in J. J. Mandler, "Developing a Concept of the Modern Family: A Proposed Uniform Surrogate Parenthood Act," *Georgetown Law Journal* 73, part 2 (June 1985): 1289–1295.

6. Chesler, *Sacred Bond*, 197.

7. R. D. Lawler, "Moral Reflections on the New Technologies: A Catholic Analysis," in *Embryos, Ethics and Women's Rights: Exploring the New Reproductive Technologies*, eds. E. Hoffman Baruch, A. F. D'Adamo, Jr., and J. Seager (New York: Harrington Park Press, 1988), 169.

8. L. Kass, "'Making Babies' Revisited," *The Public Interest* 54 (Winter 1979): 32–60.

9. H. T. Krimmel, "The Case Against Surrogate Parenting," *Hastings Center Report* (October 1983): 38.

10. Ibid.

11. Singer and Wells, *Making Babies*, 22.

12. J. Kant, *Foundations of the Metaphysics of Morals* trans. L. W. Beck (Indianapolis: Bobbs-Merrill Educational Publishing, 1959): 39.

13. D. A. J. Richards, "Commercial Sex and the Rights of the Person: A Moral Argument for the Decriminalization of Prostitution," *University of Pennsylvania Law Review* 127 (May 1979): 1257–1259.

14. R. Rosenblatt, "Baby M—Emotion for Sale," *Time* (April 6,1987): 88.

15. Ibid.

16. A. Hochschild, "The Managed Heart," *Individualism and Commitment in American Life*, eds. R. N. Bellah et al. (New York: Harper & Row, 1987), 176.

17. Krimmel, "The Case Against Surrogate Parenting," 86.

18. A. Taylor Fleming, "Our Fascination with Baby M," *The New York Times Magazine* (March 20,1987): 38.

19. "Legislator Says Massachusetts Bill for Surrogate Parents Likely," *The Boston Globe* (April 2,1987): I13.

20. L. B. Andrews, "Legal and Ethical Aspects of New Reproductive Technologies," *Journal of Clinical Obstetrics and Gynecology* 29 (1986): 190.

21. H. A. Davidson, "What Will Surrogate Mothering Do to the Fabric of the American Family?" *Public Welfare* (Fall 1983): 12.

22,. D. Gelman and D. Shapiro, "Infertility: Babies by Contract," *Newsweek* (November 4,1985): 74.

23. J. A. Robertson, "Embryos, Families, and Procreative Liberty: The Legal Structure of the New Reproduction," *Southern California Law Review* 59, no. 5 (July 1986): 1001.

24. Ibid.

25. Mandler, "Developing a Concept of the Modern Family", 1291.

26. J. A. Robertson, "Surrogate Mothers: Not So Novel After All," *Hastings Center Report* 13, no. 5 (October 1983): 29.

27. L. B. Andrews, "Alternative Modes of Reproduction," in *Reproductive Laws for the 1990s*, eds. S. Cohen and N. Taub (Clifton, NJ: Humana Press, 1989): 365.

28. Ibid, 366.

29. Ibid., 369.

30. G. Corea, *The Mother Machine* (New York: Harper & Row, 1985), 279.

31. R. H. Miller, "Surrogate Parenting: An Infant Industry Presents Society with Legal, Ethical Questions," *Ob-Gyn News* 18, no. 3 (February 1–14, 1983): 3.

32. Corea, *The Mother Machine*, 214.

33. Andrews, "Alternative Modes of Reproduction," 371.

34. Ibid.

35. Ibid.

36. "Surrogate Motherhood," *Philosophy and Public Policy*, 9, no. 1: (Winter 1989): 3–4.

37. M. Gibson, "The Moral and Legal Status of 'Surrogate' Motherhood," invited address at the winter meeting of the American Philosophical Association, December 1988.

38. L. Flourney, a district attorney with the Berkshire County Office, Pittsfield, Massachusetts, provided the details of this case. The name of the defendant and some details of the case have been altered.

39. Corea, *The Mother Machine*, 231.

40. P. A. Avery, "Surrogate Mothers: Center of a New Storm," *U. S. News and World Report* (June 6,1983): 76.

41. Andrews, "Alternative Modes of Reproduction," 369.

42. Corea, *The Mother Machine*, 276.

43. M. Atwood, *The Handmaid's Tale* (Boston: Houghton Mifflin, 1986).

44. "A Surrogate's Story of Loving and Losing," *U. S. News and World Report* (June 6, 1983): 77.

45. "Grandmother, 48, Is Surrogate for Daughter" *Boston Globe* (April 8, 1987): 17A.

46. For a complete discussion of these liberty-limiting principles, see J. Feinberg *Social Philosophy* (Englewood Cliffs, NJ: Prentice Hall, 1973), 36–55.

47. Department of Health and Social Security, United Kingdom, *Report of the Committee of Inquiry into Human Fertilization and Embryology* (London: HMSO, July 1984), 47.

48. Surrogacy Arrangements Act 1985, United Kingdom, Chapter 49, 2. (1) (a)–(c).

49. Ibid., 3. (1)–(5).

50. Ibid., 46.

51. Of pending state laws, five (in Alabama, Illinois, Iowa, Maryland, and Wisconsin) would ban surrogate motherhood altogether, whereas seven (in Florida, Kentucky, Michigan, New Jersey, New York, Oregon, and Pennsylvania) would specifically ban only paid surrogacy. See Andrews, "Alternative Modes of Reproduction." in *Reproductive Laws for the 1990s*, eds S. Cohen and N. Taub (Clifton, NJ: Humaua Press, 1989).

52. Chesler, *Sacred Bond*, 197–203.

53. S. R. Gersz, "The Contract in Surrogate Motherhood: A Review of the Issues," *Law, Medicine, and Health Care* (June 1984): 109.

54. A. M. Capron and M. J. Radin, "Choosing Family Law over Contract Law as a Paradigm for Surrogate Motherhood," *Law, Medicine, and Health Care* 16, no. 2 (Spring 1988): 3a.

55. Ibid.

56. *Maher* v. *Roe*, 432 U.S. 464 (1977).

57. Importantly, Capron and Radin ("Choosing Family Law over contract Law," 43) do not support *Maher* v. *Roe*: "Although *Maher* is thus a formidable doctrinal obstacle for those who would claim some positive right to enforcement of surrogacy contracts, we do not mean to endorse its rationale. Because state denial of freedom to choose abortion is, in the context of the current gender bias in economic and social power, a denial of equal opportunity to women, we think the right to choose abortion would be better analyzed as an equality right than as a privacy right."

58. *Doe* v. *Kelley*, 106 Mich. App. 169, 307 N. W. 2d 438 (1981), *cert. denied*, 459 U.S. 1183 (1983).

59. "Excerpts from Decision by New Jersey Supreme Court in the Baby M Case," *The New York Times* (February 4, 1988): B6.

60. Robertson, "Surrogate Mothers: Not So Novel After All," 33.

61. E. Landes and R. Posner, "The Economics of the Baby Shortage," *Journal of Legal Studies* 7 (1978): 343.

62. Ibid., 344–345.

63. Ibid., 345.

64. J. R. 5. Pritchard, "A Market for Babies?" *University of Toronto Law Journal* 34 (1981): 347.

65. Ibid., 352

66. N. Davis, "Reproductive Technologies and Our Attitudes Toward Children," *From the Center* 7, no. 1 (Summer 1988): 1–4.

67. See L. B. Andrews, "The Aftermath of Baby M: Proposed State Laws on Surrogate Motherhood," *Hastings Center Report* 17 (Oct/Nov 1987): 32. Lawmakers in Connecticut, Illinois, North Carolina, and Rhode Island have proposed statutes that would make any contracts for surrogacy void and unenforceable. Proposals in Alabama, Minnesota, Nebraska, and New York would void only contracts for paid surrogacy.

68. Ibid.

69. B. Cohen, "Surrogate Mothers: Whose Baby Is It?" *American Journal of Law and Medicine* 10, no. 3 (Fall 1984), 255

70. Andrews, "Alternative Modes of Reproduction," 383–384.

71. Ibid.

72. G. J. Annas, "Regulating the New Reproductive Technologies," 414.

73. Andrews, "Alternative Modes of Reproduction," 385–386.

74. Andrews, "The Aftermath of Baby M: Proposed State Laws on Surrogate Motherhood," 33–39.

75. "Rumpelstiltskin Revisited: The Unalienable Rights of Surrogate Mothers," *Harvard Law Review* 99 (1986): 1953 (note).

76. Ibid., 1953–1954.

77. Ibid.

78. "Surrogate Motherhood: Contractual Issues and Remedies Under Legislative Proposals," *Washburn Law Journal* 23 (1983–84): 622 (note).

79. 428 U. S. 93–95 (1975).

80. A. Kronman, "Paternalism and the Law of Contracts," *Yale Law Journal* 92 (April 1983): 780–784.

81. "Surrogate Motherhood: Contractual Issues and Remedies Under Legislative Proposals," 622 (note).

82. Ibid.

83. Chesler, *Sacred Bond*.

84. Singer and Wells, *Making Babies*, 111–112.

85. M. B. Whitehead, "A Surrogate Mother Describes Her Change of Heart—and Her Fight to Keep the Baby Two Families Love," *People Weekly* 26 (October 26, 1986): 47.

86. Capron and Radin, "Choosing Family Law over contract Law," 35.

87. Not all contracts are specifically enforceable. Martha Field ("Surrogate Motherhood: The Legal Issues," *Human Rights Annual* 12[1979]) argues that "there are some things so visceral and personal that one would not judge a person's positions on them, or change of position, by the same yardstick of rational agreement as bargains made in the workplace, and having a baby is one of those things." Field goes on to argue that "our laws concerning prostitution and childselling show we consider sex and the rearing of one's children also to be in the same realm where we as a society would "like to maintain a line between the commercial and the personal." Field points out that even if a state decriminalized prostitution, it would probably not en-

force prostitution in those cases where the prostitute changes her mind. Nor would it enforce contracts to sell babies over the changed minds of their natural parents. Nor would it enforce marriage contracts even though "promise to marry may be as certain and explicit as a promise to be a surrogate ... and "there may exist at least as great expectations and disappointment if one of the parties has a change of mind."

Despite all of her examples, Field concedes that the state has no mandate to maintain an *absolute* line between the personal and the commercial. One can marry for money or decide not to have a child because babies are expensive. Nevertheless, Field insists that "the line between natural pregnancy and pregnancy for hire is sufficiently distinct and sufficiently reasonable for a state to be permitted to use it if it makes a judgment that it wants to use it in attempting to delineate a personal sphere that is separate from the commercial sphere."

Finally, Field notes that "even in areas other than the personal, it is not foreign to contract laws for contracts to be enforceable or not at the option of areas of the parties." The Restatement of Contracts recognizes voidable contracts as contracts that are unenforceable as against public policy, and option contracts as valid contracts in which one of the parties has the right to decide whether to proceed."

88. S. A. Ketchum, "Selling Babies and Selling Bodies," Hypatia 4, no. 3 (Fall 1989).

89. M. O'Brien, *The Politics of Reproduction* (Boston: Routledge & Kegan Press, 1981), 29, 58.

90. Ketchum, "New Reproductive Technologies and the Definition of Parenthood," 120.

91. Ibid.

92. A. Rich, *Of Woman Born: Motherhood as Experience and Institution* (New York: Norton, 1976), 38–39.

93. S. Firestone, *The Dialectic of Sex* (New York: Bantam Books, 1970), 198–199.

94. M. Piercy, *Woman on the Edge of Time* (New York: Fawcett Crest Books, 1976).

95. Ibid., 102.

96. Ibid., 105–106.

97. Ibid., 183.

98. A. Donchin, "The Future of Mothering: Reproductive Technology and Feminist Theory," *Hypatia* 1, no. 2 (Fall 1986): 130.

99 A. al-Hibri, *Research in Philosophy and Technology*, 7 (1984): 266.

100. Piercy, *Woman on the Edge of Time*, 105.

101. Corea, *The Mother Machine*, 107–119.

102. G. Corea, "Egg Snatchers," in *Test-Tube Women: What Future for Motherhood?* eds. R. Arditti, R. D. Klein, and S. Minden (London: Pandora Press, 1984), 45.

103. R. Rowland, "Reproductive Technologies: The Final Solution to the Woman Question," in *Test-Tube Women: What Future for Motherhood?* eds. R. Arditti, R. D. Klein, and S. Minden (London: Pandora Press, 1984), 45.

104. Ibid., 368.

Appendix

1. I. L. Slesnick, L. Balzer, A. L. McCormack, D. E. Newton, and F. A. Rasmussen, *Biology* (Glenview, IL: Scott Foresman, 1985), chap. 3.

2. B. Alberts, D. Bray, J. Lewis, M. Raff, K. Roberts, and J. D. Watson, *Molecular Biology of the Cell* (New York: Garland, 1983), chap. 3.

3. L. Stryer, *Biochemistry*, 3rd ed. (New York: Freeman, 1988), chaps. 2, 4, 12, 14.

4. J. Darnell, H. Lodish, and D. Baltimore, *Molecular Cell Biology* (New York: Freeman, 1986), chap. 3.

5. I. L. Slesnick et al., *Biology*, chap. 4.

6. B. Alberts et al., *Biology of the Cell*, chaps. 7, 8.

7. J. Darnell et al., *Molecular Cell Biology*, chap. 5.

8. M. Pines, *Inside the Cell: The New Frontier of Medical Science*, U.S. Department of Health Education and Welfare Publication (NIH) 79-1051 (Washington, DC: U.S. Government Printing Office, 1978).

9. I. L. Slesnick et al., *Biology*, chap. 6.

10. J. Darnell et al., *Molecular Cell Biology*, chap. 5.

11. B. Alberts et al., *Molecular Biology of the Cell*, chap. 11.

12. I. W. Sherman and V. G. Sherman, *Biology: A Human Approach*, (New York: Oxford, 1983), chap. 7.

Index

RG 133.5 .K37 1994

Kaplan, Lawrence J., 1943-

Controlling our reproductive
destiny

DATE DUE

~~DEC 16 1995~~		
DEC 11 2000		
~~NOV 13 1996~~		
DEC 12 2001		

HIGHSMITH #45230   Printed in USA